THE NEW
BIRTH-CONTROL
BOOK

THE NEW
BIRTH-
CONTROL
BOOK A Complete Guide for Women and Men

HOWARD I. SHAPIRO, M.D.

PRENTICE HALL PRESS
New York London Toronto Sydney Tokyo

Figures on the following pages are reprinted with permission from the following persons and/or institutions: page 108, courtesy of Contemporary OB/GYN, Medical Economics Company; page 269, courtesy of Family Health International; pages 34 and 81 reprinted from *Making Choices: Evaluating the Health Risks and Benefits of Birth-Control Method,* The Alan Guttmacher Institute, 1983; page 257 courtesy of The Population Council; page 225 courtesy of Richard Wolf Medical Instruments Corporation; page 148 courtesy of Zetek, Inc.

Published by Prentice Hall Press
A Division of Simon & Schuster, Inc.
Gulf + Western Building
One Gulf + Western Plaza
New York, NY   10023

PRENTICE HALL PRESS *is a registered trademark of Simon & Schuster, Inc.*

An earlier version of this book, entitled *The Birth Control Book,* was published in 1977 by St. Martin's Press.

Library of Congress Cataloging-in-Publication Data

Shapiro, Howard I., 1937–
  The new birth-control book.

  New version of: The birth control book: St. Martin's
Press, 1979.
  Bibliography: p.
  Includes index.
  1. Contraception.   I. Shapiro, Howard I., 1937–
The birth control book.   II. Title.   [DNLM:
1. Contraception—popular works. WP 630 S529b]
RG136.S48 1987   613.9'4   87-7157
ISBN 0-13-611781-3

Designed by Irving Perkins Associates

Manufactured in the United States of America

10   9   8   7   6   5   4   3   2   1

First Edition

To Bette:
My love, you are truly the Renaissance woman—
actress, artist, wife, mother, lover, and friend.

ACKNOWLEDGMENTS

The author is once again indebted to Dawn Perkins for the many hours spent and the care taken in typing and preparing this manuscript.

I am especially thankful to my agent and friend, Russell Galen, for his patience, knowledge, sound advice, and most of all his wonderful letters. I look forward to many more successful projects together.

Gareth Esersky is to be congratulated for appreciating the importance of this book and for her enthusiasm and editorial skills in bringing it to its successful completion.

Finally, I am pleased I had the opportunity to devote the necessary time, effort, and research to this book. I am very proud of the finished product. Behind every successful man is a great woman, and I am especially fortunate to have had three: Bette, Suzanne, and Marjorie.

CONTENTS

PREFACE xi

1 *THE REPRODUCTIVE SYSTEM* 1
2 *BIRTH-CONTROL PILLS* 14
3 *IUDs* 78
4 *BARRIER CONTRACEPTION* 102
5 *COITUS INTERRUPTUS AND RHYTHM* 136
6 *POSTCOITAL CONTRACEPTION* 156
7 *ABORTION* 171
8 *VASECTOMY* 198
9 *TUBAL LIGATION* 208
10 *HYSTERECTOMY* 237
11 *THE FUTURE* 251

AFTERWORD 281
SELECTED BIBLIOGRAPHY 283
INDEX 299

PREFACE

Since the original publication of *The Birth-Control Book* by St. Martin's Press in 1977, and of the paperback by Avon Books in 1978, the study of contraception, abortion, and sterilization techniques has undergone exciting changes and significant advances. While much of the vital information has reached physicians via presentations in scientific journals and medical seminars, little if any has filtered down to our patients. Dr. Luella Klein, past president of the American College of Obstetricians and Gynecologists, is correct in her 1985 assessment that the public is "grossly misinformed" about birth-control methods and that commonly held notions about contraception stand in sharp contrast to the scientific evidence that has been accumulating. The radio and television industries must share some of the responsibility for this problem by maintaining their archaic policies of refusing advertisements for contraceptives until very recently and of limiting the amount of accurate information and frank discussion they allow to be presented to the public. Many physicians have also been negligent in imparting important new information to their patients.

In my own private practice, I am constantly amazed and dismayed at the misleading and outdated information that has been given to women. Many times a patient has told me she cannot take the Pill because of a family history of cancer, when it is a well-established fact that the Pill may actually help prevent certain types of cancer. This widely held misconception is evidenced in a newly released Gallup poll in which 31 percent of 1,036 women surveyed believed that the Pill posed a serious risk of cancer. Seventy-five percent of the women thought that there were substantial health risks associated with using the Pill, while two-thirds incorrectly believed that it was more dangerous to use birth-control pills than to give birth. Such misinformation has driven thousands of women away from using the Pill in favor of less effective or unproven methods of contraception. In fact, for every woman admitted to a hospital as a result of using the Pill, five others actually avoid the need for hospital care because of the Pill. Unfortunately, good news about birth-control pills just doesn't sell newspapers. Many women are still unaware of the fact that birth-control pills actually help to alleviate symptoms of ovarian cysts, rheumatoid arthritis, anemia, and premenstrual syndrome, or PMS. While consumers have been adamant in demanding less and less estrogen in their birth-control pills, most do not realize that the synthetic progesterone or progestin in certain birth-control pills may be more dangerous to them than the dose of estrogen.

Misinformation concerning the use of intrauterine devices, or IUDs, is just as prevalent. Why are so many young women who have never borne children having

IUDs inserted, with the clear risk of permanent sterility? The statistics about IUDs are frightening, but they are simply not reaching the public.

What are some of the newest findings about barrier contraception? Does one diaphragm size really fit all women, as one theory claims, or must they continue to be fitted according to individual size and pelvic shape? How effective and safe is the new TODAY contraceptive sponge, and what is its relationship to toxic shock syndrome? Is there a safe morning-after pill to replace the infamous DES? What are some of the newer abortion and sterilization techniques, and how successful are the modern microsurgical methods of sterilization reversal? I will attempt to answer these and many other difficult questions that confront today's men and women.

Times are changing! Who would have imagined ten years ago that feminists Betty Friedan and Gloria Steinem would be invited as guest speakers at the 1985 convention of the American College of Obstetricians and Gynecologists? At this meeting, Ms. Friedan aptly stated that the women's movement and the accompanying advances in modern contraceptive technology have allowed women to control their reproductive lives. "Women now want birth-control options that change according to the changing patterns and needs of their lives," she said. I believe that today's gynecologist must be responsive to these changing needs and must show the knowledge, flexibility, and willingness to help each individual find the best solution to her particular contraceptive and reproductive requirements.

Many of the health care needs of women involve not disease or illness, but education consisting of support and counsel about the anatomy and physiology of reproduction, methods of contraception, and abortion. Gynecologists must undertake to raise the level of their patients' understanding of these and other subjects.

Sexually active teenagers and women over thirty are two groups whose unique contraceptive needs continue to be neglected. Political and religious leaders in the United States appear to be obsessed with the unrealistic mission of promoting chastity and eradicating sexuality among youngsters rather than providing them with accurate contraceptive information before they become sexually active. It is no wonder that almost 60 percent of sexually active teens do not use any form of birth control during their first sexual encounter. How can we justify the fact that sexually active American teenagers wait an average of thirteen months from their initial sexual encounter to their request for contraception? In a 1985 study conducted by the Alan Guttmacher Institute, researchers found that American teenagers become pregnant, give birth, and have abortions at significantly higher rates than do adolescents in other industrialized nations. Among women fifteen to nineteen years of age there were 96 pregnancies per 1,000, compared with only 14 per 1,000 in the Netherlands; 35 per 1,000 in Sweden; 43 per 1,000 in France; 44 per 1,000 in Canada; and 45 per 1,000 in England and Wales. In the United States, 60 of every 1,000 girls will have had an abortion by the age of eighteen, compared to 7, 30, 30, 24, and 20 per 1,000, respectively, in these other countries. This sorry record reflects the inadequacy and ambivalence surrounding contraceptive education of the young in our country. While we continue to cling to the irrational fear that teaching sex education and providing contraceptive services to youngsters will encourage promiscuity, the lack of such teaching has only contributed to the more than 1 million teenage pregnancies in the United States each year. Those countries with lower pregnancy and abortion rates share more liberal attitudes toward teenage sexuality, comprehensive programs of sex education at an early age, and easily accessible and low-cost contraceptive services. Since we in this country have seen the futility and foolishness of trying to discourage teenage sexual activity, it's about time that we accept it as fact and move to end this national epidemic of unplanned pregnancies among the young.

An increasing proportion of adult women are postponing their first births until their middle or even late thirties, rather than having children in their twenties. The unique contraceptive needs of women in their thirties are far different than those of younger women. Pill use after the age of thirty-five is best avoided, while the IUD may prevent pregnancy but cause permanent sterility. Many women in this age group are avid readers in search of unbiased and accurate reading material. Unfortunately, many of the articles in popular women's magazines seem more interested in downplaying the many benefits of the Pill while promoting newer and less effective methods such as the cervical cap, TODAY sponge, and Vaginal Contraceptive Film (VCF).

It is obvious that women and men will make correct choices about the subjects of contraception, sterilization, and abortion only if accurate medical information is made available to them in language that can be easily understood. The first edition of *The Birth-Control Book* was successful because it was written for patients, not doctors. I firmly believe that there is no medical subject so complex that it can't be explained in easy-to-understand terms rather than in confusing medical jargon. The purpose of this book is to share with the reader my knowledge of the vital subjects of contraception, sterilization, and abortion. I have maintained the question-and-answer format used in *The Birth-Control Book* because I believe it helps to achieve this goal while also serving as a quick reference source for specific concerns. The vast majority of these questions represent concerns of the many women I have had the privilege of treating during the past eighteen years. This project, therefore, belongs to them as well as to me. My greatest personal pleasure will be in knowing that women who read this book will consider it the best and most accurate reference source for contraception available to them.

1

THE REPRODUCTIVE SYSTEM

Before you can understand the questions and answers about contraceptive methods and gynecological surgery in this book, some knowledge of the basic anatomy and physiology of reproduction is essential. When teaching my patients about their external, or outer, genital anatomy, I often use a magnifying mirror while indicating the different parts. Follow the diagrams in the text and compare them with your own normal anatomy (figure 1-1).

In viewing the external genitals, you can readily identify the *mons pubis* as the triangular area covered with hair. By pressing down on the lower part of the mons in direct line with the middle of the abdomen, you can touch the pubic symphysis bone.

What are the labia?

The labia are paired folds of skin on either side of the vaginal opening. There are two types: the outer, larger labia, called the *labia majora;* and the inner, more delicate, *labia minora.* The former are covered with hair and contain sweat glands and sebaceous, or

Figure 1–1. *The external genitals (vulva).*

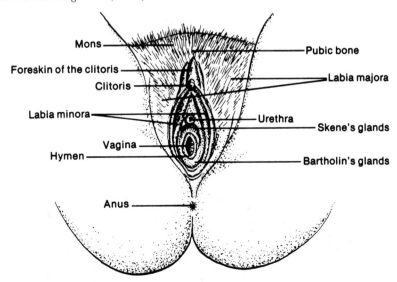

oil, glands. In women who have never had children, the labia majora often meet in the middle, but following childbirth they may remain farther apart. They protect and cushion against injury the more fragile structures of the vulva within them. The enlarged healthy size of the labia majora is dependent on hormonal factors, and women in the menopausal years who lack estrogen hormone often note a flattening and even a disappearance of these structures.

The labia minora are the hairless, more delicate folds lying inside the labia majora. They are supplied with oil glands, numerous blood vessels, and erectile tissue, which becomes swollen during sexual arousal. There are many nerve endings in the labia minora, making it very sensitive to sexual stimulation. The foreskin, or hood, of the clitoris is formed by the joining of the two labia minora.

How large is the normal clitoris?

The clitoris is a small organ of erectile tissue lying under the hood formed by the labia minora. The length of the clitoris varies from less than $\frac{1}{4}$ inch (6 millimeters) to as much as 1 inch (25 millimeters) during sexual excitation. This sensitive structure plays a most important role in female orgasm.

Why can't I find my urethra?

The urethra, or urinary opening, always seems easy to locate in textbooks, but it is difficult to find on people. Honest doctors and nurses will readily admit that they occasionally have trouble finding the urethra of a patient when inserting a catheter, or urinary tube. To find your urethra, separate and lift the labia minora with the index and middle finger of one hand while focusing a mirror in the opposite hand. You will find it between the vagina and clitoris, but closer to the vagina. If that doesn't work, passing urine while viewing with the mirror always proves successful.

Are there any other openings into the vagina?

On each side of the urethra are two tiny openings leading from two mucus-secreting glands named *Skene's.* Two other openings at the lower part of the vagina on each side enter into glands named *Bartholin's.* It is often difficult, if not impossible, to see these with a mirror. These glands have little, if any, function, but inflammation can block their openings and cause a large, painful swelling.

What is the shape of the normal hymen?

The hymen is a thin membrane lying across the opening to the vagina, and any one of many different shapes may be considered normal (figure 1-2).

It should be noted that an easily stretched hymen may be intact, or unbroken, in a sexually active woman, or may be almost totally absent in a virgin. Usually, however, initial intercourse produces tearing of the hymen. This heals quickly, leaving little tags of tissue. Childbirth produces further tearing of these tags, and following delivery they may become fewer in number and flatter in appearance. *Carunculae myrtiformes* is the name given to the appearance of hymenal remnants following childbirth.

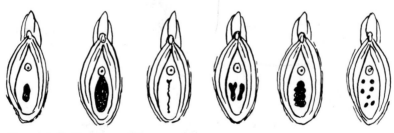

Figure 1–2. *Variations of the normal hymen.*

An *imperforate* hymen is one with no opening, which results in the trapping of menstrual blood within the vagina, and the accumulation of blood in both the vagina and the cavity of the uterus. When a young woman of menstruating age complains of monthly cramping but no bleeding, this condition should immediately be suspected. Treatment consists of opening the hymen with a small incision under anesthesia.

How can I examine my inner vagina and cervix?

You can accomplish this easily by using a viewing instrument called a *speculum.* If you can't get a speculum from a doctor or a clinic, you can buy a plastic or metal one from most surgical supply stores. The speculum may be used over and over again by the same individual, but must be rinsed with warm water after each use. When using a speculum, you must place a light and a mirror near the vulva in order to see the inner vagina and cervix. A more elaborate model with its own detachable light source is also available, which has the advantage of being prelubricated and is available in both regular and small sizes.

Can STDs (sexually transmitted diseases) be carried by a speculum?

Contrary to popular belief, it is almost impossible to contract venereal disease from a vaginal speculum that has been used several hours before by an infected individual. The organisms that cause gonorrhea and syphilis are very delicate and are unable to survive for more than a few minutes outside the body. Bacteria, viruses, and protozoa capable of causing other types of veneral disease are slightly more hardy, but most bacteriologists would agree that it would be most unusual for these organisms to survive for several hours on a speculum, especially a dry one.

This does not mean that one should abandon sensible precautions when using a speculum. If a plastic speculum is believed to have been in contact with a person with a sexually transmitted disease, it should be scrubbed with an antiseptic solution (Betadine, Phisohex) and left to dry. Metal speculums should be sterilized by placing them in boiling water for five minutes. Since sexually transmitted diseases may be present in a totally asymptomatic individual, a speculum should never be passed from woman to woman.

How do I use a speculum?

Lying on your back with your knees bent and your thighs as far apart as possible, insert the index finger of your left hand (if you're right-handed) into the vagina, exerting firm, downward pressure in the direction of the rectum. Insert the closed speculum, held in the right hand, over this finger into the vagina. Turn the handle of the speculum in the direction of your right side while it is being inserted. If you are not using a prelubricated speculum, insertion will be easier if K-Y Lubricating Jelly, available at any pharmacy without a prescription, is liberally applied to the speculum and inner labia before insertion. Gently advance the speculum as far as it can comfortably go—usually, that is its full length of 4 inches (10 centimeters). Then rotate it so that the handle faces the floor or ceiling. Open the speculum by pressing the lever with your thumb.

What do I see when using a speculum?

The slightly reddened side walls of the vagina can easily be seen, and by gently rotating the speculum back to its insertion position while it remains open in the vagina, the upper and lower vaginal walls may be examined. If you experience pressure on the urinary bladder or rectum during these maneuvers, it is only natural, since the vagina is in such close proximity to these structures, as you can see from the side view of a woman's pelvis (figure 1-3).

Figure 1–3. *Side view of a woman's pelvis.*

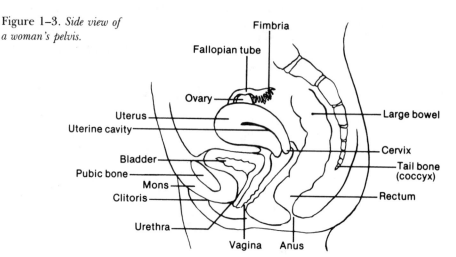

At the end of the vagina is the lower part of the uterus, called the *cervix,* and its opening, the *cervical os,* which leads into the cavity of the uterus (figure 1-4).

It is through the os that sperm pass on their journey toward fertilizing the egg in the upper, outer part of the fallopian tube. The glands within the cervix discharge mucus into the os throughout the month. The amount of mucus and its consistency is dependent upon the female hormones *estrogen* and *progesterone.* Estrogen causes an abundance of thin, watery, stretchable mucus that is very receptive to sperm as they pass through the cervix at the time of ovulation. Progesterone, on the other hand, produces a thick, nonstretchable mucus that prevents sperm from entering the os.

You can touch the cervix by first removing the speculum and then inserting the index finger as far as possible into the vagina. Notice that the cervix has the consistency of the cartilage at the tip of the nose. During pregnancy, the cervix softens

Figure 1–4. *Cervix and os as seen through the speculum.*

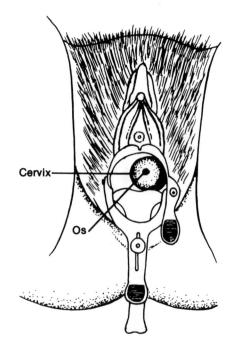

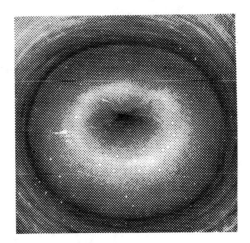

Figure 1–5. *Appearance of cervix before and after childbirth.*

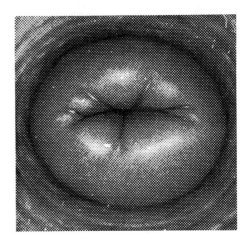

considerably, becomes swollen, and takes on a bluish color due to an increase in its blood supply. In labor, it has a tremendous capacity to dilate, or open, in order to accommodate the baby's head. After childbirth, the appearance of the cervix is changed, since the small opening has been stretched (figure 1-5).

For many women the appearance of the cervix is not perfectly smooth. On the contrary, the reddened, mucus-secreting glandular tissue of the inner cervix may actually turn outward, or *evert*. Eversion is a perfectly normal and harmless condition which produces only one symptom: an increase in mucus secretion, especially at the time of ovulation.

What is the upper part of the uterus called?

The upper part of the uterus is called *corpus,* or "body." In the adult woman this structure is smaller than her fist and weighs approximately 2 ounces (55 grams). By the end of pregnancy it may weigh $2\frac{1}{4}$ pounds (1.02 kilograms), and its muscle layer, or *myometrium,* will have stretched to a point where it can hold a huge infant or two, amniotic fluid, and a placenta. Figure 1-6 demonstrates a nonpregnant uterus as it appears from the inside, showing the myometrium and the very important *endometrium.*

Figure 1–6. *Inner anatomy of the cervix, uterus, and fallopian tubes.*

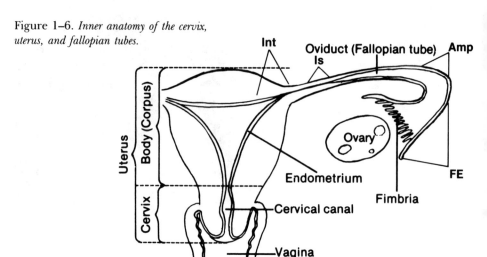

Why is the endometrium so important?

The glands in the endometrium, as in the cervix, undergo changes in response to estrogen and progesterone, which circulate in a woman's body. Though not visible to the naked eye, those changes can clearly be seen under the microscope. It is the endometrium, under the influence of progesterone, that accepts and nourishes the fertilized egg at the onset of pregnancy. When the egg is not fertilized, the upper layer of the endometrium detaches from its blood supply, and bleeding, or *menstruation,* begins.

What is the function of the fallopian tubes in the process of conception?

The two oviducts, or *fallopian tubes,* are of vital importance in grasping the egg with their fingerlike projections, called *fimbria,* as it is released from the ovary (figure 1-6). Fertilization—the uniting of the egg and the sperm—takes place shortly after the egg enters the fallopian tube. The muscles of the tube then transport the egg in the direction of the endometrium. According to the latest research, this journey takes approximately seventy-two hours. Proof of the fimbria's efficiency in conducting the egg toward the fallopian tube is demonstrated by several reports of successful pregnancy following surgical removal of the ovary on one side of the body and the tube on the opposite side.

For anatomical and medical purposes, the tube is divided into four distinct portions. The outer third, including the fimbria, is known as the *fimbriated extremity* ("FE" in figure 1-6). The wide middle portion of the tube adjacent to the fimbriated extremity is known as the *ampullary portion* ("Amp"), while the narrow part of the tube closest to the uterus is called the *isthmus* ("Is"). The interstitial portion of the tube ("Int") is contained in the muscular wall of the uterus which the tube penetrates on its way to the uterine cavity. It is technically possible to occlude any of these four areas of the tube when sterilization surgery is performed. The specific area involved and the degree of tubal destruction will be the key determinants in the success or failure of reversal operations, should a woman later change her mind and want more children (see chapter 9, "Tubal Ligation," and chapter 11, "The Future").

What are the ovaries like?

The two ovaries are white and oval-shaped. In the adult woman they measure about $1\frac{1}{2}$ inches (4 centimeters) in length and $\frac{3}{4}$ inch (2 centimeters) in breadth. They are attached to the uterus by the *ovarian ligament.* Though each ovary may contain as many as 400,000 egg cells, only one of these eggs, which is surrounded by fluid and called a *follicle,* develops to maturity each month. The follicle pushes through the surface of the ovary at the time of ovulation. Occasionally two separate eggs will do this at the same time, and if both are fertilized the result is *fraternal* (nonidentical, or dizygotic) twins. The newer fertility drugs responsible for multiple births cause several eggs to pop at once so that all the offspring are usually fraternal. (Identical twins are conceived when a single fertilized egg divides and separates into two equal parts.)

Which egg of the several thousand will next become a mature follicle is strictly a matter of chance. Contrary to popular belief, the ovaries do not alternate ovulations with each menstrual cycle. It is more like a random flip of a coin, and one ovary may get the assignment several times in a row. Furthermore, surgical removal of one ovary should not present a problem for pregnancy, since the remaining one has more than enough eggs to last for a lifetime. Under such circumstances, the single ovary works at full capacity in producing an ovulation every month. Most scientists believe that the egg cannot live beyond twenty-four hours, and its ability to be fertilized probably lasts no longer than fifteen to eighteen hours. Healthy sperm may be capable of movement for twenty-four to forty-eight hours (and on rare occasions even longer), though their ability to fertilize is believed to last considerably less time.

The ovary makes estrogen and progesterone, the two female hormones. Estrogen, which is produced in the cells of the developing follicle, is responsible for breast development, thinning of the cervical mucus, and the microscopic growth of the endometrium prior to ovulation. This growth begins after menstruation and is referred to as the *proliferative phase* of the menstrual cycle (Figure 1-7).

Following ovulation, the now-empty follicle in the ovary becomes a yellow structure called the *corpus luteum* (figure 1-8). Progesterone is produced by the corpus luteum and is responsible for turning the endometrium into a lush receptor and supporter of the fertilized egg. This is termed the *secretory phase* of the menstrual cycle (figure 1-7). If the egg is fertilized, the corpus luteum continues to produce progesterone in

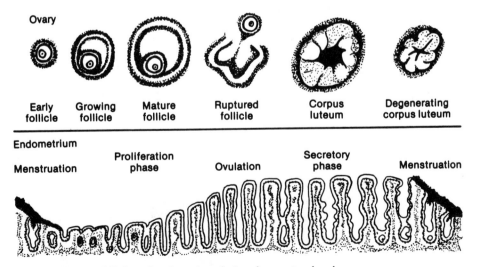

Ovary

| Early follicle | Growing follicle | Mature follicle | Ruptured follicle | Corpus luteum | Degenerating corpus luteum |

Endometrium

Menstruation | Proliferation phase | Ovulation | Secretory phase | Menstruation

Figure 1–7. *The follicle and endometrium during the menstrual cycle.*

Figure 1–8. *The control of ovulation and menstruation.*

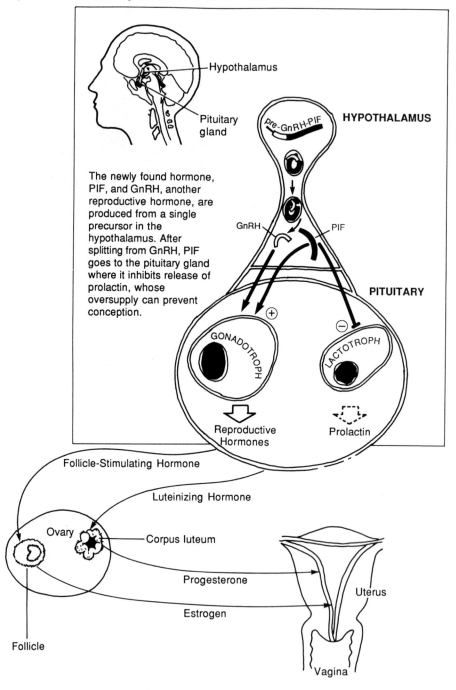

support of the pregnancy. In the absence of pregnancy, the corpus luteum dies and no more progesterone is produced. Among the more promising methods of contraceptive technology is the development of medications that prevent the action of progesterone on the endometrium, thereby making it impossible for a fertilized egg to implant (see chapter 11, "The Future").

To reiterate, when the support of the endometrium collapses, menstruation ensues.

How is the cycle regulated? What makes all this happen?

It all begins in a small but vital area of the brain called the *hypothalamus* (figure 1-8). The hypothalamus contains substances, called *releasing factors,* that travel via small veins to the pituitary gland. The releasing factor believed to be most responsible for ovulation is named *gonadotropin-releasing hormone (GnRH),* also known as *luteinizing hormone-releasing hormone (LH-RH).* Scientists have found that GnRH is released from the hypothalamus in pulses of 1 per 90 minutes, and travels to target receptor cells in the pituitary called *gonadotrophs* (figure 1-8). These, in turn, release two hormones: *luteinizing hormone* (LH) and *follicle-stimulating hormone* (FSH). If the target cells in the pituitary are exposed to GnRH continuously rather than in a pulsating manner, they fail to respond and to release LH and FSH. This bit of information and the availability of synthetic GnRH compounds or analogs is the basis for some of the new and exciting research in contraceptive technology (see chapter 11).

During the typical menstrual cycle, FSH acts by traveling through the bloodstream to the ovary, where it stimulates the follicle to grow and to produce estrogen. Immediately before ovulation a large amount of estrogen, combined with GnRH, is responsible for a sudden increase of LH. It is this surge of LH that ejects an egg from the ovary. Estimates of the interval between the LH surge and ovulation vary widely. According to a study by the World Health Organization, ovulation occurs an average of thirty-two hours after the onset of the LH surge, varying between twenty-three and thirty-eight hours. While the length of the LH surge varies from woman to woman, each woman has her own predictable and repeatable pattern.

The newest and most exciting advance in the understanding of the hormones regulating fertility was made by scientists at the University of California at San Francisco in 1985. They isolated a hormone named *prolactin-release inhibitory factor,* or PIF, which many believe will lead to the development of new contraceptive and fertility drugs. Like GnRH, it too is produced by the hypothalamus and travels to the pituitary gland where it prevents the production of *prolactin* by cells called *lactotrophs* (figure 1-8). Prolactin is responsible for stimulating milk production in nursing women. It has a somewhat effective contraceptive action due to the fact that prolactin prevents ovulation by inhibiting the pituitary gland's release of FSH and LH. When prolactin is present in excessive amounts in nonpregnant women or in men, it may cause abnormal milk secretion from the breasts and infertility. The California scientists discovered that PIF and GnRH start from the same precursor chemical in the hypothalamus and then split off to perform their individual functions on the pituitary gland (see figure 1-8).

Since I have an unlimited number of eggs, why will I stop ovulating at menopause?

It is not known why the ovary suddenly ages and is no longer able to produce mature follicles from the thousands of surplus eggs. It is also a mystery why some women menstruate into their late fifties while other women experience premature menopause before the age of forty. Menopause, by definition, is the end of menstruation. According to the latest statistics, it occurs at an average age of fifty-one years. Many women are actually unable to conceive long before menopause, however. It is only natural that

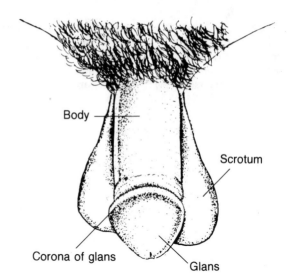

Figure 1–9. *External male genitals.*

Body

Scrotum

Corona of glans

Glans

Figure 1–10. *Penis of circumcised male.*

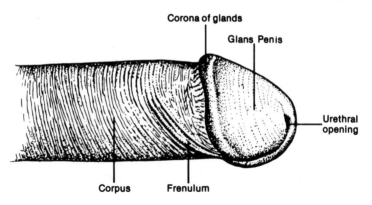

Corona of glands

Glans Penis

Urethral opening

Corpus

Frenulum

Figure 1–11. *Penis of uncircumcised male.*

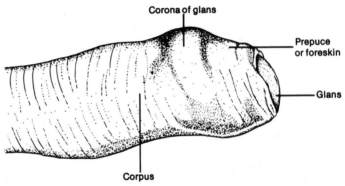

Corona of glans

Prepuce or foreskin

Glans

Corpus

women over fifty who are menstruating are deeply concerned that they might conceive, but pregnancy in this age group is rare because most such menses are preceded by inadequate follicle growth without actual ovulation. When ovulation does take place in a woman over fifty, the corpus luteum appears to be unable to sustain a pregnancy.

Practically speaking, a woman need not use contraceptives after the age of fifty, even if her periods remain regular. In addition, if she is between the ages of forty-seven and fifty and has not menstruated for one year or more, it would be nearly impossible for her to conceive. It should be mentioned that neither birth-control pills nor any other hormones are able either to accelerate or to postpone the onset of menopause. Neither are the new ovulation-stimulating drugs able to stimulate ovulation in a woman past menopause.

How does the male reproductive system function?

The external genitals of the male consist of the *penis* and the *scrotum,* which is the skin covering the two testes. The penis is composed of two parts: the *glans* and the *body* (figure 1-9).

At the undersurface of the corona of the glans in a circumcised male is a fold of skin called the *frenulum* (figure 1-10).

In an uncircumcised man, the *prepuce,* or foreskin, completely covers the corona, frenulum, and most—if not all—of the glans (figure 1-11).

Sperm cells, or *spermatozoa,* are produced by the two testes from adolescence until old age. The sperm are passed up from each testicle to a lower tube, called the *epididymis* (figure 1-12). From there, they pass through a second tube, called the *vas deferens.* The spermatozoa are then temporarily stored in the upper part of the vas deferens, or in a small sac called the *seminal vesicle.* When a man reaches orgasm, the sperm and other secretions are pushed out from these two locations and into the urethra. From there, they are ejaculated from the tip of the erect penis.

The fluid ejaculate is called *semen* and usually equals about a tablespoon in volume. A normal ejaculate contains between 40 million and 400 million sperm—not an excessive amount, since many are lost on their long journey, and only a few survivors reach the outer part of the fallopian tube. Of these, only one sperm fertilizes the egg, by breaking through its protective coating.

Figure 1–12. *Internal male anatomy.*

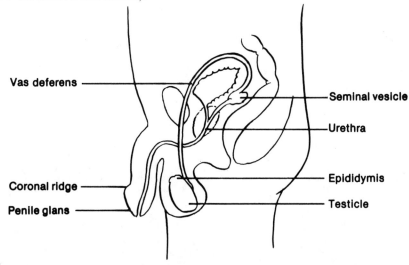

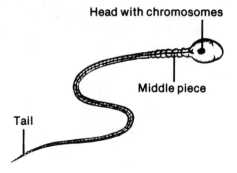

Figure 1–13. *Appearance of sperm under the microscope (enlarged).*

Testosterone is the hormone produced by the testes that is responsible for masculine characteristics, libido, and sexual potency. The production of testosterone is under the influence of the pituitary hormone LH, the same as that found in women. The other pituitary hormone, FSH, is also found in men. Scientists believe that its major function is to initiate sperm formation during adolescence and maintain sperm production in adulthood. In 1977, Belgian endocrinologists isolated *inhibin,* a key male hormone produced by the testes. Inhibin has the unique ability to inhibit or prevent FSH release without altering LH levels. Researchers throughout the world are cautiously optimistic that inhibin may be the long-sought male contraceptive, capable of preventing sperm formation while maintaining libido (see chapter 11, "The Future").

What do normal sperm look like under the microscope?

Spermatozoa look like small, wormlike creatures. The head is oval and it contains the chromosomes that will determine half the traits of the potential child. The tail is vital for forward movement of the sperm. Even the slightest changes in the shape or movement of the sperm adversely affect a man's fertility (figure 1-13).

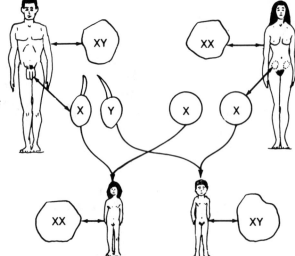

Figure 1–14. *Sex chromosomes of sperm and egg.*

What determines the sex of a fetus?

The sex of a fertilized egg is determined by the type of sex chromosome present in the head of the sperm. The adult male has two sex chromosomes in his body cells: They are called X and Y (figure 1-14).

Each sperm can carry either an X or a Y. The adult woman contains two X chromosomes in each of her body cells, but no Ys. Therefore, her egg always contributes an X to the future offspring (figure 1-14). If a sperm cell carrying a Y chromosome fertilizes the X egg, the result is XY, a male. If a sperm cell carrying an X gets there first, the result is XX, a female.

What does all this basic anatomy have to do with contraception?

Throughout this book I will refer to this chapter when describing how the various contraception, sterilization, and abortion techniques work. In addition, much of the new information presented in chapter 11 is based on the principles mentioned in this section of the book.

2

BIRTH-CONTROL PILLS

Until recently, birth-control pills had been the most popular form of contraception in the United States. As a result of adverse publicity about the Pill's safety, however, its use has declined precipitously from a high of over 10 million women in 1974 to its present level of approximately 6 million women. While many of the serious complications and unpleasant side effects in the past occurred with dangerously high hormonal formulations that are no longer in use, skepticism about Pill safety remains prevalent. In fact, despite recent favorable reports about the contraceptive and non-contraceptive benefits of birth-control pills, three out of four American women continue to cling to the mistaken notion that the Pill creates substantial health risks.

Is there one birth-control pill that is better than the others?

Manufacturers of the sixty birth-control pills on the market have spent billions of dollars in an effort to prove that their particular product is better than any other. In reality, many of the pills are similar and occasionally identical to others, differing only in the promotional schemes and advertising gimmicks used to sell them to physicians. Friendly sales representatives from competing pharmaceutical companies pay frequent visits to your gynecologist with the specific mission of supplying him or her with as many free samples as possible. The motive behind this goodwill gesture is to get your doctor into the habit of dispensing these free "starter" samples and writing prescriptions for that particular birth-control pill.

The table that follows lists all the birth-control pills currently available in the United States as well as the amounts of estrogen and progestogen in each pill. All these products, with the exception of the minipills, contain estrogen, in the form of either mestranol or ethinyl estradiol. The progestogen is either norethynodrel, norethindrone, norethindrone acetate, ethynodiol diacetate, levonorgestrel, or norgestrel. A description of each pill, along with a breakdown of its ingredients, is given in the table. As you can readily see, switching from Ortho-Novum 1/35/21 to Norinyl 1/35/21 or from Modicon to Brevicon could not possibly relieve an unpleasant side effect as the contents of the pills are identical.

14

THE PILLS: WHAT'S IN THEM?

BRAND NAME	NUMBER OF TABLETS	DESCRIPTION (Combinations)	ESTROGENS (milligrams)*		PROGESTOGENS (milligrams)*					
			Mestranol	Ethinyl Estradiol	Norgestrel	Levonorgestrel	Norethindrone	Norethindrone Acetate	Ethynodiol Diacetate	Norethynodrel
Brevicon (Syntex)	21	In brown "Wellette"; 21 blue tablets		0.035			0.5			
Brevicon-28 (Syntex)	28	Same as above plus 7 orange placebos		0.035			0.5			
Demulen 1/35-21 (Searle)	21	In blue-green compact; 21 white tablets		0.035					1.0	
Demulen 1/35-28 (Searle)	28	In blue-green compact; 21 white tablets and 7 blue placebos		0.035					1.0	
Demulen 1/50-21 (Searle)	21	In yellow compact; 21 white tablets		0.05					1.0	
Demulen 1/50-28 (Searle)	28	In yellow compact; 21 white tablets and 7 pink placebos		0.05					1.0	

THE PILLS: WHAT'S IN THEM? (Continued)

BRAND NAME	NUMBER OF TABLETS	DESCRIPTION (Combinations)	ESTROGENS (milligrams)*		PROGESTOGENS (milligrams)*					
			Mestranol	Ethinyl Estradiol	Norgestrel	Levonorgestrel	Norethindrone	Norethindrone Acetate	Ethynodiol Diacetate	Norethynodrel
Enovid 5 (Searle)	20	White calendar pack or sold separately; light pink pill with "51" on one side	0.075							5.0
Enovid 10 (Searle)	20	White calendar pack or sold separately; dark pink pill with "101" on one side	0.15							9.85
Enovid-E 21 (Searle)	21	White compact; white tablets with "131" on one side	0.1							2.5
Levlen-21 (Berlex)	21	Beige case; 21 light-orange tablets		0.03		0.15				
Levlen-28 (Berlex)	28	Same as above plus 7 pink placebos		0.03		0.15				
Loestrin 21-1/20 (Parke-Davis)	21	Yellow compact; 21 white pills with "PD" on one side		0.02				1.0		

	#	Description					
Loestrin Fe-1/20 (Parke-Davis)	28	Light yellow compact; 21 white pills with "PD" on one side and 7 brown iron tablets		0.02			1.0
Loestrin 21-1.5/30 (Parke-Davis)	21	Light blue compact; 21 green tablets with "PD" on one side		0.03			1.5
Loestrin Fe-1.5/30 (Parke-Davis)	28	Beige compact; 21 green tablets with "PD" on one side and 7 brown iron tablets		0.03			1.5
Lo/Oval (Wyeth)	21	In pink oval case; 21 white tablets with "7-8" on one side		0.03	0.3		
Lo/Oval-28 (Wyeth)	28	In pink oval case; 21 white tablets and 7 pink placebos		0.03	0.3		
Modicon 21 (Ortho)	21	In aqua dial pack; 21 white tablets with "Ortho" on each side		0.035		0.5	
Modicon 28 (Ortho)	28	Same as above plus 7 green placebos		0.035		0.5	
Norinyl 1 + 50-21 (Syntex)	21	In brown "Wallette"; 21 white tablets with "1" on one side	0.05			1.0	
Norinyl 1 + 50-28 (Syntex)	28	Same as above plus 7 orange placebos	0.05			1.0	
Norinyl 1 + 80-21 (Syntex)	21	In brown "Wallette"; 21 yellow tablets with "3" on one side	0.08			1.0	

THE PILLS: WHAT'S IN THEM? (Continued)

Combinations

BRAND NAME	NUMBER OF TABLETS	DESCRIPTION	ESTROGENS (milligrams)*		PROGESTOGENS (milligrams)*					
			Mestranol	Ethinyl Estradiol	Norgestrel	Levonorgestrel	Norethindrone	Norethindrone Acetate	Ethynodiol Diacetate	Norethynodrel
Norinyl 1 + 80-28 (Syntex)	28	Same as above plus 7 orange placebos	0.08				1.0			
Nordette-21 (Wyeth)	21	In silver oval case; 21 light-orange tablets with "75" on one side		0.03		0.15				
Nordette-28 (Wyeth)	28	Same as above plus 7 pink placebos		0.03		0.15				
Norinyl 1 + 35-21 (Syntex)	21	In brown "Wallette"; 21 lemon-colored pills with "111" on one side		0.035			1.0			
Norinyl 1 + 35-28 (Syntex)	28	Same as above plus 7 orange placebos		0.035			1.0			
Norinyl 2 (Syntex)	20	No packet; white tablets with "2" on one side	0.1				2.0			

Norlestrin 21-1/50 (Parke-Davis)	21	Light-green compact; 21 yellow pills with "PD" on one side	0.05			1.0
Norlestrin Fe-1/50 (Parke-Davis)	28	Pea-green compact; 21 yellow pills with "PD" on one side and 7 brown iron pills	0.05			1.0
Norlestrin 21-2.5/50 (Parke-Davis)	21	Pink compact; 21 pink pills with "PD" on one side	0.05			2.5
Norlestrin Fe-2.5/50 (Parke-Davis)	28	Light purple compact; 21 pink pills with "PD" on one side	0.05			2.5
Ortho-Novum 1/35-21 (Ortho)	21	Peach-colored dial pack; 21 peach-colored tablets		0.035	1.0	
Ortho-Novum 1/35-28 (Ortho)	28	Same as above plus 7 green placebos		0.035	1.0	
Ortho-Novum 1/50-21 (Ortho)	21	Yellow dial pack; 21 yellow tablets		0.05	1.0	
Ortho-Novum 1/50-28 (Ortho)	28	Same as above plus 7 green placebos		0.05	1.0	
Ortho-Novum 1/80-21 (Ortho)	21	Pink dial pack; 21 white tablets		0.08	1	
Ortho-Novum 1/80-28 (Ortho)	28	Same as above plus 7 green placebos		0.08	1	

THE PILLS: WHAT'S IN THEM? (Continued)

BRAND NAME	NUMBER OF TABLETS	DESCRIPTION Combinations	ESTROGENS (milligrams)* Mestranol	Ethinyl Estradiol	PROGESTOGENS (milligrams)* Norgestrel	Levonorgestrel	Norethindrone	Norethindrone Acetate	Ethynodiol Diacetate	Norethynodrel
Ortho-Novum 7/7/7/-21 (Ortho)	21	Peach-colored dial pack; 7 white tablets, 7 light peach tablets, 7 peach tablets		0.035 in all tablets			0.5(7W) 0.75(7LP) 1.0(7P)			
Ortho-Novum 7/7/7/-28 (Ortho)	28	Same as above plus 7 green placebos		0.035 in all tablets			0.5(7W) 0.75(7LP) 1.0(7P)			
Ortho-Novum 10/11/-21 (Ortho)	21	Blue dial pack; 10 white tablets and 11 peach-colored tablets		0.035 in all tablets			0.5(10W) 1.0(11P)			
Ortho-Novum 10/11-28 (Ortho)	28	Same as above plus 7 green placebos		0.035 in all tablets			0.5(10W) 1.0(11P)			
Ortho-Novum 2 mg-21 (Ortho)	21	Purple dial pack; 21 white tablets	0.10				2			

Product (Manufacturer)	Days	Description						
Ovcon-35 (Mead Johnson)	21	Gray pack; 21 pink tablets with "MJ" on one side		0.035			0.4	
Ovcon 35-28 (Mead Johnson)	28	Same as above plus 7 green placebos		0.035			0.4	
Ovcon-50 (Mead-Johnson)	21	Blue pack; 21 beige tablets with "MJ" on one side		0.05			1.0	
Ovcon 50-28 (Mead-Johnson)	28	Same as above plus 7 green placebos		0.05			1.0	
Ovral (Wyeth)	21	In white oval case; 21 white tablets with "56" on one side		0.05	0.5			
Ovral-28 (Wyeth)	28	Same as above plus 7 pink placebos		0.05	0.5			
Ovulen-21 (Searle)	21	White case; 21 white tablets with "401" on one side	0.1					1.0
Ovulen-28 (Searle)	28	Same as above plus 7 pink placebos	0.1					1.0
Tri-Levlen-21 (Berlex)	21	Gray case with blue stripes; 6 brown tablets, 5 white tablets, 10 light-yellow tablets		0.03(6B) 0.04(5W) 0.03(10Y)		0.05(6B) 0.075(5W) 0.125(10Y)		
Tri-Levlen-28 (Berlex)	28	Same as above plus 7 light-green placebos		0.03(6B) 0.04(5W) 0.03(10Y)		0.05(6B) 0.075(5W) 0.125(10Y)		

THE PILLS: WHAT'S IN THEM? (Continued)

BRAND NAME	NUMBER OF TABLETS	DESCRIPTION (Combinations)	ESTROGENS (milligrams)*		PROGESTOGENS (milligrams)*					
			Mestranol	Ethinyl Estradiol	Norgestrel	Levonorgestrel	Norethindrone	Norethindrone Acetate	Ethynodiol Diacetate	Norethynodrel
Tri-Norinyl-21 (Syntex)	21	Brown "Wallette"; 7 blue tablets, 9 green tablets, and 5 more blue tablets		0.035 in all tablets		0.5(7B) 1.0(9G) 0.5(5B)				
Tri-Norinyl-28 (Syntex)	28	Same as above plus 7 peach-colored placebos		0.035 in all tablets			0.5(7B) 1.0(9G) 0.5(5B)			
Triphasil-21 (Wyeth)	21	White rectangular case; 6 brown tablets, 5 white tablets, 10 light-yellow tablets		0.03(6B) 0.04(5W) 0.03(10Y)		0.05(6B) 0.075(5W) 0.125(10Y)				
Triphasil-28 (Wyeth)	28	Same as above plus 7 light-green placebos		0.03(6B) 0.04(5W) 0.03(10Y)		0.05(6B) 0.075(5W) 0.125(10Y)				

Progestins Only (Minipills)

Micronor (Ortho)	28	In green dial pack; 28 green tablets		0.35
Nor-Q.D. (Syntex)	42	In cardboard package; 42 yellow tablets		0.35
Ovrette (Wyeth)	28	In blue compact; 28 yellow tablets marked "Wyeth" and "62"	0.075	

* .05 milligrams = 50 micrograms
SOURCE: *Compiled by the author.*

How do birth-control pills prevent pregnancy?

Birth-control pills that combine estrogen and progestogen are thought to prevent conception by inhibiting the release of GnRH from the hypothalamus. That in turn stops FSH from stimulating an ovarian follicle to grow and stops LH from triggering ovulation. In addition, both components of combination pills change the endometrium in such a manner that even if ovulation were to take place, implantation of the fertilized egg would be unsuccessful. Furthermore, the progestogen in each of those pills produces a thick cervical mucus that is hostile to sperm trying to penetrate and migrate through the cervical os. Minipills, which contain only progestogen, do not always prevent ovulation, but they exert the dual action of thickening the cervical mucus and making the endometrium unreceptive.

Is one of the two types of estrogen in the Pill stronger than the other?

Both mestranol and ethinyl estradiol are synthetic estrogens, many times more potent than those produced naturally by the body. A variety of rat experiments has suggested that mestranol is the weaker hormone. In terms of equivalents, 0.05 milligrams of ethinyl estradiol was found comparable to 0.08 milligrams of mestranol. But most researchers now believe that in the human body there is little if any difference in potency between the two. One exception is the effect that the two estrogens have on the endometrium, or lining of the uterus. Breakthrough bleeding (endometrial bleeding that occurs on days when the Pill is taken rather than at the normal time, during the days when the Pill is not in use) is more likely to occur as the dose of estrogen is decreased below 0.05 milligrams. Ethinyl estradiol is far better than mestranol in preventing breakthrough bleeding, as evidenced by the fact that it is used in all pills containing 0.035 milligrams of estrogen or less (see the table on pages 15–23). Therefore, if you are experiencing annoying breakthrough bleeding with a pill that contains mestranol, ask your doctor to switch you to an ethinyl estradiol product with the same number of milligrams.

Whether ethinyl estradiol is more potent than mestranol in areas of the body other than the endometrium remains an unanswered question due to a lack of conclusive data.

What are some of the undesirable side effects and complications associated with the estrogen in birth-control pills?

Pill formulations containing less than 0.05 milligrams of estrogen were introduced in 1975, and only recently have epidemiologists confirmed that the incidence of minor side effects and major complications has been reduced dramatically. Today, 65 percent of all oral contraceptives prescribed in the United States contain 0.030 to 0.035 milligrams of estrogen. The public's awareness of pill-related complications is based on earlier studies in which much higher doses of estrogen were evaluated, and this misunderstanding, more than any other factor, is responsible for the 40 percent decline in Pill use since 1979.

Nor is the Pill totally innocuous. While side effects and serious complications occur less frequently today, they do exist but they can be remedied. The following list shows all the minor and major problems that may be associated with the estrogen component of birth-control pills.

SIDE EFFECTS AND COMPLICATIONS OF ESTROGEN IN BIRTH-CONTROL PILLS

Minor Side Effects

1. Nausea and vomiting
2. Fluid retention and bloated feeling

3. Cyclic weight gain
4. Cyclic nonmigraine headaches
5. Breast tenderness
6. Increased mucus discharge from glands of cervix; cervical erosion
7. Depression
8. Dizziness
9. Hay fever and allergic nasal congestion
10. Galactorrhea (clear-to-white nipple discharge)
11. Confusing but harmless changes in thyroid function tests and tests measuring cortisone levels
12. Increased skin pigmentation (chloasma) or "mask of pregnancy" on face
13. Vision changes caused by changes in the contour of the cornea; contact lens discomfort

Major Complications

1. Worsening of migraine headaches
2. Increase in blood pressure
3. Changes in sugar tolerance in both diabetics and nondiabetics
4. Increased growth of benign (noncancerous) fibroid tumors of the uterus
5. Increased growth rate of estrogen-dependent cancers of the breast and uterus (estrogen will not create new ones, however)
6. Vitamin deficiencies
7. Urinary tract changes and infections
8. Increased incidence of benign liver tumors
9. Jaundice or yellowing of the skin due to altered liver function and bile excretion
10. Gallbladder disease
11. Abnormalities in blood clotting factors
12. Thrombophlebitis (inflamed blood clot in a vein)
13. Pulmonary embolism (passage of blood clot to the lung)
14. Cerebral thrombosis stroke (presence of blood clot in a vessel in the brain)
15. Cerebral hemorrhage stroke (bursting of a blood vessel in the brain)
16. Myocardial infarction (heart attack caused by blockage of an artery in the heart)

Are the progestogens associated with any side effects or serious complications?

Progestogens, or progestins, as they are called, are synthetic hormones more closely related to the male hormone testosterone than to the female hormone progesterone. Until recently, doctors were obsessed with lowering the estrogen dose in birth-control pills while paying little attention to the potential problems created by the progestins. It is now realized that progestins in too high a dose may be responsible for a host of side effects and serious metabolic derangements. For example, all six progestins can increase a person's risk of atherosclerosis and heart disease by lowering plasma levels of protective high density lipoprotein-cholesterol (HDL-C). The progestins' newly discovered role in altering glucose metabolism is also of great significance. The list that follows presents some side effects and complications from the progestin component of the Pill.

SIDE EFFECTS AND COMPLICATIONS OF PROGESTINS

Minor Side Effects

1. Acne
2. Oily skin and scalp
3. Increase in facial hair
4. Thinning and loss of scalp hair
5. Increased appetite and noncyclic weight gain
6. Reduction in size of breasts
7. Fatigue
8. Increased predisposition to monilial vaginitis (yeast)
9. Diminished sex drive
10. Nervousness
11. Vaginal dryness
12. Absent or shorter periods

Major Complications

1. Change in sugar tolerance and insulin requirements in both diabetics and nondiabetics
2. Alterations in liver function and cholesterol concentration in the bile
3. Along with estrogen, may contribute to formation of rare liver tumor
4. Altered lipid metabolism and increased risk of atherosclerosis, heart attack, and stroke
5. Increase in blood pressure
6. Increase in blood clotting factors

How do the progestins differ in strength?

There are six progestins: norethindrone, norethynodrel, norethindrone acetate, ethynodiol diacetate, norgestrel, and levonorgestrel. Determining the relative strengths of the progestins has intrigued and confounded scientists since 1960. One method is based on how small an amount of a given progestin or progestogen, combined with a fixed amount of estrogen, can delay the start of a healthy woman's period for two weeks. Others have used its ability to prevent ovulation and to thicken a woman's cervical mucus as measurement of a progestin's strength. Based on these criteria, norethindrone and norethynodrel have been found to be the weakest progestins, while levonorgestrel is the strongest, followed by norgestrel, ethynodiol diacetate, and norethindrone acetate. Levonorgestrel is the active component of norgestrel. Half of the norgestrel in Lo-Ovral is in this hormonally active levo form. Even though Pills such as Levlen and Nordette contain only 0.15 milligrams of progestin, the fact is that they contain the metabolic equivalent of 0.3 milligrams of norgestrel found in Lo-Ovral.

Since ethynodiol diacetate, norethindrone acetate, and norethynodrel are all converted to norethindrone in a woman's body, many scientists believe that these four progestogens are essentially of equal strength. Further research is needed to confirm this theory. All investigators agree, however, that norgestrel and levonorgestrel are stronger progestins than the others.

Since progestins are derived from the male hormone testosterone, they can, in high doses, cause a woman to develop androgenic, or masculinizing, traits such as facial hair, acne, and oily skin. Of all the formulations, levonorgestrel is believed to be the most androgenic, followed closely by norgestrel. It would thus be inappropriate for a doctor to prescribe a Pill such as Ovral, containing 0.5 milligrams of norgestrel, to a woman who is particularly concerned about a problem with acne or facial hair.

A portion of each progestin is metabolized to estrogen compounds in the body. This conversion to estrogen varies in degree among the different progestins and probably among individuals using the same Pill formulation. Ethynodiol diacetate, in contrast to the more androgenic levonorgestrel and norgestrel, is considered by some scientists to be the most estrogenic. For this reason, products such as Demulen and Demulen 1/35 may be more suitable than Ovral for acne sufferers. Norethynodrel is considered to have estrogenic properties that are similar to those of ethynodiol diacetate.

Though it is difficult if not impossible to match each individual woman perfectly with a birth-control pill, a doctor can often overcome the side effects of oral contraceptive use by changing a woman's prescription. The following table lists methods of dealing with a wide variety of Pill side effects. It should be pointed out, however, that doctors are not in the practice of matching the Pill to the patient. A doctor's primary concern should always be to prescribe the lowest possible dose of estrogen and progestin to avoid serious side effects and complications. This would mean a maximum dose of 0.05 milligrams of ethinyl estradiol or of mestranol, and a limit of 1.0 milligrams of norethindrone, norethindrone acetate, ethynodiol diacetate, or norethynodrel. And no more than 0.30 milligrams of norgestrel or 0.15 milligrams of levonorgestrel should be prescribed. Any doctor who currently prescribes Enovid, Enovid-E, Loestrin 1.5, Norinyl 1+80, Norinyl 2, Norlestrin 2.5, Ortho-Novum 1/80, Ortho-Novum 2, or Ovulen solely for contraception is practicing outdated medicine.

Are there any advantages to using the new triphasic birth-control pills?

The aim of the new triphasic birth-control pills is to lower the total amount of progestogen in each pill cycle and thereby reduce progestogen-related side effects and complications. This is done by maintaining the lowest possible dose of progestogen early in the cycle, and then increasing the amount toward the middle of the cycle in order to prevent ovulation and breakthrough bleeding which is most likely to occur between the eighth and sixteenth pill.

There are currently four triphasics on the market: Triphasil, Tri-Levlen, Tri-Norinyl, and Ortho-Novum 7/7/7. Triphasil contains the progestin levonorgestrel in progressively increasing doses: 0.05 milligrams for six days; 0.075 milligrams for five days; and 0.125 milligrams for ten days. In addition, the dose of ethinyl estradiol changes from 0.30 milligrams to 0.40 milligrams for five days in the middle of the cycle (see table earlier in the chapter, "The Pills: What's in Them?"). The newest, highly touted triphasic product named Tri-Levlen is actually identical to Triphasil. Tri-Norinyl and Ortho-Novum 7/7/7 maintain the same dose of 0.035 milligrams of ethinyl estradiol throughout the cycle. Both products contain norethindrone, but with Ortho-Novum 7/7/7 the amount increases progressively every seven days from 0.5 milligrams to 0.75 milligrams to 1.5 milligrams, respectively. In contrast, the dose of norethindrone in Tri-Norinyl is 0.5 milligrams for the first seven days, followed by 1.0 milligrams for nine days, and a return to 0.5 milligrams during the last five days of the cycle.

As far as total progestogen reduction per Pill cycle is concerned, a woman taking Triphasil will ingest 1.925 milligrams of levonorgestrel each month. Lo-Ovral, produced by Wyeth, as is Triphasil, contains the lowest progestogen dose of all standard or monophasic Pills the company manufactures. A Lo-Ovral user ingests 0.3 milligrams of norgestrel each day, for a total of 6.3 milligrams per cycle. As previously stated, 1.925 milligrams of levonorgestrel equals 3.85 milligrams of norgestrel. Therefore, 6.3 milligrams minus 3.85 milligrams equals a reduction equivalent to 2.45 milligrams of norgestrel or 1.23 milligrams of levonorgestrel for each month that a woman uses Triphasil rather than Lo-Ovral. Ortho-Novum 7/7/7 contains a total of 15.8 milligrams of norethindrone each cycle, compared to 15 milligrams with Tri-Norinyl. The lowest monophasic Pill produced by their respective companies—

MANAGING SIDE EFFECTS OF ORAL CONTRACEPTIVES

RECOMMENDED CORRECTION OF SIDE EFFECT

Side Effect	Estrogen Dose Correction	Progestin Dose Correction	Other Suggestions
Nausea or vomiting	Decrease	No Change	Take after full meal; Minipill
Bloating and fluid retention	Decrease	No Change	Minipill
Breast tenderness	Decrease	No Change or Increase	Minipill
Cyclic weight gain	Decrease	No Change or Decrease	
Noncyclic weight gain and increased appetite	No Change or Decrease	Decrease	Avoid norgestrel and levonorgestrel
Dizziness	Decrease or Stop	No Change	
Increased skin pigmentation	Decrease or Stop	No Change	Minipill
Cervical eversion and increased mucus	Decrease	No Change	
Headache, migraine	Decrease or Stop	Decrease or Stop	
Increased blood pressure	Decrease or Stop	Decrease or Stop	
Thrombophlebitis	Stop	Stop	
Varicose veins	Decrease	No Change	
Contact lens discomfort	Decrease or Stop	No Change	Minipill

Blind spots	Stop	Stop	
Increased growth of benign fibroids	Decrease or Stop	No Change or Decrease	
Breast or uterine cancer	Stop	Stop	
Change in thyroid function tests	No Change	No Change	
Decrease of HDL-C	Decrease or Stop	Decrease or Stop	Triphasic pill
Heart attack or stroke	Stop	Stop	
Pulmonary embolus	Stop	Stop	
Liver disease, jaundice, or benign liver tumor	Stop	Stop	
Gallbladder disease	Stop	Stop	
Decreased breast milk in nursing mothers	Stop	No Change or Decrease	Minipill
Increased sensitivity to light	Decrease or Stop	No Change or Decrease	Minipill
Ovarian cysts	No Change	No Change	
Rheumatoid arthritis	No Change	No Change	
Pelvic inflammatory disease	No Change	No Change	
Anemia	No Change	No Change or Increase	
Menstrual flow too heavy	Decrease	Increase	

MANAGING SIDE EFFECTS OF ORAL CONTRACEPTIVES (Continued)

RECOMMENDED CORRECTION OF SIDE EFFECT

Side Effect	Estrogen Dose Correction	Progestin Dose Correction	Other Suggestions
Urinary tract infection	Decrease	No Change	
Light or absent menses	Increase	Decrease	
Acne	Increase	Decrease	
Increased facial hair and thinning of scalp hair	Increase	Decrease	
Decreased size of breasts	Increase	Decrease	
Yeast infections	No Change	Decrease	
Decreased sex drive	Decrease or Stop	Decrease or Stop	
Depression	Decrease or Stop	Decrease or Stop	Vitamin B_6?
Breakthrough bleeding	Increase	No Change or Increase	
Decreased vaginal secretion (dry vagina)	Increase	Decrease	
Worsening of diabetes	Decrease or Stop	Decrease or Stop	
Nervousness	No Change	Decrease or Stop	

SOURCE: *Compiled by the author.*

namely, Norinyl 1+35 and Ortho-Novum 1+35—contains a total of 21 milligrams per cycle of norethindrone.

Whether these small reductions in total monthly progestin dose make triphasics safer than low-dose monophasics is unknown. Epidemiologists believe it will take years before this question can be answered. Preliminary studies, however, while somewhat contradictory, are still encouraging. In one 1985 report from Frankfurt, published in the *American Journal of Obstetrics and Gynecology,* doctors found that the estrogen and progestogen combination in Triphasil actually increased high density lipoprotein-cholesterol (HDL-C) levels in the blood without altering those of low density lipoprotein-cholesterol (LDL-C) and very low density lipoprotein-cholesterol (VLDL-C). Since high levels of HDL-C are believed to be protective against atherosclerosis and heart disease (see page 35), the authors concluded that this triphasic Pill may actually exert beneficial effects on these conditions. In another 1985 study, researchers in Denmark noted no change in HDL-C when women used Triphasil for two to six months. In addition, glucose tolerance tests remained normal among all women studied, including those with a previous history of gestational or pregnancy-related diabetes (see page 41). In his 1987 review of triphasic contraceptives, Dr. Jeffrey W. Ellis concluded that triphasics offer considerable advantages over combination products. Based on available research to date, Dr. Ellis concluded that triphasics containing norethindrone, such as Ortho-Novum 7/7/7 and Tri-Norinyl, are less likely to adversely affect cholesterol and carbohydrate metabolism than are products containing the stronger levonorgestrel.

Triphasic manufacturers have claimed that their products are more "natural" and closer to a woman's normal menstrual cycle than are monophasic birth-control pills, equating the progestogen increase to the normal progesterone rise that follows ovulation in women who are not on the Pill. Most experts, however, do not agree, since both triphasics and monophasics work by preventing ovulation and altering the endometrium and cervical mucus. Manufacturers have also stated that the incidence of breakthrough bleeding is significantly less with triphasics. Several studies comparing Triphasil with Lo-Ovral, however, have shown that just the opposite is true. When Ortho-Novum 7/7/7 and Tri-Norinyl were compared with Ortho-Novum 1/35 and Norinyl 1/35, the incidence of breakthrough bleeding was equal in some studies and reduced in others.

Though much remains to be learned about the new triphasics, it would seem prudent for doctors to prescribe them, as they all contain less than 0.05 milligrams of ethinyl estradiol and the lowest possible total dose of progestogen per cycle. As we have learned from unpleasant experiences with oral conceptives in the past, less is better and healthier than more.

If less is better than more, why don't doctors prefer the Minipill for their patients?

The Minipill, or progestin-only pill, was introduced in the early 1970s to eliminate the risk of the old-fashioned high-dose estrogen formulations. At that time it was not yet known that progestogens play the key role in adversely altering lipid and carbohydrate metabolism. No one realized that these harmful progestogen changes could be lessened or totally reversed simply by lowering, rather than eliminating, the estrogen dose in the Pill.

There are currently three Minipills sold in the United States: Ovrette (0.075 milligrams of norgestrel); NorQD (0.35 milligrams of norethindrone); and Micronor (0.35 milligrams of norethindrone). Unlike other birth-control pills, the Minipill must be taken every day without interruption. If a day is missed, the chances of pregnancy are much greater than when one combination pill is missed. For 100 women using the Minipill diligently for one year, there will still be approximately two to eight pregnancies, or a success rate of 92 to 98 percent. The combination pill, on the other hand, is 99.3 percent effective. The reason for this difference is that the Minipill does not always inhibit ovulation. Instead, it exerts its contraceptive effect by creating a cervical mucus that is hostile to sperm and a uterine lining that is unreceptive to a fertilized egg. Because the Minipill contains no estrogen, at least half the women using it experience unpredictable bleeding. Is it any wonder that Minipills make up only 1 percent of the oral contraceptive sales in the United States?

Of the progestogens present in Minipills, norgestrel (Ovrette) exerts a more profound change in body metabolism than does norethindrone acetate (NorQD and Micronor). In one study from the University of Florida, doctors noted an abnormal or borderline glucose tolerance test in 16 percent of previously healthy women who used Ovrette for twelve months. While both progestogens are capable of causing unfavorable changes in lipid metabolism (see page 35), the changes from norgestrel are greater than those from norethindrone. If an identical dose of either progestogen is combined in a birth control pill with 0.30 to 0.035 milligrams of the estrogen ethinyl estradiol, however, both glucose tolerance and lipid metabolism will revert to normal. This shows the protective effect that small doses of estrogen have on these metabolic indicators.

Data from eighteen separate studies strongly suggests a higher incidence of ectopic pregnancy among women who accidentally conceive while using the Minipill (see page 61). One group of researchers suggested that the progestin norgestrel, the type found in Ovrette, was more likely than other progestins to be the culprit. From the information available, it is clear that a doctor should always consider the possibility of an ectopic pregnancy in a woman who develops lower abdominal pain while she is on a progestin-only oral contraceptive. Why the Minipill makes a woman more susceptible to ectopic pregnancy is unknown. It is theorized that the progestin slows down the transport of the fertilized egg by the fallopian tube. As a result, the egg attaches itself within the tube rather than in its normal location in the endometrium of the uterus.

The estrogen contained in the combination birth-control pills is capable of reducing the quantity of breast milk in nursing women. The progestin-only Minipill, on the other hand, does not appear to affect adversely the quantity of milk produced. As a result, many obstetricians prescribe the Minipill as contraception for nursing women. Other doctors are reluctant to do so because no large-scale studies have been conducted to prove that small amounts of progestin ingested in the milk over a long period of time are harmless to a nursing infant. While Minipills do not appear to reduce milk quantity, statistics show that they do alter the basic composition of breast milk—decreasing the total protein content, milk fat, lactose, phosphorous, calcium, magnesium, and zinc, among other changes. It is for these reasons that Minipills are not usually a doctor's first choice of contraception for the nursing woman.

Chemists have found that a small percentage of the norethindrone in Micronor and NorQD is converted to estrogen in the body, so it is not possible to prescribe Minipills for women whose medical problems absolutely preclude the use of pills containing estrogen.

How effective is the biphasic pill Ortho-Novum 10/11?

Ortho-Novum 10/11 is called a biphasic (two-phase) formulation because the dose of the progestogen norethindrone changes from 0.5 milligrams during the first ten days to 1.0 milligrams during the last eleven days of the cycle. The estrogen dose of 0.035 milligrams remains the same in all twenty-one pills. Since norethindrone is probably the weakest progestin, the increase to 1 milligram on the eleventh day is necessary to prevent excessive breakthrough bleeding. Nevertheless, several studies have suggested that there is a higher incidence of breakthrough bleeding with this product than with many other low-dose combination pills. The effectiveness in pregnancy prevention is the same for Ortho-Novum 10/11 as it is for triphasics and other estrogen-progestogen formulations. Though it offers no clear-cut advantages over other birth control pills, its introduction several years ago led to the development of the newer triphasic pills.

Can a woman really die from taking birth-control pills?

The so-called bottom line for cold and calculating statisticians means something they can accurately measure. Certainly the number of women who die from using a particular contraceptive method is an endpoint we can all readily appreciate. The following chart (figure 2-1) estimates the number of deaths, per 100,000 women, associated with various methods of birth control, abortion, and pregnancy. The groups are listed in four-year blocks of time between the ages of seventeen and forty-four. The risks of dying from Pill use, IUDs, and abortion result from complications caused directly by each method. The risks associated with rhythm and barrier methods, however, stem entirely from complications of untended pregnancy, whether it be abortion, ectopic pregnancy, or death in childbirth.

Though these statistics were published in 1983, they are based on data accumulated between 1972 and 1978 when most women used birth-control pills of a higher dose than they do now. With current lower dose formulations, the death rate from Pill use today will undoubtedly prove to be much lower than that presented here. Nevertheless, the extreme safety of the Pill for nonsmokers under the age of thirty-five is impressive. The death rate soars to 14.1 per 100,000, however, between the ages of thirty-five to thirty-nine, and 32 per 100,000 between forty and forty-four. If you believe that statistics don't lie, you are probably best advised to use a method other than the Pill after the age of thirty-five, even if you are in excellent health and a nonsmoker.

For women under the age of twenty-five who do not smoke, Pill use carries the lowest risk of any method except barrier contraception (diaphragm, condom, spermicides) backed up by early abortion. Even if a teenager or a woman under twenty-five does smoke, her risk of dying from Pill use is still fairly equal to the risk with all other methods and much lower than the risk of dying from pregnancy complications.

The most important and frightening lesson to be learned from these statistics is the danger of smoking and using birth-control pills if you are more than thirty. The dramatic rise from 13.7 deaths per 100,000 women between the ages of thirty and thirty-four to an astonishing 117.6 per 100,000 deaths after the age of forty is just too high a price to pay for effective contraception. Based on the statistics in this chart, it is estimated that approximately 500 of the more than 8 million women who use the Pill will die each year as a direct result of this method.

What are the main causes of Pill-related deaths and hospitalizations?

Heart attack and stroke account for the overwhelming majority of the estimated 300 fatalities associated with Pill use each year. This number is based on the statistic that there are approximately six million Pill users in the United States. A small number of deaths are associated with pulmonary embolism, or the passage of blood clots to the lung from the lining of veins deep in the legs and pelvis.

The risk of both fatal and nonfatal heart attacks and strokes rises with age from an estimated 4 per 100,000 users under the age of twenty-five, to 13 per 100,000 for those aged twenty-five to thirty-four, and to 54 per 100,000 for those thirty-five and older. It has been estimated that there are about 600 Pill-related hospitalizations annually from heart attacks and strokes.

Deep vein clotting and pulmonary embolism are believed to account for about 72 hospitalizations per 100,000 Pill users, for a total of approximately 4,200 per year. While this may sound like a large number, it is really very low, considering how many American women take the Pill.

The most optimistic report to date about the safety of the Pill was published in *Obstetrics and Gynecology* in July 1985 and based on Pill use from 1980 to 1982. Researchers from Boston and Seattle studied 6,500 women and found no difference in the incidence of myocardial infarction or of stroke between Pill users and nonusers, although the Pill users did have a slighly higher risk of pulmonary embolism. Many of the women in the study were using the newer low estrogen and progestogen combinations—encouraging news for women using today's safer Pills.

Estimated annual number of deaths associated with unintended fertility and fertility control methods per 100,000 nonsterile women, by age group

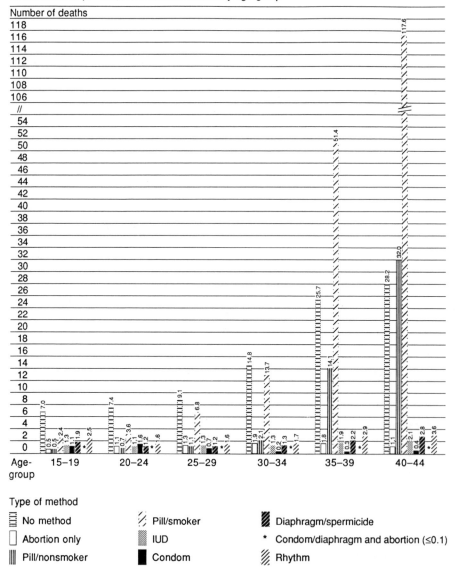

Figure 2–1. *Mortality rates associated with various methods of fertility control. (Reprinted with permission from* Making Choices: Evaluating the Health Risks and Benefits of Birth Control Method, *The Alan Guttmacher Institute, 1983.)*

Epidemiologists have determined that an estimated 86 percent of deaths associated with oral contraceptive use result from the combined effects of the Pill and smoking, and from reliance on the Pill by women aged thirty-five and older. The 300 deaths attributed to Pill use each year could be reduced to about 42 if all Pill users quit smoking and none used the Pill after their thirty-fifth birthday. Furthermore, if doctors screened patients more carefully for abnormalities of lipid and glucose metabolism, prescribed Pills with no more than 0.030 to 0.035 milligrams of estrogen and the lowest progestogen dose possible, and immediately investigated potentially serious symptoms such as disturbances in vision, severe headache, chest pain, cough, and shortness of breath, the number of yearly deaths would undoubtedly be reduced to less than 15. It is somewhat disconcerting to note that 12 percent of all women on the Pill take formulations that contain more than 0.050 milligrams of estrogen. A 1985 survey revealed that 30 percent of oral contraceptive users were still taking Pills containing 0.050 milligrams or more of estrogen despite the availability of the safer preparations. Even more alarming is the fact that older Pill users, who are at the highest risk, are more than five times as likely to be taking a high-dose pill as women in the youngest age group.

Does the Pill alter lipid content (cholesterol, triglycerides, etc.) in the blood, believed to be associated with heart disease?

Lipids refer to a wide variety of potentially harmful chemical substances in the body, including fatty acids, cholesterol, phospholipids, triglycerides, and lipoproteins. It has been theorized that changes in the concentrations of these substances in the blood help to accelerate the development of atherosclerosis—the formation of lipid plaques lining the walls of arteries. Atherosclerosis narrows the blood vessels that carry oxygen to the body's vital organs, sometimes resulting in a heart attack if arteries going to the muscles of the heart become completely blocked by atherosclerotic plaques or blood clots. Angina, or chest pain, precipitated by exertion is often a symptom of impending occlusion. When the blood supply to a portion of the heart muscle is completely shut off, the muscle dies or becomes infarcted. Survival from a myocardial infarction (heart attack) depends on how great an area of myocardium has been destroyed by this lack of oxygen.

Atherosclerosis is more likely to develop among individuals with a family history of heart disease and abnormal lipid metabolism. Obesity, diabetes, hypertension or high blood pressure, smoking, and diets rich in animal fat and cholesterol all contribute to this condition.

Of the two components in the Pill, the progestogen is clearly the culprit in causing heart attack. Several recent studies have shown that the incidence of this condition drops significantly when the progestogen dose is lowered while the estrogen concentration remains unchanged.

Lipid metabolism is a complex subject, but the important part to remember is that there are two major lipid fractions of cholesterol in the blood: HDL-C, or high density lipoprotein-cholesterol, and LDL-C, or low density lipoprotein-cholesterol. HDL-C is known as the protective or "good" cholesterol because high levels in the bloodstream are known to protect against atherosclerosis. LDL-C, or the "bad" cholesterol, has just the opposite effect and is the main component of a person's total blood cholesterol. Although all progestogens in high enough doses will lower HDL-C and raise LDL-C, the strongest progestogens, such as ethynodiol diacetate, norgestrel, and levonorgestrel, will do so to a greater degree. A 1983 article published in *The New England Journal of Medicine* reported that users of Pills containing high doses of progestogen—such as Norlestrin (1.0 to 2.5 milligrams of norethindrone acetate), Ovral (0.5 milligrams of norgestrel), and Demulen (1.0 milligrams of ethynodiol diacetate)—had a 24 percent higher average concentration of LDL-C than did women not on the Pill, emphasizing the importance of using the lowest possible progestogen dose to help prevent potentially harmful changes from taking place. Levonorgestrel (Nordette, Levlen, and Triphasil) and norgestrel (Lo-Ovral) products will not alter LDL-C and HDL-C levels if doses are left below 0.15 and 0.30 milligrams, respectively. I would, however, be less willing to say the same about a product such as Ovral, which contains 0.5 milligrams of norgestrel.

The biggest news in oral contraceptive research is that the estrogen component of the Pill is not all that bad, and the progestogen is not as good as we once thought. Lipid metabolism is a perfect example of this discovery, with estrogens increasing HDL-C and lowering LDL-C, thereby balancing the harmful changes induced by progestogens. The progestin-only Minipill was initially developed to protect women from the undesirable complications associated with estrogen and oral contraceptives (see page 31). Now scientists are questioning whether this unopposed progestogen might not in the long run have a more negative than positive influence on lipid metabolism.

Dr. Ronald M. Krauss and his associates at the University of California compared HDL-C and LDL-C levels in women before and seven weeks after they were started on either Lo-Ovral (0.3 milligrams norgestrel and 0.03 milligrams ethinyl estradiol) or Ovcon-35 (0.4 milligrams norethindrone and 0.035 milligrams ethinyl estradiol). The women using Lo-Ovral showed no changes in lipoprotein levels, while those in the Ovcon-35 group had a significant elevation in HDL-C levels. The reason for this difference was most likely because norethindrone is a weaker progestogen than norgestrel, and therefore the estrogen effect of raising HDL-C became dominant over the progestogen influence of lowering HDL-C. The study did not conclude that Ovcon-35 was a safer birth-control pill than Lo-Ovral in reducing the risk of heart disease, since it was also associated with slightly higher increases of LDL-C (the "bad" cholesterol) as well as the HDL-C ("good" cholesterol).

Another recent study showed that women using oral contraceptives with the highest amounts of estrogen and lowest amounts of progestogen, such as Enovid, had the most favorable levels of HDL-C. Too much of a good thing can be dangerous, however, as high estrogen doses can create other serious problems, such as blood clots (see page 37).

If you have a family history of high cholesterol, diabetes, heart disease, hypertension, or stroke, and if you are 50 percent or more above your ideal weight, do not exercise regularly, are close to thirty-five years of age, or smoke fifteen or more cigarettes per day, you should have your blood lipids analyzed before starting the Pill. Have them checked annually for as long as you use the Pill. It is imperative that you use a Pill with the lowest and weakest progestogen dose combined with no more than 0.035 milligrams of estrogen.

How is stroke related to birth-control pills?

A stroke is a circulatory disorder of the brain which may result in paralysis, loss of consciousness, and even death. For Pill users, stroke was originally thought to be an estrogen-induced complication, but some of the latest research suggests that it is related to the progestogen component as well. While stroke is responsible for 5 to 10 percent of deaths caused by the Pill, its risk is almost nonexistent if a woman is a nonsmoker, has a normal blood pressure, is under thirty-five years of age, and is using a Pill with 0.035 milligrams or less of estrogen in combination with a minimal progestogen dose.

There are two major types of strokes: thrombotic, resulting from a blood clot blocking an artery in the brain; and the more deadly hemorrhagic, which occurs when an artery in the brain bursts. The latter group includes subarachnoid hemorrhage, the most common type of stroke among women of reproductive age. Though somewhat controversial, the majority of studies have concluded that Pill users are 4 to 5 times more likely than nonusers to experience a subarachnoid hemorrhagic stroke, often the result of both elevated blood pressure and atherosclerotic change. Its cause, therefore, may be attributed to both the estrogen and the progestogen components of the Pill.

Eighty to 90 percent of strokes among men and women of all ages are of the thrombotic type and are precipitated by hypertension and atherosclerotic narrowing of the arteries leading to the brain. The mechanism by which the narrowing takes place is identical to the atherosclerotic changes that cause heart disease, namely, an elevation of harmful LDL-C and a lowering of the protective HDL-C—changes that in Pill users are most likely caused by the more potent progestogens.

The degree of disability that a person experiences following a stroke will depend on how great an area in the brain has been deprived of oxygen. Occasionally, occlusion of a small blood vessel or partial occlusion of a larger vessel produces subtle warning signs such as tiny blind spots in the field of vision in one eye, inability to focus, double vision, numbness on one side of the face or in the extremities, severe headache especially if accompanied by dizziness, nausea, vomiting, or stiff neck. It is the astute physician who quickly evaluates such symptoms and immediately stops the Pill if there is even a remote possibility of an impending stroke.

How can birth-control pills cause blood clots?

Let's first define some essential terms. A *thrombus* is a plug, clot, or solid piece of blood attached to the wall of an artery or a vein. When in a vein *(phleb-)*, it is often accompanied by inflammation *(-itis)*. *Thrombophlebitis* is most common in the veins of the legs and pelvis, and may be either superficial or deep. The superficial variety is located just beneath the surface of the skin in the varicose veins that may develop with childbirth. Few women have serious complications from superficial thrombophlebitis, but thrombophlebitis of the veins deep in the legs and pelvis often presents a real threat to a woman's life. Unfortunately, deep vein thrombophlebitis may occur without any warning symptoms at all. When one of these deep clots becomes dislodged from the wall of the vein, it may circulate through the bloodstream and is then called an *embolus.* If this embolus reaches the lung, it is called a pulmonary embolus. There, it may block the opening of an oxygen-carrying blood vessel, causing severe respiratory distress and occasionally instant death.

Women who use birth-control pills increase their chances of developing thrombophlebitis and pulmonary embolism. Investigators have proven beyond a doubt that the estrogen in the Pill stimulates the liver to produce proteins called clotting factors. The most important of these, Factors II, VII, and X, then enter the circulatory system where they enhance the formation of thrombi, or clots. As the dose of estrogen in the Pill increases, the level of clotting factors and the risk of thrombophlebitis will also increase. In addition to clotting factors, blood platelets are also involved in the normal clotting process. Estrogen has the power to make platelets adhere, or stick together, more readily. This in turn enhances the formation of blood clots.

Antithrombin III is known as a coagulation inhibitor because it prevents clot formation from taking place. Gauging its level is considered one of the most important laboratory tests for measuring and predicting a person's susceptibility toward developing a thrombus. Unfortunately, as the estrogen dose in birth-control pills increases, the blood values of Antithrombin III decrease proportionately. Similar findings have been reported with plasminogen, an enzyme involved in dissolving clots once they are formed.

Though the mechanism is unknown, research suggests that the progestogen in the Pill may modify and even intensify the abnormalities in blood clotting factors created by estrogen.

Should a woman with a history of deep vein thrombophlebitis or pulmonary embolus take the Pill?

If a woman has even a questionable history of a previous deep vein thrombophlebitis or pulmonary embolus, birth-control pills must never be prescribed. Though the Minipill might appear to be a safe alternative for such women, some doctors remain skeptical about using it (see page 31). Symptoms such as calf swelling or pain, cough, chest pain, or shortness of breath in a woman on the Pill must be investigated immediately. Unlike other cardiovascular complications associated with Pill use, smoking and a woman's age appear to have no influence on her risk of suffering from deep vein thrombophlebitis or pulmonary embolism.

Are there any blood clot risks in surgery for women using birth-control pills?

Your immobility immediately following a major surgical procedure, combined with detrimental effects of the Pill on blood clotting factors, will increase your risk of blood clots following surgery fourfold. For this reason, when surgery is elective or nonemergency it is best to stop the Pill for thirty days before the operation is performed. Some doctors even recommend a pause of eight weeks prior to surgery since a small percentage of women will continue to show an elevation of clotting factors until this time. If you are taking a Pill formulation with 0.030 to 0.035 milligrams of estrogen, however, thirty days should be more than sufficient. It is important not to resume Pill use for at least two weeks after you are fully ambulatory.

In the case of emergency surgery or immobilization due to serious trauma or bone fracture, you should immediately stop the Pill in order to normalize your clotting factors. Under such conditions, many doctors advise heparin injections every twelve hours during the postoperative period of immobilization in order to thin the blood and prevent clotting.

Minor surgery does not usually require an interruption of Pill use, provided that you are not immobilized for more than a day or two.

Are certain blood types more prone to blood clots?

For some unknown reason, women with blood type A appear to be three times more susceptible than other women to thrombophlebitis, whereas those with blood type O are more resistant. Women with type B and type AB have a risk somewhere between these two extremes. The significance of these findings is minimal at best and should not deter a woman of blood group A from using birth-control pills. However, the lowest possible dose of estrogen, or the Minipill, should be prescribed.

Should a woman with varicose veins or hemorrhoids take the Pill?

If use of the Pill were limited only to women who were free of varicose veins and hemorrhoids, it would never be prescribed for any woman who had previously given birth.

Varicose veins are previously straight veins just below the skin surface that become twisted and dilated, forming areas of bluish discoloration on the legs, feet, and inner thighs. They are formed when the valves that connect one vein to another fail to propel the blood fully from the legs to the heart. As a result, circulation slows and the veins become stretched and filled with blood. Hemorrhoids are varicose veins located around the anus.

Many factors, including heredity, obesity, and pressure from an enlarged uterus can precipitate the formation of varicosities, and repeated pregnancies tend to intensify the problem.

An infection of the superficial varicose veins is called superficial thrombophlebitis, and is characterized by redness and tenderness over the skin where the vein is inflamed. Fortunately, superficial thrombophlebitis is not a serious condition (as is deep vein thrombophlebitis), and it readily responds to conservative management such as hot soaks and elevation of the leg. Two recent studies involving thousands of women have clearly demonstrated that there is no association between oral contraceptive use and the development of varicose veins or hemorrhoids. Furthermore, no evidence exists that oral contraceptive users with varicose veins are at increased risk of developing the more dangerous deep vein thrombophlebitis.

If you have varicose veins that have not been chronically inflamed, you can use birth-control pills without concern. Even if your superficial varicose veins have caused some problems in the past, it is unlikely that the use of a low-dose birth-control pill will aggravate this condition.

Can the Pill cause high blood pressure?

Abnormal elevation of the blood pressure, or hypertension, occurs in 5 percent of the U.S. population. Even after a complete medical workup on their patients, doctors will be unable to uncover a cause for the hypertension in 90 percent of all cases. Mild hypertension is usually not accompanied by symptoms, while the presence of headache, dizziness, blurred vision, nosebleeds, and ringing noises in the ears may indicate the need for immediate medical intervention. Since hypertensive individuals are more susceptible to both heart attack and stroke, early detection and treatment is vital.

A blood pressure reading is recorded as two numbers. The first, higher number is called the *systolic* pressure; the second, lower number is the *diastolic* pressure. A normal reading for a young healthy woman may range from 90 (systolic)/60 (diastolic) to 130/80. Doctors consider the reading of 140/90 as the borderline between normal and hypertensive.

Many studies involving thousands of women have demonstrated that hypertension may occur in 3 to 5 percent of all Pill users. Your doctor should not prescribe the Pill if your blood pressure is 140/90 or greater. Furthermore, if your once-normal blood pressure rises to 140/90 while you are taking the Pill, stop it immediately and use alternative contraception. Many physicians recommend that the Pill be discontinued even if your blood pressure remains within normal limits but increases by 20 systolic or 10 diastolic points while you are taking it. Normally, a woman's blood pressure reverts to normal within six weeks after stopping the Pill.

The rise in blood pressure accompanying use of oral contraceptives is directly related to the strength of estrogen they contain and the number of years the individual has been taking the Pill. Even the newest low-dose formulations containing 0.030 to 0.035 milligrams of estrogen have the capacity to raise the systolic blood pressure an average of 2 to 4 points and the diastolic blood pressure 1 to 2 points after one year of use. These increases continue gradually so that after three to four years the systolic pressure may be elevated an average of 6 to 7 points, and the diastolic 2 to 3 points. Pills containing 0.050 milligrams or more of estrogen will increase the systolic pressure an average of 5 to 7 points, and the diastolic by 3 to 5 points after the first year. In one survey, this average rose dramatically to 14 and 8.5 points, respectively, after four years of continual Pill use. Though the blood pressures of all of these women remained within the normal range, it is not known at the present time whether these small but significant changes will prove to be harmful to the cardiovascular system. Certainly, these statistics point out the necessity of using the lowest possible estrogen dose in the Pill you take.

Only very recently have scientists come to learn that the progestogen strength and dosage also affect a woman's blood pressure, but to a lesser degree than the estrogen component. A low dose of progestogen, as found in the progestogen-only Minipills, is a logical alternative for women who experience an increased or borderline blood pressure while using the combination Pills. Dr. William Spellacy and his associates noted no elevation in blood pressure among women using a Minipill containing 0.075 milligrams of norgestrel (Nordette).

Are some women more susceptible to hypertension than others?

Women with a family history of hypertension have a significantly higher tendency to develop this problem while using oral contraceptives. Other susceptible women are those more than thirty-five, and those who are obese. Individuals with certain preexisting kidney diseases accompanied by borderline elevations in blood pressure are especially at risk and should not take the Pill. In the past, it was believed that women with a history of pre-eclampsia—hypertension found only during the last three months of pregnancy—were more prone to develop a rise in blood pressure on the Pill. Recent studies suggest that this is not true. Despite this reassurance, it is best to be on the safe side, and a woman with a history of pre-eclampsia should have her blood pressure monitored every six months, rather than every year, while she is on the Pill. To date, there is no evidence linking Pill-related hypertension with smoking habits, number of children, or social class of the woman using the Pill.

Is it true that certain black women can't take birth-control pills?

The incidence of hypertension is twice as common among blacks as it is in the general population. Based on this information, doctors at Emory University recently conducted a study to prove that black women are more likely than white women to experience blood pressure elevations while using birth-control pills. After studying thousands of women over a period of six months to two years, they were surprised to reach just the opposite conclusion. Not only were blood pressure elevations less dramatic among blacks on the Pill, but those with higher blood pressures prior to starting on the Pill actually experienced a slight decline once they were on it for a few months.

Until recently it was believed that both pregnancy and birth-control pills predisposed women with sickle-cell disease, an inherited blood disorder, to life-threatening crises. While this still applies to pregnancy, recent and extensive clinical research has shown that women with sickle-cell disease do not have a greater incidence of clotting problems or sickle-cell crises when using oral contraceptives. In fact, birth-control pills are currently the most common method of contraception used by women with sickle-cell disease.

Can women with mitral valve prolapse take the Pill?

The mitral valve lies between the left atrium and left ventricle of the heart. Under normal conditions, this valve closes to prevent regurgitation or backup of blood from the ventricle into the atrium when the ventricle's muscles contract to pump blood into the arteries throughout the body. Weakening of the mitral valve causes it to balloon out or to prolapse into the left atrium when the ventricle contracts, instead of remaining firmly in its position between the atrium and the ventricle. Mitral valve prolapse (also known as floppy-valve syndrome and systolic click-murmur syndrome) is by far the most commonly diagnosed cardiac condition of the 1980s. It is more likely to occur in women between the ages of fourteen and thirty, with an estimated incidence of 15 percent among women in their twenties, although it has been reported in both men and women of all ages. There may be a familial inheritance pattern to this defect. Many individuals learn they have this condition only after their doctors tell them that they have the characteristic "click," heard with the stethoscope. Most people, however, experience varying degrees of symptoms such as dizziness, palpitations, irregular or rapid heart beat, chest pains, faintness, or shortness of breath. Mitral valve prolapse is practically always an innocuous condition, but it should be monitored by a physician.

If a woman with mitral valve prolapse is relatively free of symptoms, there is no reason why she can't take low-dose birth-control pills. Individuals with severe mitral valve prolapse are particularly at risk for thromboembolism, however. Since a rare but serious side effect associated with the use of birth-control pills includes an increased chance of thromboembolism, many cardiologists would consider it prudent to recommend alternative methods of contraception to women with severe mitral valve prolapse.

Does the Pill affect blood sugar?

A small number of both healthy and diabetic women will experience abnormalities in blood sugar tests while using birth-control pills. This "chemical diabetes" produces no symptoms, and usually reverts to normal when the birth-control pill is stopped. Other women maintain normal glucose tolerance tests while on the Pill, but demonstrate elevated levels of insulin in the bloodstream. The cause is unknown, but the most popular theory is that the progestogen in the Pill prevents the body from properly absorbing insulin. This resistance to insulin stresses the pancreas to produce even more insulin in its attempt to remove glucose from the bloodstream. Scientists do not know the long-term effects of such stress on the body, but it certainly can't be beneficial.

It has been proven that the progestogen, even in lower amounts found in the Minipill, is the culprit in worsening glucose metabolism and plasma insulin levels. Several researchers over the past five years have discovered to their surprise that the oft-maligned estrogen component of the Pill can ameliorate and even totally reverse the harmful changes in glucose and insulin levels caused by progestogens. This protective effect will occur only with the lowest doses of 0.030 and 0.035 milligrams of ethinyl estradiol, and not with amounts above 0.05 milligrams. Furthermore, the estrogen will have a greater counterbalancing effect against a weak progestogen such as norethindrone (Ovcon-35, Brevicon, Modicon) than against a stronger progestogen such as norgestrel (Lo-Ovral).

The newest and most highly touted combination birth-control pill contains a mixture of 0.015 milligrams of the powerful progestogen named levonorgestrel and 0.03 milligrams of ethinyl estradiol (Nordette, Levlen). Despite normal glucose tolerance tests among women using this Pill, it has been found that it is still capable of causing a significant elevation of a woman's plasma insulin levels.

Can you develop diabetes while taking the Pill?

There are certain women who are at greater risk than others for developing abnormal glucose tolerance while on birth-control pills. If you are over thirty-five, are grossly overweight, have a strong family history of diabetes, have given birth to a child weighing more than nine pounds, or have experienced an unexplained stillbirth or the birth of a baby with abnormalities, you should have a screening blood test for diabetes before and six months after you are started on the Pill. Gestational diabetes occurs during pregnancy as a result of the stress caused by the hormonal changes taking place. Women with gestational diabetes will have normal glucose tolerance when tested six weeks following delivery, but 40 percent will go on to develop overt diabetes years later. The majority of endocrinologists believe that women with a history of gestational diabetes should be encouraged to use alternative methods of contraception, since the Pill is more likely to provide the stress needed to make the glucose tolerance test abnormal. Stopping the Pill usually brings all these values back to normal, but if you have experienced gestational diabetes and are on the Pill it is vital that your doctor check your blood sugars periodically and that you immediately stop the Pill if abnormalities are noted.

Can I take birth-control pills if I am diabetic or borderline diabetic?

If you are a diabetic who takes insulin, it is in your best interest not to use birth-control pills. Though your doctor could easily adjust your insulin dose while you are on the Pill, of greater concern is that the progestogen might help accelerate other metabolic problems and lead to heart disease.

Too many doctors are unaware of the fact that some birth-control pills are far better than others at normalizing blood sugar and insulin values. The combination pill containing a low dose of norethindrone and 0.030 to 0.035 milligrams of ethinyl estradiol, such as Ovcon-35 and Modicon, would be a perfect choice for the concerned diabetic woman. Because of the low dose of estrogen combined with the weak progestogen norethindrone, however, one must be prepared to accept the trade-off of a higher incidence of breakthrough bleeding (see page 54). Combination pills with strong progestogens (Ovral, Lo-Ovral, Levlen, Nordette) and those with estrogen concentrations of 0.05 milligrams or more (see page 15, "The Pills: What's in Them?") are best avoided. Based on the available research, progestogen-only Minipills would appear to be less than ideal for the woman concerned about glucose tolerance and plasma insulin abnormalities. Of the three Minipills, Ovrette, which contains norgestrel, would be the most undesirable.

Preliminary research has demonstrated that the new triphasics might not adversely affect glucose and insulin levels because they contain a lower total dose of progestogen in each cycle. Of the four triphasics currently being marketed, Ortho-Novum 7/7/7 and Tri-Norinyl, which contain norethindrone, would have a lesser effect than the norgestrel in Levlen and Nordette. Either of these triphasics would be an excellent choice for a woman needing birth control and considered to be at greater risk than average for developing chemical diabetes.

What effects can the Pill have on the breasts?

The estrogen in the Pill may be responsible for tenderness and increased fullness of the breasts, but these symptoms can usually be minimized by using Pills with the lowest possible estrogen content. In the unusual situation where tenderness persists beyond the first two months, either a progestogen-only Minipill or a progestogen-dominant formulation such as Lo-Ovral, Nordette, or Levlen should be tried.

Despite the overwhelming evidence showing that the Pill does not cause breast cysts or breast cancer, misconceptions about its supposed harmful effects remain widespread and persistent. In one recent survey, one-third of the women interviewed mistakenly believed that the Pill was responsible for a higher incidence of breast cancer. Doctors are particularly responsible for many of the misconceptions their patients hold. For example, a highly publicized 1983 study from the University of Southern California claimed that there was nearly a fivefold increased risk of breast cancer in women who used oral contraceptives for six years or more before the age of twenty-five. The findings implicated Pills that the researchers noted as being high in progestogen potency. This study, known as the Pike Report after its chief author, Malcolm C. Pike, M.D., has been analyzed extensively by several highly respected research groups including the Food and Drug Administration Advisory Committee and the Centers for Disease Control. All have found the Pike Report to be totally inaccurate in its statistical methods, procedures for studying patients, determination of progestogen potency in the Pills studied, and conclusions. But such denunciations have received fewer headlines than the original damaging report.

Several studies have demonstrated that 50 to 75 percent of women with cystic breasts will experience a significant reduction in the size of their cysts while using birth-control pills. Furthermore, the longer a woman uses the Pill, the greater will be its protective effect, particularly if used for longer than four years. According to two recent reports, fibroadenoma, a benign, solid breast nodule, is also noted to diminish in incidence when a woman uses birth-control pills.

Since women with cystic breasts are at greater risk than others for developing breast cancer, it has been theorized that birth-control pills may actually reduce a woman's chances of contracting breast cancer. This, however, has not proven to be true since the rates of breast cancer among Pill users and nonusers are equal. The currently held view is that the Pill has the capacity to decrease benign breast cysts but will not alter those destined to turn malignant.

Breast cysts that do not disappear after a short period of observation often require a biopsy to be sure that they are benign. Breast biopsies are usually performed in doctors' offices or outpatient ambulatory facilities within hospitals. Epidemiologists have calculated that if 100,000 women on the Pill are compared with the same number using other forms of contraception, the former group will require 235 fewer hospitalizations for the diagnosis and treatment of benign breast disease. Assuming that there are six million American women currently on the Pill, this would represent approximately 14,000 averted hospitalizations each year.

Is it true that breast cancer can worsen if birth-control pills are taken?

At least 50 percent of breast cancers appear to be estrogen-dependent. This means that once the cancer is present, estrogen could make it grow faster. Proof of this is the marked improvement many women experience when their estrogen-producing ovaries are removed as treatment for advanced breast cancer. Thus, birth-control pills (or any estrogen for that matter) should never be taken by a woman who has premalignant or malignant breast disease. If the diagnosis of breast cancer is made while a woman is on the Pill, she should stop taking it immediately.

If my mother had breast cancer, is it safe for me to take birth-control pills?

A woman who has a mother, sister, or aunt with breast cancer has a much greater chance of developing this disease than does a woman without such a history. Taking the Pill does not make these women more susceptible to breast cancer, however. A 1984 study from the Centers for Disease Control demonstrated that women with a strong history of breast cancer will have the same chance of developing this disease whether they take the Pill or not.

Since the oral contraceptive does not cause breast cancer, there is no reason for a doctor to refuse to prescribe the Pill to a woman with a family history of breast cancer, provided that she has a breast exam at least once a year. Women more than thirty-five should also have a mammography or breast X ray at least every two years. It is probably wiser for women to stop taking the Pill at this age because of other risks that may be involved (see table on page 34).

What effects do birth-control pills have on the cervix?

Women using birth-control pills tend to have a greater incidence of cervical eversion than nonusers (see chapter 1), probably because of the estrogen component in the Pill. It is not unusual for these everted glands to be covered over by the cells from the outer surface of the cervix. When this happens, the mucus in the gland can't be released and small yellow *Nabothian* cysts are formed. They produce no symptoms, are harmless, and need not be treated. Too many doctors cauterize (burn), freeze, or cut out Nabothian cysts and everted glands that should be left alone.

(Erosion of the cervix is an actual defect or sore often associated with inflammation on the surface of the cervix. It should not be confused with eversion, although it often is. An erosion will often bleed following direct contact, such as intercourse. A doctor should be able to demonstrate the bleeding from an erosion by touching a cotton-tipped applicator to the eroded spot. Cervical erosion is more inconvenient than serious, and is often treated in the office by either cauterization or cryosurgery [freezing] of the area.)

It has long been known that the hormonal stimulation of both pregnancy and birth-control pills causes the growth and secretion of endocervical glands, or those located within the cervix. This benign condition, known as *microglandular hyperplasia,* reverts to normal once the pregnancy or Pill taking has ended.

Cancer originating in the endocervical cells is called *adenocarcinoma* of the cervix. It comprises approximately 10 percent of all cervical cancers and, unlike the more common type of cervical cancer (see below), is not associated with a woman's sexuality and has an unknown cause. Since 1982 there have been three reports linking prolonged use of oral contraceptives to the development of adenocarcinoma of the endocervix. The most recent study, published in *Obstetrics and Gynecology* in 1986, noted adenocarcinoma of the endocervix in seven women who had used the Pill from four and a half to nine years. In another study, thirty-four of forty women with this disease were long-term Pill users. Though the incidence of adenocarcinoma of the endocervix among the millions of current and former Pill users remains extremely low, further epidemiologic studies on the effect of oral contraceptives on the endocervical glands appear warranted.

Are birth-control pills ever responsible for an abnormal Pap smear or the more common type of cancer of the cervix?

At least 90 percent of all cases of cancer of the cervix originate in the outer cells of the cervix rather than the inner glands. These cells are known as *epidermoid,* or *squamous,* cells, and the cancer that originates in them is named epidermoid- or squamous-cell carcinoma. At least twenty scientific investigations conducted over the past ten years have failed to demonstrate whether there is a relationship between use of birth-control pills and the incidence of abnormal Pap smears, *epidermoid carcinoma* of the cervix, or precancerous conditions of the cervix called *dysplasia.*

Epidermoid cancer of the cervix is truly a venereal disease related to a woman's age at first coitus as well as to coitus with multiple sexual partners. It is virtually nonexistent among nuns and the lesbian population. The sexual revolution brought with it an epidemic among young women of dysplasia and *carcinoma-in-situ*—cancer limited to the upper surface of the cells of the cervix. This condition, if left untreated, may progress over a period of years to the invasive and dangerous stage of this disease.

Epidemiologists looking for the cause of cervical cancer have implicated a variety of agents including certain bacteria, proteins in the semen of some men, and the herpes virus. The most likely culprit, based on the latest research, appears to be the human papilloma virus, or HPV. HPV strains also cause *condyloma acuminata,* or "venereal warts," while other types are believed most responsible for precancerous and cancerous changes of the cervix.

It is the opinion of most experts that the use of birth-control pills happens to coexist with, but is not the cause of, these changes of the cervix. For this reason, they do not believe that the use of birth-control pills should be restricted if a woman is diagnosed as having dysplasia or carcinoma-in-situ. There have been several studies carried out to support this position. In contrast, other researchers have concluded that Pill use for longer than five years is more likely to be associated with dysplasia, carcinoma-in-situ, and invasive carcinoma.

Unfortunately, these and other studies concerning this subject have failed to carefully consider the sexual habits, age at first intercourse, and the many other variables of women using the Pill and those with whom they were compared. Certainly the cervix of a woman on the Pill will be continually exposed to the papilloma virus in her partner's semen, while those using the condom and diaphragm will be protected to a great extent (see chapter 4, "Barrier Contraception").

There is not yet convincing evidence of a direct link between oral contraceptive use and cervical cancer. While some recent epidemiologic studies suggest a risk for long-term oral contraceptive users, it is probably of borderline statistical significance. Peter E. Schwartz, M.D., Director of Gynecologic Oncology at Yale, remarked in 1987: "There's absolutely no evidence that oral contraceptives are associated with cervical neoplasm [cancer]." At the present time, the best advice for all women on the Pill is to have a Pap smear at least every twelve months. For women with a history of dysplasia or carcinoma-in-situ, a Pap smear every six months would be more appropriate.

Is there a relationship between Pill use and uterine cancer?

Amid misinformation about the dangers of oral contraception use, no one seems to be aware of the fact that the Pill exerts a powerful protective effect against cancer of the uterus.

Cancer of the uterus is known as endometrial adenocarcinoma because it has its origins in the glands of the endometrium, the lining of the uterine cavity. There are approximately 39,000 new cases of this disease reported in the United States each year, resulting in over 3,000 deaths. Ninety percent of such cases begin at or after the onset of the menopause. Though no woman is immune, endometrial carcinoma is more prevalent among women with a long history of irregular periods, infrequent ovulation, and infertility. Early symptoms of abnormal bleeding or watery vaginal discharge require immediate study of the endometrium either as an outpatient biopsy or a hospital dilatation and curettage (D and C). The Pap smear, so important in the diagnosis of cervical cancer, is of little aid in the diagnosis of endometrial disease.

Though the exact cause of endometrial adenocarcinoma is unknown, there is no doubt that the main precipitating factor is excessive stimulation of the endometrial glands by estrogen without the counterbalancing protective influence of progesterone. A woman with irregular periods frequently does not ovulate and as a result her endometrium receives excessive estrogen stimulation from the developing ovarian follicle without benefit of progesterone from the corpus luteum which develops after ovulation (see chapter 1). As a result, the endometrial glands increase in number and in the activity of their cells. This microscopic condition, known as *endometrial hyperplasia,* may initially be mild, but following prolonged unopposed estrogen stimulation, a cancer may eventually ensue among susceptible individuals.

There is no doubt that the progestogens in birth-control pills provide almost continuous protection against the stimulation of the endometrial glands by the estrogen component of the Pill. At least six recent epidemiologic studies have demonstrated that women on the Pill for at least one year have half the likelihood of developing adenocarcinoma of the endometrium than woman using other birth-control methods. This protective effect increases with prolonged Pill use and is most likely to benefit those at greatest risk, namely, women who have never borne children.

The most remarkable finding of these studies is that birth-control pills continue to prevent endometrial adenocarcinoma for at least ten years after the Pill is stopped. Often, this protective effect extends well into a woman's forties and fifties. In a 1987 study from the National Institute of Child Health and Human Development, researchers found that this protection lasted for more than fifteen years, provided that the combination pill had been used for a period of at least one year. Examinations of the eight most frequently used pill formulations revealed little difference in their protective effects. Epidemiologists have calculated that for every 100,000 women on the Pill, five hospitalizations for cancer are prevented each year. All in all, it is estimated that 2,000 hospitalizations and 100 deaths from endometrial adenocarcinoma are averted annually among the approximately 40 million current and former Pill users between the ages of twenty and fifty-four. Why hasn't this good news about the Pill been given extensive media coverage?

Does the Pill cause ovarian cysts?

Though there are many types of ovarian cysts, most of those that develop in menstruating women are not cancerous. In fact, the large percentage of those benign cysts form within the ovarian follicle prior to ovulation or in the corpus luteum following ovulation (see chapter 1). Follicle and corpus luteum cysts are usually not larger than 5 to 6 centimeters (2 to $2\frac{1}{2}$ inches) in diameter, and always disappear within one to two months. Most often, they produce no symptoms and are only discovered during a routine gynecological exam. On occasion, however, they can cause severe pain, especially if they leak their contents of fluid and blood into the abdominal cavity.

Since combination birth-control pills prevent both follicle development and ovulation, they protect women from forming these two types of cysts. As a result, many expensive diagnostic procedures, such as ultrasound, and many hospitalizations for laparoscopy and exploratory surgery are averted by Pill users each year. One estimate is that 35 out of every 100,000 women on the Pill will be saved each year from hospitalization related to follicle and corpus luteum cysts. This translates to 2,100 annual hospitalizations averted among the six million women currently using oral contraceptives.

Many gynecologists actually prescribe birth-control pills for one to two months for women who are not on the Pill but are suspected of having a follicle or corpus luteum cyst on examination. The reasoning is that the Pill inhibits the release of FSH and LH (see chapter 1), the pituitary hormones most responsible for stimulating the cells within these cysts. As a result, it is theorized that the cysts will disappear faster when the Pill is used in this manner.

If you are a young woman who is not using birth-control pills, beware of any doctor who rushes you into an operation for an ovarian cyst after only one vaginal examination. Too often, unnecessary surgery is performed on women with follicle or corpus luteum cysts when all that is required is one to two months of observation while the cyst shrinks in size (see chapter 10, "Hysterectomy"). Such a delay causes no harm, since practically all cysts in young women are benign, but it does prevent many unnecessary operations.

Does the Pill cause ovarian cancer?

While cancer of the ovary is less common than cervical or uterine cancer, with 18,000 new cases reported each year, it is far more deadly. Approximately two-thirds of all women who contract ovarian cancer will die of the disease, making it the leading cause of gynecological cancer death and the fourth cancer-killer overall. Unlike cancer of the cervix and endometrium, which can be diagnosed at an early stage by Pap smear and endometrial biopsy, respectively, ovarian cancer is a silent killer for which there is no early diagnostic test. Vague symptoms such as increasing abdominal girth, bloating, heartburn, and indigestion are often misdiagnosed and mistreated by internists and family physicians for weeks or months before the diagnosis becomes evident. One can only agree with a famous gynecologic surgeon who said, "Too many ovarian cancers have been bathed in a sea of antacids." Early referral to a gynecologist for a thorough pelvic exam will help avert some of these tragedies. Women between the ages of fifty and seventy are most susceptible to ovarian cancer. Especially at risk are those who have never borne children. As noted with the overwhelming majority of other malignancies, the exact cause of ovarian cancer remains an enigma although scientists refer to "incessant ovulation" or "ovulatory age" as an important precipitating factor. This means that the total number of months that a woman ovulates in her lifetime is a powerful predictor of her ovarian cancer risk. Conversely, time spent pregnant or on oral contraceptives, with the resultant blockage of ovulation, is now established as being protective against ovarian cancer. No less than ten different studies have concluded that women on the Pill will decrease their risk of developing ovarian cancer by about 40 percent when compared to nonusers. As with endometrial cancer, the Pill's protective effect improves with duration of use and lasts for ten or more years after it has been discontinued. It is estimated that 4 per 100,000 Pill users will avoid hospitalization for ovarian cancer each year. Even more encouraging, 1,700 hospitalizations and 850 fatalities from ovarian cancer are averted each year among the approximately 40 million current and former Pill users in the United States aged twenty to fifty-four.

Does the Pill affect the pigment of the skin?

Chloasma or *melasma* is the presence of dark brown pigmented areas on the face, believed to be caused by sensitivity to the marked increase in estrogen hormone during pregnancy and to the estrogen component of the Pill. Melasma involving the cheeks, upper lip, and forehead is commonly called "the mask of pregnancy." It is often accompanied by brown coloration of the nipples and *linea nigra,* a dark, thin line that runs from the navel to the pubic hairline. Freckles and brown moles (*nevi*) on the skin also darken as a result of these hormonal changes. The incidence of chloasma among Pill users varies. Estimates have ranged from 4 to 37 percent, with the incidence increasing gradually with each month of Pill use.

It has been theorized that hyperpigmentation occurs when estrogen stimulates the pituitary gland to release large amounts of melanocyte-stimulating hormone, or MSH. MSH in turn induces cells on the skin's surface called melanocytes to increase in number and to secrete greater amounts of the skin pigment named melanin. Exposure to sunlight intensifies chloasma, especially among fair-skinned individuals.

Though many women with chloasma are often distressed by their appearance, the condition is harmless and improves once the Pill is stopped. Women who switch from a high to a lower estrogen formulation will also notice improvement. The effect of sunlight on chloasma can be reduced to some degree by applying a sunscreen. Once chloasma is well established, the pigmentation can safely be lightened with Eldoquin bleach products. Another product, RV paque, is recommended for women who have lightened their hyperpigmentation but still need protection from the sun while they are on the Pill.

Of far greater concern than melasma is the question of whether the Pill increases a woman's risk of malignant melanoma. This often fatal form of cancer originates in the melanocytes within a pigmented mole on the skin and then reproduces at an abnormally rapid rate, followed by spreading to other parts of the body. Its incidence in the general population is 9 to 13 per 100,000 and is more common among fair-skinned individuals and those exposed to excessive amounts of sunlight over a period of years.

To date, the majority of the studies link Pill use to malignant melanoma, but investigators have not adequately accounted for a host of variables such as a woman's personal and family history of cancer, her skin and hair coloring, the climate in which she lives, and the amount of time she spends in the sun. Until further research is carried out, the relationship between use of birth-control pills and a woman's predisposition to malignant melanoma will remain inconclusive. To be safe, anyone with a history of this disease, even if it occurred years before, should use alternative methods of contraception. Similarly, if a woman develops melanoma while using birth-control pills, she should discontinue the Pills immediately and forever.

Can you describe other skin changes that might occur from using birth-control pills?

If you have a tendency toward acne, oily skin and scalp, or significant facial and body hair, these problems will intensify if your doctor puts you on a Pill with strong androgenic (male hormone) dominance. Therefore, it is best to avoid Pills containing the progestogens norgestrel or levonorgestrel, such as Ovral, Lo-Ovral, Nordette, Levlen, Triphasil, Tri-Levlen, and Ovrette. Increasing the estrogen content of the Pill while lowering the progestogen dose will usually improve a woman's complexion. However, the benefits of using an oral contraceptive with amounts of estrogen exceeding 0.050 milligrams are far outweighed by the potential risks of more serious complications. Birth-control pills that will not adversely affect your complexion and may actually help it include Demulen, Demulen 35, Norinyl 150, Norinyl 1+35, Ortho-Novum 10/11, Ortho-Novum 1+35, Ortho-Novum 1+50, Ortho-Novum 7/7/7, Tri-Norinyl, Ovcon 35, and Ovcon 50.

Women with a strong history of allergies to various foods and medications may experience itching or a rash while on birth-control pills because of the hormones, the coloring, or the inner filler in the Pill. Rashes caused by allergy of this type are symmetrical and cause significant itching, but usually do not affect the face. Switching to a different Pill formulation will often solve the problem. Generalized itching and a rash may also occur in women who are allergic to milk, since lactose is used as a filler in many Pills. It is wise to check with your pharmacist if you have a history of milk allergy and are contemplating using the Pill.

Intense generalized itching occasionally associated with jaundice or yellowing of the skin has been reported in a small number of women on the Pill. This condition, known as *cholestatic pruritis* and *jaundice,* is the result of the accumulation of bile in the circulatory system. While the progestogen is probably the main culprit, the estrogen component has also been implicated in this problem; the only known method of treating it is to stop using the Pill. It is interesting to note that women with cholestasis note its recurrence if they become pregnant because the same hormonal stimulation is again present.

Telangiectasias, also known as spider nevi or liver spots, are tiny red spots occasionally found on the upper chest, neck, and face of fair-skinned Pill users. They are due to the dilatation and fragility of tiny skin capillaries and are totally harmless. Switching to a Pill with a lower estrogen dose will usually decrease the number of spider nevi.

Can birth-control pills cause the adrenal and thyroid glands to become overactive?

Oral contraceptives cause characteristic changes in some tests that measure adrenal and thyroid gland function. These changes are also noted during pregnancy and are believed to be due to an increase in binding globulins or carrier proteins in the blood as the result of estrogen stimulation. Binding globulins serve an important role in transporting hormones throughout the body in their bound or inactive forms, and each hormone has its own specific binding globulin. For example, cortisol, the main adrenal gland hormone, is bound to cortisol-binding globulin, while thyroxine, the main hormone of the thyroid gland, attaches to thyroxine-binding globulin.

Though laboratory tests of the adrenal and thyroid glands may give falsely high readings for women on the Pill, the actual functioning of the glands has not been affected. If your doctor is not aware that you are taking birth-control pills, the test results may initially confuse him or her into thinking something is wrong. But other, more specific tests will easily confirm the fact that the thyroid is functioning normally, and this should not present a problem in either diagnosis or treatment. Once you stop using birth-control pills, the altered tests will return to normal within a few days. The progestogen-only Minipill will not cause these changes.

Is it true that the Pill can protect women from developing rheumatoid arthritis?

Initial reports from Europe and the United States created great optimism because they concluded that women on birth-control pills experienced a 50 percent reduction in their incidence of rheumatoid arthritis when compared to women not using the Pill. This finding was based on still unexplained data showing a significant decline in rheumatoid arthritis rates following introduction of the Pill in 1964. Several larger and more selective studies since 1983 have refuted this claim. In a 1985 report, published in *The Journal of the American Medical Association,* doctors at the University of Texas School of Public Health and the Mayo Clinic interviewed 182 women with rheumatoid arthritis and an equal number of healthy women with comparable backgrounds. The results showed that Pill use exerted no protective effect on the incidence or severity of arthritis.

Do birth-control pills affect the gallbladder?

Bile passes from the liver to the gallbladder and then into the intestine via the bile ducts. Stones form when the composition of the bile is altered by chemical substances such as cholesterol. The presence of stones is called *cholelithiasis,* while *cholecystitis* refers to an inflammation of the gallbladder usually caused by stones. Cholelithiasis is a fairly common and often asymptomatic condition, as evidenced by the fact that it may be found in anywhere from 4 to 11 percent of all healthy pregnant women. When symptoms are present they often include digestive disturbances and pain in the right upper abdomen which may radiate or travel to the back and right shoulder. Eating fried and fatty foods seems to precipitate attacks of pain. Cholecystitis is a more painful condition which is often associated with the above symptoms as well as with fever, nausea, vomiting, and occasionally jaundice if the major bile duct is blocked.

Some investigators have claimed that both the estrogen and the progestin in birth-control pills can change the bile's composition and thereby increase a woman's risk of cholelithiasis and cholecystitis. Closer analysis of recent data, however, suggests that most cases of painful and symptomatic gallbladder disease occur during the first one to three years of Pill use. After that, the incidence is equal to or even lower than that in the general population. The conclusion to be drawn from this data is that oral contraceptives probably do not cause gallbladder disease but they will accelerate the condition among women who already have stones. Certainly, if you have a history of food intolerance that suggests gallbladder disease, or if you have been found on a previous X ray or ultrasound examination to have gallstones, it is best that you not use any oral contraceptives, including the Minipill.

Are women on the Pill more susceptible to PID (Pelvic Inflammatory Disease)?

One of the most tragic consequences of the sexual revolution has been the epidemic of *salpingitis* (fallopian tube infections) and PID (pelvic inflammatory disease). These sexually transmitted infections are responsible for the hospitalization of over 200,000 American women and the outpatient treatment of another 1 million sufferers annually. Salpingitis and PID have long been considered synonymous with gonorrhea because the bacterium *Neisseria gonorrhoeae* was believed to be the only offending organism. In recent years other bacteria, including *Chlamydia trachomatis,* have been found to be responsible for as many, if not more, cases of this disease. Both gonorrhea and chlamydia bacteria are introduced into the vagina during intercourse, ascend through the cervical os, and travel along the endometrial lining and up into the fallopian tubes (see chapter 1). There they can cause inflammation or salpingitis, scarring, destruction of the tube, and subsequent infertility. It is not unusual for the ovaries to become involved in the inflammatory process, producing a serious infection known as a tubo-ovarian abscess. PID is the term used when the infection spills from the fallopian tubes to the adjacent pelvic structures. For some women, the infection becomes a chronic, smoldering disease with frequent bouts of incapacitating pain. Chronic PID occasionally requires surgical drainage of abscesses and even removal of the uterus, tubes, and ovaries in order to control the infection and relieve the unrelenting pelvic pain.

Sadly, at least one out of every five women who recover from a first episode of PID are infertile, while chronic PID may be associated with an infertility rate approaching 90 percent. Compared with PID caused by gonorrhea, chlamydia-associated PID usually exhibits milder symptoms but its effects on tubal damage and infertility are often worse. When pregnancy does occur, it has a far greater likelihood of being ectopic—located in the fallopian tube, rather than in its normal location within the uterus. This occurs because tubal damage and scarring prevent passage of the fertilized egg down the tube. The soaring ectopic pregnancy rates in this country have closely paralleled those of the PID epidemic.

There is a commonly held misconception in our society that birth-control pills impair a woman's future fertility. If anything, the opposite is true, as evidenced by the fact that at least twelve studies over the past ten years have concluded that the Pill actually offers some protection against salpingitis and PID. The protective effect against gonorrhea is well established, while that for chlamydia remains controversial. Researchers at the Centers for Disease Control estimate that use of the Pill for at least one year by women with no history of PID reduces the expected incidence of PID by more than two-thirds. Prolonged use beyond one year may offer even greater protection.

It has been noted that *Chlamydia trachomatis* is more likely to be cultured from the cervix of a woman on the Pill than from the cervix of a woman using other contraceptive methods. This had led to the false conclusion that Pill users are more susceptible to this infection. A more likely explanation is that women on the Pill, unlike those relying on diaphragms, condoms, and spermicides, are not afforded the barrier necessary to prevent the entry of bacteria into the cervix. Once *Chlamydia trachomatis* and *Neisseria gonorrhoeae* get inside the cervix, the organisms will be half as likely in a woman on the Pill compared to other women to ascend from there and damage the fallopian tubes. The reason for this tendency is not fully understood, but one theory suggests that the progestin component of the Pill thickens the cervical mucus and makes it less permeable to bacteria. Another hypothesis is that decreased flow and duration of menstruation among Pill users reduces the number of infective organisms that can use the blood as a growth medium as they ascend and reproduce in the endometrial cavity.

A 1984 report from Sweden, published in *The Journal of the American Medical Association,* found that even when Pill users contract salpingitis or PID, the severity of the infection is lessened considerably when compared to women using other methods of contraception. In this study, doctors viewed the fallopian tubes of over 500 women hospitalized for PID and found the mildest infections and those least likely to incur permanent sterility to be among women using oral contraceptives. While the mechanism of this beneficial effect remains unknown, the reduction of salpingitis, PID, and ectopic pregnancy is particularly beneficial to those women who are most susceptible—teenagers, women with multiple sexual partners, blacks, and women with a previous history of PID.

One should not conclude from these remarks that I am advocating use of birth-control pills as a preventive against gonorrhea and chlamydia infections. In fact, a significant number of doctors remain unconvinced that oral contraceptives protect against these infections. Certainly condoms, diaphragms, and spermicides offer far greater protection against PID than do birth-control pills. Regardless of the type of contraception used, it is vital that women become aware that the early symptoms of salpingitis include abdominal pain, fever, and a yellowish vaginal discharge. For the majority of women, the infectious organisms will reside in the cervix and cause no symptoms. Unfortunately, these so-called asymptomatic carriers can transmit their bacteria to their sexual partners who, in turn, will infect others. Even if you have no symptoms, but have more than one sexual partner, or suspect your partner has more than one partner, it is a good idea to be tested periodically for chlamydia and gonorrhea. If your gynecologist tells you that he or she is not equipped to run these tests, find a new gynecologist. Aggressive antibiotic treatment of asymptomatic and symptomatic women and men is vital if young, sexually active men and women are to avoid the devastation caused by chlamydia and gonorrhea.

Can't the Pill cause infertility by delaying the return of normal periods and ovulation once it is discontinued?

Even though more than 98 percent of all women will ovulate within three months after stopping the Pill, fertility rates will be significantly lower during this time. Beyond three months, and certainly within six months, there is no difference in fertility between former Pill users and women who used other methods of contraception. So don't panic if you are trying to conceive and are unsuccessful for the first few months after you stop the Pill.

Approximately 2 percent of women will experience prolonged absence of menstruation, called *amenorrhea*, after they stop the Pill. This will happen regardless of the strength of the oral contraceptive formulation or the length of time one has used it. In the past this condition, termed post-Pill amenorrhea, was believed to be caused by the lingering effects of the suppression of the hypothalamus by the Pill (see chapter 1). It is now believed that this small percentage of young women probably would have developed amenorrhea, absence of ovulation, and infertility even if they had never taken the Pill. Careful questioning will usually reveal a markedly irregular menstrual pattern long before the Pill was started.

A small number of women with post-Pill amenorrhea also experience a thin, clear-to-milky discharge from the nipples caused by tumors of the pituitary gland known as *prolactinomas*. They inhibit the action of the hypothalamus in suppressing lactation. A new drug, bromocriptine mesylate, corrects this problem as well as restoring ovulation, menstruation, and fertility.

The notion that the Pill can permanently damage a woman's ovulatory mechanism just isn't true, and infertility following Pill use is undoubtedly no more than a coincidental occurrence.

Does a woman's prolactin level change when she is on the Pill?

It is important for you and your doctor to know that 30 percent of women on the combination Pill will show a slight increase in their serum prolactin levels. Two percent will experience a mild degree of galactorrhea, clear nipple discharge, while taking the Pill. While this condition is harmless, you should be tested at yearly intervals to be sure that prolactin secretion does not rise to levels associated with the presence of a prolactinoma.

Why do some doctors advise their patients to stop using the Pill for two or three months every three years?

If your doctor believes that you should take a temporary break from the Pill at periodic intervals, take a permanent break from that doctor. The reasoning behind this outdated ritual is supposedly to cleanse the body of the Pill's synthetic hormones and assure women that they are capable of reestablishing ovulation and menstruation. Since we now know that duration of contraceptive use is unrelated to a woman's future fertility (see above), arbitrarily stopping the Pill for two or three months without replacing it with another effective method will only lead to an unnecessary number of unwanted and unplanned pregnancies. In addition to the risk of pregnancy, there are no health benefits to be derived by pursuing this policy.

Are birth-control pills a good treatment for women in their thirties who have irregular periods?

The term "irregular periods" encompasses a wide range of menstrual patterns from frequent, prolonged, and heavy, to infrequent, short, and light. The cause of the irregularity should be determined before any medication is taken.

For a woman with heavy and frequent periods or vaginal staining between periods, an endometrial biopsy should be performed to be sure there is no evidence of a cancerous or precancerous condition. While this may be done by having a D and C (dilatation, opening of the cervix, and curettage, scraping of the endometrium) in a hospital, one of several inexpensive office procedures of almost equal accuracy and not requiring anesthesia is recommended. Some women, especially those who have previously given birth, find these office procedures almost painless; the majority, however, experience a great deal of discomfort. A paracervical anesthetic block (see chapter 7, "Abortion") may be helpful in relieving severe degrees of pain. If your doctor uses a suction device such as a Vabra Aspirator, the procedure can be performed in seconds and the pain will be gone as soon as it is completed.

Although birth-control pills taken by women over thirty-five years old present very definite hazards and are best avoided if possible, they have proven to be of great benefit for women in their thirties who suffer from totally unpredictable, heavy, and prolonged periods. This type of menstrual pattern is often characterized by infrequent or absent ovulation and too much stimulation of the glands of the endometrium by an abundance of estrogen and not enough progesterone. This may cause hyperplasia, or overgrowth of the glands, and a predisposition to cancer of the endometrium. Studies have convincingly shown that women in their thirties with irregular periods will be protected from endometrial hyperplasia and cancer and will be far less likely to require a D and C or a hysterectomy for uterine hemorrhage if they stay on the Pill. One can certainly understand the difficult decisions to be made by doctors for their patients who are thirty-five years of age and older who enjoy light, predictable menses on the Pill but fear the rare though serious consequences of Pill use after the age of thirty-five.

How about younger women?

Younger women, especially teenagers who experience heavy or frequent menstruation, rarely need to have an endometrial biopsy. The usual cause of such bleeding is the immaturity or malfunctioning of the hypothalamus (see chapter 1). Unpredictable release of GnRH causes production of estrogen by the ovarian follicle, but not enough LH is released from the pituitary to trigger ovulation. Without ovulation, a corpus luteum can't develop and secrete progesterone. Characteristically, these young women may go for months without a period, and then suddenly, without any premenstrual symptoms, experience a tremendously heavy flow with blood clots which may last for several days. The heavy bleeding takes place because the endometrium, which is stimulated only by estrogen and not by progesterone, sheds its lining unpredictably. These periods are practically always painless but they can create severe anemia due to the amount of blood loss.

A complete gynecological exam is in order for such young women to ascertain whether any serious abnormality is present. A test measuring thyroid function is often helpful, since occasionally an underactive thyroid gland may be responsible for this type of bleeding problem. In addition, if there is heavy bleeding, blood coagulation studies should be done to be sure that a clotting or platelet deficiency is not the source of the problem. If all these tests are normal, birth-control pills may be given for several months simply for the sake of allowing lighter, more predictable periods and preventing severe anemia. Some degree of anemia may result, and iron tablets are often helpful in building up the hemoglobin levels. The Pill will *in no way correct* the hypothalamus problem, however. After approximately three to four oral contraceptive cycles, the Pill may be stopped and future menses observed. If the hemorrhage recurs, the Pill should be started again. In time, the hypothalamus will function more efficiently and more predictably. Often the first sign of this maturity is an unusually painful period lasting less than one week and indicating that ovulation probably had taken place two weeks earlier.

When a young woman with previously normal periods notes that they are now several months apart and very light, most likely the hypothalamus is again responsible. In stressful situations, it fails to release any of its factors, including GnRH. Women in college dormitories, prisoners, dieters, heroin addicts, and thousands of other women under pressure have this hypothalamus defect in common. Menses usually return to normal when the woman's lifestyle changes for the better.

Until recently, medical authorities believed that it was dangerous to use birth-control pills solely to regulate menses. In addition, women with marked menstrual irregularities were denied the Pill for fear that it would further inhibit the hypothalamus's already inadequate functioning. These beliefs are no longer held. It is now known that a woman's prior menstrual history is the key predictor of the nature of her periods after she stops the Pill. Use of the Pill for months or years does not change the functioning of her hypothalamus or pituitary gland.

For the adolescent with irregular menses, the Pill is definitely the most logical choice of contraception. Predictable monthly cycles will eliminate the fear of wondering whether the delay of a period is the result of hypothalamus immaturity or of an early unplanned pregnancy.

Should I be concerned if I don't get periods while taking birth-control pills?

One of the great obstacles to the widespread use of the new low-dose birth-control pills has been amenorrhea—failure to experience bleeding during the week when the Pill is not taken and the hormones are withdrawn. The incidence of this phenomenon during a woman's first year on the Pill is 1 percent, but it may rise to 6 to 8 percent after three years. Most women will notice periods becoming progressively lighter and shorter in the months before they stop altogether.

Failure to experience withdrawal bleeding while taking birth-control pills is a totally innocuous condition, unrelated to the post-Pill amenorrhea that can develop after a woman stops using the Pill (see page 51). Despite reassurances, many patients continue to express concern that the absence of menses means that toxic blood products are accumulating in the body. The truth of the matter is that the dose of estrogen in the new Pill formulations is so low that it is incapable of stimulating the growth of the glands in the endometrium, or lining of the uterine cavity. In addition, the progesterone in these Pills dominates the estrogen effect to a degree that a shallow endometrium is produced. As a result, there is an insufficient amount of tissue capable of bleeding during the week that the hormones are withdrawn. So, contrary to the idea of a buildup of tissue that is retained, there is actually no tissue buildup when the 0.030 to 0.035 milligram estrogen dose in the newer oral contraceptive formulations is taken. These changes are temporary and subside soon after the Pill is stopped.

Obviously, pregnancy is another major fear of the woman who fails to have withdrawal bleeding. If all the Pills have been taken during the cycle, the possibility of pregnancy would be highly unlikely. Despite this, all Pill manufacturers recommend a pregnancy test if you fail to have withdrawal bleeding for two cycles in succession.

Since it can become an intrusive and expensive proposition to take pregnancy tests every two months, a more economical and practical solution is to take your basal body temperature (see chapter 5) immediately upon awakening on any morning of the week you are off the Pill. If your temperature is less than 98°F you don't have to worry about pregnancy since your temperature would always be higher if you were pregnant.

While some women welcome the absence of a period each month, the vast majority prefer the assurance of experiencing some menstrual flow. This may be achieved in several ways. One solution is for the physician to increase the estrogen dose from a 0.030 or 0.035 milligram formulation to one with 0.050 milligrams for a few cycles. This will build up the endometrium, induce withdrawal bleeding, and offer assurance that all is well. But, switching back to the lower dose Pill will usually result in the recurrence of amenorrhea within a few months. Many doctors keep their patients on the higher 0.050 milligram formulations permanently in order to avoid this situation. My opinion is that the many benefits of the lower estrogen dose far outweigh the mere reassurance of menstruating monthly. Rather than change birth-control formulations, some gynecologists have reported success by giving 0.020 milligrams of ethinyl estradiol with each birth-control pill for a period of one to three months. This has the effect of building up the endometrium to a thickness that is sufficient to induce withdrawal bleeding on the 0.035 milligram birth-control pill even for several months after the ethinyl estradiol is stopped. These doctors believe that the health risks of using the extra dose of ethinyl estradiol for a short period of time are far milder than permanently switching to the 0.050 milligram birth-control pill.

The new triphasic birth-control pills have a monthly progestin dose that is lower than the combination Pills (see triphasics, discussed earlier in the chapter). Researchers have theorized that these Pills will be associated with lower rates of amenorrhea because of the lessened growth-inhibiting effect on the endometrium. Long-term studies are needed to confirm or refute this belief.

It is important for doctors to warn their patients that their periods may become scanty or even disappear altogether on the Pill and that this is a welcome sign that they are on a safe, low-dose formulation. Permanently raising the estrogen content merely for the sake of eliciting withdrawal bleeding should be discouraged.

What is the significance of breakthrough bleeding and how should it be managed?

Bleeding between normal periods is referred to as breakthrough bleeding or spotting, depending on the amount of flow. Though breakthrough bleeding is of no medical consequence, it is often alarming and annoying for the women who experience it, and it remains the single most frequent reason for discontinuing birth-control pills. The incidence of breakthrough bleeding may be anywhere from 2 to 3 percent with Pill formulations containing 0.050 milligrams or more of estrogen, to 6 to 15 percent among women on 0.030 to 0.035 milligram Pills. Minipills (progestogen-only pills) are responsible for the high breakthrough bleeding rate of almost 50 percent (see Minipill, page 31). Over 90 percent of all Pill-related calls to doctors' offices concern breakthrough bleeding. This number could be reduced significantly if doctors took the time to explain to their patients that breakthrough bleeding or spotting is a harmless condition most likely to occur during the first three months of Pill use, after which it will usually disappear, and that breakthrough bleeding will not increase a woman's chances of conceiving.

Breakthrough bleeding and spotting occur because of an inadequate buildup of the endometrium, which breaks down and bleeds earlier in the cycle than expected. Breakthrough bleeding can be minimized by taking the Pill at approximately the same time each day, rather than haphazardly. Skipping one Pill in the pack will increase your chances of breakthrough bleeding significantly, especially if it occurs in the second half of the cycle.

It is suspected that when breakthrough bleeding occurs early in the Pill cycle, it is probably the result of inadequate stimulation of the endometrium. Bleeding in the second half of the cycle is usually attributed to too little endometrial support by the progestin. Based on this reasoning, doctors have successfully treated early break-through bleeding by temporarily switching from a 0.030 or 0.035 milligram estrogen formulation to a 0.050 milligram formulation for three to four months, or by prescribing 0.020 milligrams of ethinyl estradiol with each of the first seven to fourteen birth-control pills for two Pill cycles. Bleeding in the second half of the cycle can be remedied by switching to a birth-control pill with a stronger progestin. For example, if you are taking Ortho-Novum 1/35, it might be helpful to change to a Pill such as Lo-Ovral since the progestin norgestrel is many times stronger than norethindrone (see progestins, page 26). Doubling up, or taking two birth-control pills per day during the spotting days, is not recommended, nor is the use of the new triphasic birth-control pills. Recent studies have shown that triphasics show the same or even a higher incidence of breakthrough bleeding than the low-dose monophasic Pills.

Before you or your doctor assume that your breakthrough bleeding can be attributed solely to the Pill, an examination at the time you are bleeding can help eliminate other possible causes unrelated to the Pill, such as cervical erosion (see earlier in this chapter and chapter 1) or a benign polyp or growth on the cervix. If your examination and Pap smear are both normal, it is perfectly safe to ignore one to two days of harmless spotting each month rather than to switch to a more potent pill. If the breakthrough bleeding continues for several days of each cycle, however, it is probably a good idea to take the steps outlined above. When breakthrough bleeding persists despite these measures, your doctor should instruct you to stop taking the Pill for one or two months to see if the problem corrects itself. If it doesn't, the next step would be to obtain a sampling of the endometrium to be sure that there are no other reasons for this abnormal bleeding pattern (see irregular menses, page 52).

If I use birth-control pills and don't want my period on the expected date, how can I alter the date?

This can easily be done with the standard monophasic pills by stopping them five days or sooner before the full supply is diminished, and discarding the remainder of the Pills in the pack. A normal period will follow, and the next new box of pills may be started as usual. An alternative method is to prolong the cycle by using additional pills from another pack for up to twenty-one days. If you are using a triphasic pill, such as Ortho-Novum 7/7/7, Tri-Norinyl, Triphasil, or Tri-Levlen, it becomes a bit trickier because the hormonal contents of the Pills differ. Stopping early may result in incomplete sloughing of the endometrium, and this can cause the prolonged bleeding you are trying to avoid. A better idea is to prolong the cycle by taking as many of the last seven pills from another pack as your plans require. Keep an extra pack of pills on hand for such circumstances.

If I forget to take a Pill, what should I do?

The standard advice in the past has been to take the forgotten Pill when you remember it even if it meant taking two Pills at the same time. But your risk of pregnancy will be no greater if you discard the forgotten Pill and complete the cycle without it. Missing one standard monophasic Pill during the cycle will rarely result in pregnancy. To avoid that remote possibility as well as the threat of breakthrough bleeding, however, it is obviously best not to miss a Pill and to take it at approximately the same time each day. It is widely believed that the most important Pill not to forget is the first one of the pack, since most accidental pregnancies on the Pill occur when the interval between the last combination pill of one pack and the first of the next exceeds seven days. The reason for this is that a follicle in the ovary begins to develop during the week you are off the Pill and a so-called "escape ovulation" may occur if the follicle is allowed to grow. While this may be true for some low-dose estrogen formulations, it is especially significant with the new triphasic Pills which contain minimal amounts of progestin during the first seven days of the cycle. For this reason, many doctors advise only a six-day hiatus between packs of Pills.

Not all authorities share this concern about the risk of escape ovulation when the first Pill is not taken on time. Researchers at the University of Manchester Medical School in England contend that pregnancy is unlikely to occur even when the length of time between one pack of Pills and the next is extended to eleven days. In their 1986 report, they tested the efficacy of both monophasic and triphasic birth-control pills used in this manner. Though follicles of potentially ovulated eggs were more likely to develop by the eleventh Pill-free day, their growth was successfully halted once the first Pill was taken. Though no one should alter her Pill-taking habits based on these preliminary findings, it is encouraging to note that you will most probably not conceive even if you start your new Pill pack one or two days later than you should have.

If you do miss one Pill in the pack, it is not a bad idea to use backup contraception such as a condom, a diaphragm, the TODAY sponge, or foam during that cycle. This is especially sound advice for users of the progestin-only Minipill, who are at significantly greater risk of pregnancy even when they don't miss a Pill.

Missing two consecutive Pills during a cycle should be treated in the same fashion as missing one, and so-called "makeup Pills" are unnecessary and can be discarded. Backup contraception becomes more important when two Pills are missed. However, even then the risk of pregnancy is minimal. In one 1982 study, thirty-two women using Nordette were instructed to deliberately omit taking Pills for two consecutive days at varying times of the cycle. In all cases, the Pill was still able to inhibit ovulation regardless of when the two Pills had been omitted. The reason for this outcome may very well be the fact that Nordette contains the strong progestin levonorgestrel. No studies have been conducted on the omission of three or more consecutive Pills in a pack, but if this has been your situation on more than one occasion, I would strongly advise that you use another method of contraception. If your problem is forgetfulness, it is a good idea to get into the habit of taking a Pill daily by using a twenty-eight-day formulation that contains seven placebos. If you miss three or more Pills in succession it is best to stop the cycle at that point, await withdrawal bleeding, and restart a fresh pack no later than one week after the last Pill was taken even if you are still bleeding. Until ten Pills of the new pack are taken, it is important that you use alternative contraception.

In a 1985 survey of members of the American College of Obstetricians and Gynecologists, 20 percent reported that the problem of omitting a Pill or taking the wrong Pill was most likely to occur with triphasic formulations. The reasons cited were confusion over the different-colored Pills and the poor design of the Pill package.

Can the Pill cause an abnormal Pap?

Long-term use of birth-control pills may be associated with slightly lower levels of important vitamins and minerals (see birth-control pills and vitamins, page 57). Folic acid is a vitamin that plays a key role in cell metabolism. Cervical cells obtained with a Pap smear may appear grossly abnormal in the presence of a folic acid deficiency, but this can be corrected with folic acid supplements.

In a 1980 study from the University of Alabama School of Medicine, Birmingham, doctors gave 10 milligrams of folic acid daily to forty-seven women with proven mild and moderate dysplasia of the cervix. In seven women, the cervical abnormality completely reverted to normal. Furthermore, none of the forty-seven women progressed to the more ominous carcinoma-in-situ.

Before folic acid is considered to be an acceptable adjunct to the treatment of precancerous disease of the cervix, larger and more complete studies will be required.

Can a folic acid deficiency cause other medical problems?

Some interesting, though preliminary, research from Europe over the past five years has suggested that use of folic acid supplements in the month prior to conception may decrease a woman's risk of giving birth to a baby with a neural tube defect such as anencephaly and spina bifida. Theoretically, this bit of information sounds like it would be of great importance to the woman who is contemplating pregnancy shortly after stopping the Pill. There is no evidence, however, to show that women who conceive shortly after stopping the Pill are at a greater risk of giving birth to a baby with neural tube defect (see page 61).

The longer a woman is on birth-control pills the more likely she is to experience a decline in her folic acid levels. For this reason, nutritionists suggest that women on the Pill for longer than a year eat foods rich in folic acid such as liver, veal, kidney, beans, lean meats, yeast, raw green leafy vefetables, and citrus fruit juices.

Are there other deficiencies associated with Pill use?

Several studies have suggested that the estrogen in oral contraceptives prevents the intestine from absorbing certain important vitamins and minerals, including vitamin B_6 (pyridoxine), vitamin B_2 (riboflavin), vitamin B_{11} (folic acid), vitamin B_1 (thiamine), vitamin B_{12} (cobalamin, cyanocobalamin), vitamin C (ascorbic acid), vitamin E (alphatocopherol), and zinc. Regardless of unfounded reports and speculation, there has never been a definitive scientific study demonstrating that use of oral contraceptives causes any clinically apparent vitamin deficiency in a woman who is on an adequate diet. There is no real evidence that oral contraceptive users need to take vitamin supplements; vitamin and mineral supplements are indicated only when deficiency symptoms become apparent and can't be corrected through dietary adjustments.

Though adverse psychological effects of the Pill such as depression, fatigue, and irritability have been associated with the progestins (see page 65), some authors have attributed these symptoms to a deficiency of vitamin B_6. In one report of fifty-eight Pill users suffering from depression, administration of a high daily dose of vitamin B_6 resulted in a marked improvement of symptoms in forty-four of these women. Subsequent studies, however, have not confirmed these findings. A severe vitamin B_6 deficiency can also impair glucose and insulin metabolism. In one report, doctors corrected abnormal glucose tolerance in some Pill users simply by prescribing supplemental B_6.

The Recommended Daily Allowance, or RDA, for vitamin B_6 is 2 milligrams for adult women not using oral contraceptives. Some nutritionists believe that a daily dose of more than ten times that amount, or 25 milligrams, is recommended for Pill users. This can easily be obtained by eating foods rich in B_6 such as yeast, wheat germ, meats, liver, bananas, fish, whole-grain cereals, soy beans, peanuts, and corn.

Vitamin B_2, riboflavin, levels also decrease with the use of oral contraceptives. The need for riboflavin is often closely related to B_6, since both vitamins are used by the body in a similar fashion. Symptoms of a riboflavin deficiency include glossitis, or inflamed tongue, dryness of the skin, cracks in the corners of the mouth, and irritation of the eyes. There has never been a case of riboflavin deficiency associated with Pill use, and the RDA of 1.2 milligrams can easily be met with a minimum daily intake of foods such as milk, cheese, eggs, liver, kidney, and green leafy vegetables.

Though the levels of vitamin B_{11} may decline when you are on the Pill, it is of no clinical significance.

Levels of both vitamin B_1, thiamine, and vitamin B_{12}, cyanocobalamine, decline when a woman is on the Pill. In the case of B_{12}, this decline is noted soon after the Pill is started and does not progress with further oral contraceptive use. Foods rich in B_1 are pork, ham, and wheat germ, while B_{12} sources include liver, kidney, and milk.

A deficiency of vitamin C, secondary to use of birth-control pills, has also been reported. No clinical significance of this alteration has been observed, however, and there's no need to take supplements if citrus fruits, raw leafy vegetables, and tomatoes, all excellent sources of vitamin C, are eaten frequently. In a 1981 study from England, doctors found that if a woman took one gram of vitamin C with her birth-control pill, it had the effect of increasing the amount of circulating estrogen in her body and possibly adding to the efficacy of the low-dose Pill formulations.

Opinions differ as to the effect of birth-control pills on vitamin E levels. Increases as well as decreases have been reported, and it is generally concluded that supplements of vitamin E are of little, if any, value. Though vitamin E is thought of as an exotic and rare vitamin, in fact it is found in essentially every food. Its wide distribution in vegetable oils, cereal grains, corn, peanuts, eggs, and animal fats make a deficiency of vitamin E extremely unlikely.

Though very little is known about zinc requirements, it is vital to the body's metabolism. Some doctors have recommended increased zinc intake if a woman plans to be on birth-control pills for a long period of time. Fish, oysters, meat, eggs, and milk are all excellent sources of zinc.

Does the Pill cause an increase in any of the body's important vitamins and minerals?

One of the great benefits of using birth-control pills is that a woman's dietary requirements for iron will be significantly diminished because periods are lighter, so less iron-containing blood is lost each month. The average blood loss during a period is approximately 20 cubic centimeters (cc.) among Pill users, compared to 35 cc. among women not using oral contraceptives. This decreased blood loss reduces the risk of iron deficiency anemia by 50 percent among women on the Pill. And the protective effect persists long after the Pill is stopped, because a woman on the Pill for a prolonged period of time has built up her iron stores which will not usually be depleted for several years. In practical terms, if we assume that there are currently six million Pill users in the United States, approximately 19,000 cases of iron deficiency anemia can be averted each year.

The absorption of calcium from the intestine into the body tissues is enhanced because of the estrogen in the Pill, so the requirements for this mineral are reduced among Pill users. It has long been known that estrogen prevents loss of calcium from bones and prevents osteoporosis in menopausal women. It is the prevention of osteoporosis and accompanying vertebral and hip fractures that has made estrogen replacement therapy so popular. However, recent medical research has clearly demonstrated that calcium loss from the bones may begin in a woman's thirties. Therefore, use of the Pill until the mid-thirties may help retard this process.

It has also been reported that a woman's need for vitamin A (retinol), vitamin K, niacin, and copper may be reduced if she is on birth-control pills. Further studies are needed to confirm this. In the case of vitamin A, the increase may be not in the vitamin itself but in the so-called carrier protein to which vitamin A is attached.

Of interest is the fact that certain clotting factors in the blood are dependent on the presence of vitamin K. Since vitamin K levels will be increased among some Pill users, researchers have suggested that it is this phenomenon that may contribute to the increased incidence of thrombus formation among oral contraceptive users (see discussion of thrombus and emboli, page 38).

How effective is the Pill in helping women who are suffering from PMS?

PMS, premenstrual syndrome, may be defined as the cyclic recurrence of a wide variety of distressing physical, psychological, and behavioral changes during the week to ten days prior to each period. It is estimated that 10 to 12 million menstruating women in this country—30 percent—suffer from PMS. For many, PMS destroys interpersonal relationships, creates great unhappiness, and makes coping with even the simplest of tasks very difficult. Statistics prove that suicides, accidental deaths, and even deaths from natural causes are more likely to occur during the premenstrual phase of the cycle. While PMS has been rejected as a contributing factor in the commission of a crime in the United States, French and British courts have acknowledged its existence and importance in such acts.

The cause of PMS remains an enigma since studies have shown no differences in estrogen or progesterone levels between PMS sufferers and other women. It is known, however, that PMS occurs exclusively among women who ovulate each month. Symptoms are often as varied as the women who have them, and include irritability, depression, breast tenderness, acne, weight gain, anxiety, insomnia, fatigue, headaches, bloating, diminished sexuality, aggressiveness, and clumsiness. Because the symptoms are often so diverse, no one method of treatment has been successful for all women with PMS. Special diets; vitamins; exercise; progesterone in the form of a pill, injection, or vaginal suppository; and diuretics have all been tried with limited success. As with other conditions that are difficult to define, even placebos have achieved temporary improvement in as many as one-third of all PMS sufferers. Despite claims to the contrary, to date no method has been scientifically proven to cure or relieve this condition.

Since PMS is a condition that affects ovulating women, it is theorized that a logical treatment would be to inhibit ovulation with birth-control pills. Surprisingly, this has proven to be quite disappointing. In one study, oral contraceptives decreased physician visits for PMS by only 29 percent, a result not any better than those achieved with placebos. Other reports have shown that birth-control pills have the effect of delaying the onset of the same symptoms until the week when the Pill is not taken. Complete suppression of the menstrual cycle with continual oral contraceptive therapy over a period of several months has been suggested as a form of treatment but has not yet been evaluated.

What is the relationship between birth-control pills and diseases of the liver?

There is no doubt that the estrogen and, to a lesser extent, the progestin in the Pill are capable of altering the results of certain laboratory tests that measure liver function. This may occur in anywhere from 10 to 30 percent of women who use Pills containing more than 0.050 milligrams of estrogen, and to a much lesser degree when the 0.030 to 0.035 milligram formulations are used. These test results revert to normal when the Pill is stopped, and this phenomenon appears to be harmless.

If you currently have liver disease, don't take birth-control pills. This warning applies to the Minipill as well, since the progestin in it could activate certain enzymes in the liver.

Hepatitis is an inflammation of the liver in which bile pigments that would normally be destroyed circulate in the blood, producing jaundice or yellowing of the skin and the whites of the eyes. While hepatitis may result from exposure to chemical or environmental agents, most cases are caused by one of three viruses, appropriately named Hepatitis A virus, Hepatitis B virus, and non–A and –B virus. Hepatitis B is known as serum hepatitis and for years believed to occur only in individuals who received blood transfusions from others with the disease or in drug-addicted persons using contaminated needles. Epidemiologists now know that Hepatitis B is frequently transmitted sexually, while Hepatitis A may follow a similar route on rare occasions. The Hepatitis B virus has a long incubation period—two to six months—and while some individuals with the disease experience few if any symptoms, the majority are quite ill with jaundice, fever, extreme lethargy, loss of appetite, nausea, vomiting, and sometimes generalized body itching and joint pain. Over 90 percent of those who contract Hepatitis B recover within a few weeks, but a significant percentage remain long-term carriers. Though the overwhelming majority of doctors would not prescribe the Pill in the presence of hepatitis, a report in a 1977 issue of the *Journal of the American Medical Association* demonstrated that thirty-four women with the disease took the Pill without apparent ill effect or worsening of liver function tests. The small number of patients involved, however, makes any favorable conclusion suspect until more impressive data is available. Once recovery from hepatitis is complete, as measured by normal blood tests, it is perfectly safe to prescribe the Pill. Too often I have seen healthy women unnecessarily denied the Pill because of a history of hepatitis several years earlier.

As previously mentioned (see page 48, skin diseases), a small percentage of women will suffer from cholestasis on the Pill. This occurs because the estrogen and progestin make it difficult for the liver to rid itself of the bile it produces. As a result, the bile backs up into the circulatory system and causes severe itching of the skin and occasionally jaundice. If this should occur while you're on the Pill, see your doctor; the Pill should be stopped immediately.

Since 1973, doctors have become aware of a relationship between Pill use and an increased incidence of two rare and benign liver tumors called *hepatocellular adenoma* and *focal nodular hyperplasia*. The Centers for Disease Control have estimated that women who have never been on the Pill or who have used it for twenty-four months or less have only one chance in a million of developing these tumors. However, if you have been a Pill user for seven or more years, are over thirty years old, and are using a Pill formulation with 0.050 milligrams or more of estrogen, your risk increases 500 times. Though this sounds frightening, it is important to remember that your overall risk of contracting hepatocellular adenoma or focal nodular hyperplasia will still be no greater than 3 to 4 out of every 100,000 women on the Pill. In terms of actual numbers, of the 6 million American Pill users, there will be approximately 200 tumors and 25 deaths annually. This risk is so low that it would be offset by the Pill's well-documented protective effects against ovarian and uterine cancers (see pages 45–46).

It was originally believed that these liver tumors were more common in women whose birth-control pills contained the estrogen mestranol rather than ethinyl estradiol. Recent data, however, suggest that both forms of estrogen are equally to blame. In addition, the progestins may also play a role. Since these tumors can rupture and cause severe intra-abdominal hemmorrhage, it is vital that your doctor discontinue your Pill use as soon as the diagnosis is made.

What are the risks of liver cancer among Pill users?

Two separate studies published in the *British Medical Journal* in 1986 claim that there is a link between oral contraceptive use and liver cancer. In one of the studies, eighteen of twenty-six women who developed liver cancer had used oral contraceptives for an average of eight years. Pill use beyond eight years was associated with an almost fivefold increase in the risk of this rare cancer. In the second report, doctors from Radcliffe Infirmary in Oxford, England, described nineteen women aged twenty to forty-four who died of liver cancer. They estimated that the risk of liver cancer for oral contraceptive users was twenty times greater than for nonusers.

Both reports have been severely criticized by epidemiologists and researchers throughout the world, and larger studies are presently under way to confirm or refute these claims. Even if we assume that these reports are accurate, the excess risk of liver cancer for long-term oral contraceptive users would be no more than four cases per million compared to less than one case per million in the general population. This would translate to less than twenty-five deaths annually among the six million oral contraceptive users in this country.

If a pregnancy occurs while I am on the Pill, is it more likely to be in the tube rather than in the uterus?

This depends on the type of birth-control pill you take. A pregnancy located outside the uterus is called an ectopic pregnancy (see chapter 3). By far the most common type of ectopic pregnancy is one in the fallopian tube, called a tubal pregnancy. Rupture of the wall of the tube by an ectopic pregnancy can result in severe intra-abdominal hemorrhage and even death. Tubal pregnancies may also pass out the end of the tube. This condition is known as a tubal abortion. In extremely rare circumstances, the fetus will implant in the abdominal cavity and continue to grow after it has been passed out of the tube. An abdominal pregnancy may go to term.

No reports suggest that users of combination-type oral contraceptives are more likely than other women to suffer from an ectopic pregnancy if they accidentally conceive. However, data from at least eighteen separate studies strongly suggest a higher incidence of ectopic pregnancy among women who conceived while using the progestin-only Minipill. One group of researchers suggested that the progestin norgestrel, the type found in Ovrette, was most likely to be responsible; other studies have implicated norethindrone, which is found in both NorQD and Micronor. In contrast, a progestin named lynestrenol, which is manufactured in Europe, has not been found to increase a woman's risk of ectopic pregnancy. The mechanism by which a Minipill makes one more susceptible to an ectopic pregnancy is unknown, but it is theorized that the progestin slows down the transport of the fertilized egg through the fallopian tube. As a result, it attaches itself within the tube rather than in its normal location within the endometrium of the uterus.

Your doctor should always consider the possibility of an ectopic pregnancy if you develop lower abdominal pain while on a progestin-only Minipill.

Is it true that if I continue to take birth-control pills without realizing I am pregnant, there is a chance that the genitals of my female fetus may be masculinized?

Yes. This has not been reported frequently but it is a very real possibility. The reason is that the progestin in the Pill is a synthetic hormone more closely related to the male hormone testosterone than to the female hormone progesterone. The formation of a grossly enlarged clitoris, resembling a male penis, and of labia majora resembling a male scrotum is believed to be caused by the passage of progestins across the placenta at the time when these organs are being formed, between the seventh and twelfth weeks of pregnancy. If you stop the Pill before the seventh week, you can be assured that your female offspring will not be masculinized.

As previously mentioned, the more potent progestins such as norgestrel and levo-norgestrel are much more likely to cause this problem than the other four progestins which are not as androgenic (see progestins, page 26).

To avoid fetal anomalies, isn't it best for a woman to wait three months from the time she stops the Pill to the time she conceives?

Among the many misconceptions surrounding the use of birth-control pills, this is undoubtedly one of the most prevalent. It is based on one outdated 1970 report showing an increased incidence of chromosomal defects in spontaneously aborted fetuses of women who had conceived within three months after stopping the Pill. Several subsequent studies have not shown this to be true, nor is there an increased likelihood of spontaneous abortion, ectopic pregnancy, or congenital anomalies when a woman conceives immediately after she stops taking the Pill. Unfortunately, many doctors continue to believe and to disseminate this misinformation.

Are birth defects more common among women who inadvertently use birth-control pills early in pregnancy?

Though there is a great deal of controversy about this subject, the majority of today's authorities are far more optimistic than earlier researchers. Between 1973 and 1980 several reports concluded that inadvertent use of birth control pills early in pregnancy predisposed the fetus to a wide variety of congenital anomalies of the heart, limbs, and other organs. Many of these studies were flawed because they lumped all hormones together instead of distinguishing between birth-control pills and other estrogen and progestin preparations. Furthermore, it has been impossible to document statistically the findings of these earlier reports.

The current prevailing opinion is that inadvertent use of the Pill early in pregnancy may increase your risk of giving birth to a baby with a congenital heart defect. Fortunately, this risk is probably no greater than 1 per 1,000 births above the usual incidence of 7 to 8 per 1,000 births. Your risk of giving birth to a baby with other defects is no higher than that of the general population. The most recent and optimistic article dealing with this question was published in the *Journal of the American Medical Association* in 1986. Doctors at The Centers for Disease Control in Atlanta, Georgia, studied first-trimester hormone exposure among mothers of 1,091 infants with Down's syndrome and eleven other major malformations. They concluded: "There is no statistically significant association between any malformation category and oral contraceptive exposure." In another article, published in the *International Journal of Fertility* in 1985, doctors actually found a lower risk of minor malformations among former Pill users.

Most experts would agree that the risk of a birth defect is so low for a woman who accidentally took birth-control pills early in pregnancy that it is not necessary for her to consider abortion. The problem can be avoided completely if the absence of pregnancy is confirmed before oral contraceptives are started. This may sound like a simple suggestion, but it is violated repeatedly by women and their doctors. Second, hormones should no longer be used as pregnancy tests or as a method of bringing on periods and should rarely, if ever, be used to support a pregnancy in jeopardy. In the rare cases where the last is necessary, pure progesterone preparations given intramuscularly appear to be safest for the developing fetus. If you miss one or more Pills during a cycle, then skip a period after the last birth-control pill is taken, get a pregnancy test before starting a new box of Pills. Some studies actually conclude that women who conceive soon after stopping the Pill have lower miscarriage and stillborn rates and a greater likelihood of giving birth to fraternal, or nonidentical, twins. In one report from Israel, doctors found that the number of infants born with heart defects was 1.7 per 1,000 for recent Pill users, compared with 3.7 per 1,000 for nonusers. Thousands of newborns were studied to determine whether the type of contraception the mother had used earlier influenced the development of congenital malformations in her offspring. Their findings, published in the *International Journal of Fertility* in 1985, showed that the incidence of major congenital malformations was 17.2 per 1,000 among former Pill users, compared with 15 and 20 per 1,000, respectively, in the groups using other methods or no method at all. Statistically, these differences are not significant. The incidence of major abnormalities among those who had conceived in the first month after having stopped the Pill were actually slightly lower than those who had conceived later.

The only justification for waiting to conceive after you stop the Pill is that it will be easier for your doctor to determine your date of conception, since periods tend to be irregular for the first three months after stopping the Pill. Today, however, this should present no great problem since ultrasound is readily available for accurately determining fetal age.

Can a woman with fibroids take birth-control pills?

Fibroids, or *leiomyomas,* are benign tumors of the uterus (see chapter 10) which grow under the influence of the high levels of estrogen during the reproductive years and diminish in size once the menopause is reached. Symptoms of fibroids include heavy periods with clotting as well as pressure symptoms on the bladder and rectum.

A large 1982 epidemiologic study clearly demonstrated that birth-control pills do not cause fibroids. Many gynecologists discontinue oral contraceptive use once the diagnosis of fibroids is made, however, because they fear that the estrogen in the Pill will stimulate fibroid growth. There is now evidence to show that the progestin in birth-control pills more than counterbalances this estrogen effect. In a 1986 report from The University of Southern California School of Medicine, Dr. Don Ross and his associates compared the medical records of 535 women with fibroids to those of an equal number of women without fibroids. The surprising and encouraging conclusion was that with each five years of oral contraceptive use, the risk of developing fibroids actually declined by 17 percent. Dr. Ross further noted that high progestin and low estrogen formulations were the most successful.

If you have fibroids and are on the Pill, your doctor should carefully monitor the size of your uterus every six months and possibly more often if your periods become heavier or longer while you are on the Pill. At the first sign of an increase in the size of the fibroids, the Pill should be discontinued. The estrogen dose of the Pill should not exceed 0.035 milligrams, combined with a strong progestin such as norgestrel or levonorgestrel. Despite its drawbacks, the progestin-only Minipill may be the preferred method of oral contraception for women with fibroids (see discussion of Minipill earlier in the chapter).

Can taking birth-control pills stunt the growth of an adolescent girl?

If a young girl is given estrogen prior to achieving her full adolescent growth, premature closure of her long bones may occur. This can result in the reduction of final height by about 1 inch, but occasionally by as much as 3 inches. Doctors have used estrogen treatment in reducing the final height of girls destined to be abnormally tall.

Once she has had her first period, a sexually active adolescent need not worry about taking birth-control pills. A woman's growth spurt always precedes the onset of menarche, the first period. The amount of additional growth following menarche is only 1 to $1\frac{1}{2}$ inches at the most. The low dose of estrogen in currently prescribed pills is not enough to stop any additional growth that might follow the onset of menses.

What effect do birth-control pills have on the menopause?

Birth-control pills can't accelerate or postpone the onset of the menopause, or cessation of menses. But because of the estrogen they contain, oral contraceptives usually mask or hide the symptoms that accompany the menopause, such as the characteristic hot flashes. Though the average age of the menopause is fifty-one years, a small percentage of women experience premature menopause prior to the age of forty. Most birth-control pills, including the latest formulations, contain 50 to 100 times the dose of estrogen usually needed to control hot flashes. Therefore, it is not surprising for a woman with premature menopause to experience symptoms within days after she stops using the Pill.

How does the use of birth-control pills affect a woman's athletic performance?

Only one scientific study has attempted to accurately compare a woman's athletic performance on and off the Pill. In his 1987 report, Dr. Morris Hotelovitz and his associates at the University of Florida performed blood tests measuring the cardiorespiratory fitness of six women three and six months after using a low-dose oral contraceptive. Two measurements of aerobic capacity, the oxygen uptake and volume of oxygen consumed per heart beat, were found to worsen by 7 and 8 percent respectively after six months of regular exercise. In contrast six women using alternative methods of contraception increased their oxygen values by 7 and 9 percent after six months of exercise. The authors concluded that low-dose oral contraceptive use is associated with a significant decrease in aerobic capacity. For the serious athlete, use of alternative birth-control methods is advised.

The majority of testimonials and letters written by long-distance runners and other athletes seem to support the belief that times are faster and performance is better among women who do not use birth-control pills. Athletes tend to prefer alternative methods of contraception, citing bloating, water retention, weight gain, fatigue, and mood swings as reasons for not using birth-control pills. In a 1983 study published in *Fertility and Sterility,* John C. Jarrett II, M.D., and William N. Spellacy, M.D., studied the contraceptive practices of 70 runners. Only 9 of the 70 used birth-control pills, compared with 31 diaphragm users. In another 1982 report, only 6 percent of 394 marathon runners used the Pill.

Obviously, if you are a woman who suffers from severely painful periods, dysmenorrhea (see page 71), irregular periods, heavy periods, or anemia secondary to heavy menstrual flow, the predictability of light and painless periods afforded by the Pill can only improve your athletic performance.

Is it safe for obese women to take birth-control pills?

There is no medical evidence to show that obesity poses an increased risk with oral contraceptive use. However, since obesity is often associated with other medical problems such as hypertension, abnormal lipid metabolism, abnormal glucose tolerance, and phlebitis, it is a good idea for a doctor to test for these conditions before prescribing the Pill and to examine obese women at least every six to twelve months.

Obese women should use the lowest estrogen and progestin Pill formulations. Since weight gain and abnormalities in lipid metabolism are most pronounced when a strong progestin is used, a Pill containing norethindrone, norethynodrel, norethindrone acetate, or ethynodiol diacetate is preferable to one with norgestrel or levonorgestrel (see progestins and lipids).

How do birth-control pills influence a woman's sexual response?

Though many medical publications have attempted to evaluate the effect of oral contraceptives on a woman's sexual response, the conclusions reached have been contradictory and confusing. The difficulties encountered in trying to study such a subject are readily apparent. For example, how does one determine whether a woman's increased libido is due to the specific ingredients of a birth-control pill or to the security of knowing that an unwanted pregnancy is unlikely? In a 1980 study, Princeton University researchers were able to demonstrate a direct relationship between frequency of intercourse and the effectiveness of the contraceptive method a couple used. Highest coital rates were reported by women who used the Pill or IUD, or whose husbands had had vasectomies.

Despite the difficulties in conducting such studies, some meaningful conclusions do emerge. The most important statistic is that the majority of women using oral contraceptives experience no major psychosexual changes. Approximately 70 percent of all Pill users, regardless of age or marital status, will note no change in libido. Of the 30 percent who do experience a change, it is usually for the better. In one interesting study of over 200 women on the Pill, single women were much more likely to experience enhanced libido, while married women were as likely to increase as to decrease their sexuality. Several studies have demonstrated an increase in coital frequency among women using the Pill over a prolonged period of time, but other studies have failed to confirm these findings.

Despite all the research, sexologists are still not sure whether there is a particular time in the menstrual cycle when women are most sexual. Some say it is at midcycle, others that it is immediately prior to the period. Two studies have purported to show that Pill use influences the time in the menstrual cycle when intercourse takes place. In one report, researchers found that coital rates increased premenstrually among Pill users, possibly because they were less likely to suffer from symptoms associated with PMS. Another study done by psychologists at Wesleyan University used interviews with thirty-five women in order to determine when during the menstrual cycle "female-initiated sexual behavior" was most likely to occur. It reported that for the twenty-three women not using the Pill, "autosexual" (masturbation) and "female-initiated heterosexual behavior" peaked at ovulation, or midcycle. This corresponds to the maximum estrogen production by the ovaries. The women using oral contraceptives did not show a rise in female-initiated sexual behavior at the corresponding times in their menstrual cycles.

Most researchers believe that loss of libido experienced by a small percentage of women using oral contraceptives is unrelated to the specific type and amount of estrogen or progestin that they contain. Others, however, believe that estrogen-dominant Pills are less likely than progestin-dominant Pills to decrease libido. If sexuality is adversely affected while a woman is using a progestin-dominant Pill, switching to one with a greater relative amount of estrogen may occasionally be helpful. But more often than not, another form of contraception or sexual counseling are probably better alternatives.

Can birth-control pills be responsible for causing depression?

Mood changes such as depression, lethargy, listlessness, anxiety, and pessimism have been observed in approximately 5 percent of oral contraceptive users. But, the subjective nature of our understanding of mental disturbances makes it impossible to determine whether the Pill is actually to blame. A survey of the literature shows as many studies in which women report either no change or improvement of mood while using the Pill as studies claiming that it causes depression. In a 1985 report from England, published in *The British Journal of Psychiatry,* Martin P. Vessey and his associates evaluated the incidence of psychiatric problems among almost 10,000 women on birth-control pills compared to 7,000 others using alternative methods of contraception. He found no differences between the two groups. All researchers agree, however, that women with a previous history of depression and psychiatric illness are more likely than others to see these problems intensified while using oral contraceptives. Some doctors therefore prefer alternative methods of contraception for a woman who has a history of depression or mental illness. Others will prescribe the Pill for one or two months to ascertain whether adverse mood changes will occur. While low-dose formulations are always preferred, there are no studies that conclusively prove that certain brands are better than others in averting depression.

In trying to explain why some women become depressed while using birth-control pills, scientists have theorized that the Pill causes a reduction of serotonin, a body chemical that affects mood. Tryptophan is a protein needed to produce serotonin, and its metabolism is in turn dependent upon the body's supply of vitamin B_6, pyridoxine. Theoretically, a Pill user who takes vitamin B_6 supplements can correct disturbed tryptophan and serotonin metabolism and prevent depression (see vitamins). This theory has never been subjected to large-scale objective scientific scrutiny.

How long does it take after starting on birth-control pills until I will be safe from pregnancy?

Contrary to the popular belief that the Pill must be taken for one or two months before it becomes effective, you will be safe after taking ten Pills from the first pack. To ensure against pregnancy, it is usually recommended that you take your first Pill no later than the seventh day after the start of the period. As previously mentioned, however (see page 56), doctors at the University of Manchester Medical School in England have found that birth-control pills are effective in preventing pregnancy even when the Pill-free phase between one pack and the next is extended to eleven days. Though these researchers found that follicle development of an egg was likely to begin with a greater number of Pill omission days, it ceased once the new Pill pack was started. But until further studies are available, I would not endorse this method.

Do birth-control pills interact with other drugs and medications taken at the same time?

There are several commonly used drugs that alter the body's metabolism of estrogen to such a degree that the effectiveness of an oral contraceptive may be diminished. When the Pill is taken concurrently with one of these drugs, extensive breakthrough bleeding is a good indication that contraceptive efficacy is less than optimal. The potential for an unwanted pregnancy, though unlikely, is then theoretically possible, especially when Pills with the lowest amounts of estrogen are used. Barbiturates, used as sleeping pills and anticonvulsants, are examples of drugs that accelerate estrogen metabolism, thus reducing its biological effectiveness. A small number of pregnancies have been reported among women using birth-control pills and barbiturates concurrently. Phenylbutazone (trade name Butazolidin), a medication often used in the treatment of arthritis, phlebitis, and traumatic joint injuries, may also reduce oral contraceptive efficacy. Phenacitin (APC) is an anti-inflammatory and analgesic agent that has also been cited as reducing oral contraceptive efficacy, though I know of no reports of accidental pregnancies associated with its use.

Miltown and Equanil, two popular brands of meprobamate, a drug used in the treatment of anxiety and nervous tension, may also exert this type of effect. Other psychiatric medications, known as tricyclics, similarly alter contraceptive metabolism: Elavil, Amitril, Norpramin, Sinequan, Aventyl, and Pomelor.

Phenytoin (trade name Dilantin), aminopyrine, primidone, and carbamazepine are medications used to treat epilepsy. All can increase the failure rate of oral contraceptives by altering estrogen metabolism. In a review of this subject published in the *Journal of the American Medical Association* in 1986, Dr. Richard H. Mattson and his associates at Yale University School of Medicine pointed out that women who experience a high incidence of breakthrough bleeding while using one of these anti-epileptic drugs were more likely than other Pill users to ovulate and to experience an accidental pregnancy. They recommended that the dose of the estrogen in the Pill be progressively increased until the bleeding stopped. They also suggested that an additional barrier method of contraception be used during any cycle in which breakthrough bleeding occurred.

Rifampin, an important drug in the treatment of tuberculosis, also appears capable of altering estrogen metabolism. To date there are several reports of women who have become pregnant while taking a combination of rifampin and oral contraceptives. It has also been demonstrated that ampicillin and tetracycline, probably the two most commonly prescribed antibiotics, diminish the excretion of estrogen in the urine.

There have been infrequent reports of pregnancy in women concurrently taking oral contraceptives and ampicillin. The widespread use of low-dose oral contraceptives may mean that women on such Pills who are taking ampicillin should be told to use alternative birth-control methods as long as they are on this antibiotic. Similarly, when prescribing tetracycline in the treatment of acne, physicians are obligated to discuss with their patients the possibility that this antibiotic might reduce the effectiveness of oral contraceptives. In 1981, British investigators reported thirty-six cases of oral contraceptive failure that were associated with the use of tetracycline and ampicillin. One pregnancy has been reported with oxacillin, a synthetic penicillin. Rifampin, tetracycline, ampicillin, and oxacillin are all believed to accelerate the metabolism of estrogen in the Pill, leaving too little estrogen in the bloodstream. The latest addition to the list of potentially troublesome drugs is the very popular antifungal agent griseofulvin (trade name Fulvicin, Grisactin). European doctors reporting in the *British Medical Journal* in 1984 noted two pregnancies among women using griseofulvin and birth-control pills concurrently. In addition, fifteen of the twenty women studied experienced breakthrough bleeding, believed to be the result of rapid breakdown and metabolism of the estrogen in the Pill.

In a very important report published in *The New England Journal of Medicine* in 1982, doctors at Tufts University School of Medicine and the New England Medical Center Hospital compared the effects of diazepam (trade name Valium) on long-term Pill users and nonusers. Diazepam remained in the bloodstream for longer and at significantly higher levels among women on the Pill, prompting the authors to caution women taking both diazepam and the Pill that they may risk an overdose of the diazepam if it were not lowered. Chlordiazepoxide (trade name Librium) is another very popular tranquilizer that, in an earlier study, was shown to have similarly prolonged activity among women on the Pill.

Acetaminophen (trade name Tylenol, Pamprin) is the most commonly used nonprescription pain medication in the United States. In a 1982 study reported in *Obstetrics and Gynecology,* Dr. Darrell R. Abernethy and his associates found that women on oral contraceptives metabolized acetaminophen more rapidly than women not using the Pill. Therefore, to obtain optimal pain relief, Pill users may require a more frequent dosage schedule of this medication, as well as of lorazepam, oxazepam, and morphine—prescription analgesics that are metabolized in the same way as acetaminophen.

How does the Pill affect alcohol and caffeine metabolism?

Whether or not the Pill affects alcohol metabolism is a controversial issue. Doctors at the Oklahoma Center for Alcohol reported that women using birth-control pills are more likely to feel the effects of a drink for a longer period of time than women who do not use birth-control pills. Blood alcohol levels of twenty-two women were measured following a stiff drink, and it was found that the eleven women who were not on the Pill had no alcohol in their blood after an average of four hours and fifteen minutes; the eleven women on the Pill took five hours and thirty minutes to eliminate all the alcohol in their blood. In contrast with this study is a 1985 report from Australia in which doctors found that women using oral contraceptives showed a better tolerance for alcohol than did women not on the Pill, while blood levels, metabolism, and elimination of the alcohol from the body were equal in both groups.

Coffee drinkers should take note of a study conducted at the Vanderbilt University Medical Center and the Veterans Administration Medical Center in Nashville, Tennessee in which women on the Pill were found to retain caffeine for longer periods of time and to accumulate higher levels of caffeine than women not on the Pill. If you are on the Pill, your morning cup of coffee may keep you going for longer than women not on the Pill.

Can vomiting or diarrhea prevent the Pill from working effectively?

If you vomit within thirty minutes after taking a birth-control pill, take another pill, since there is a good chance that not all the hormones have been absorbed into the body. Vomiting that occurs later than that does not require another pill because the formulation will have been absorbed and metabolized at that point. If vomiting is prolonged during any Pill cycle, it is probably best to use alternative contraception.

In instances of severe diarrhea, the intestinal tract will not adequately absorb the full hormonal content of the Pill. This may happen in a perfectly healthy woman who has an attack of stomach flu, traveler's diarrhea, or food poisoning while using the Pill. In one report, eight healthy women using oral contraceptives for periods ranging from two to thirty-six months became pregnant after experiencing diarrhea lasting from one to five days. In all the cases, symptoms were present between days 3 and 16 of the cycle, and no Pills had been missed. Therefore, if you have an attack of severe diarrhea during the Pill cycle, use a different method of contraception until after your next period, when a new cycle of pills can be started.

Even when the lowest pill formulations are used, a small number of sensitive individuals will still not be able to use the Pill because it makes them ill. Others with chronic intestinal disorders and prolonged diarrhea will be poor candidates for the Pill. Though other methods of contraception are usually recommended for these women, two recent studies suggest that daily intravaginal insertion of the Pill may provide contraception without unpleasant side effects. In the first study, published in *Fertility and Sterility* in 1982, doctors instructed women to insert either one or two birth-control pills vaginally for twenty-one days followed by a week without pills. Of the twelve women studied, no pregnancies occurred and it was clearly demonstrated that the hormones in the Pill were effectively absorbed through the vaginal wall and into the bloodstream. Those women given one Pill daily were more likely to experience breakthrough bleeding, though all of the women experienced a normal menstrual flow during the week that the Pill was not being taken. In the second study, published in the *British Journal of Sexual Medicine,* doctors instructed ten women to insert one Pill vaginally in the same cyclic fashion. In all ten cases, there were no reported nausea, vomiting, or, most important, pregnancies. While this simple solution to the problem sounds harmless and effective, more research on greater numbers of women will be required before this method of using the Pill can be endorsed.

What is the effect of birth-control pills on women suffering from intestinal ailments such as colitis, ulcers, and appendicitis?

Oral contraceptives do not appear to have a detrimental effect on the overwhelming majority of women with these intestinal conditions. In one early study, the Pill was actually found to decrease a woman's incidence of duodenal ulcers. Rare cases of occlusion of blood vessels in the intestinal wall have been reported, attributed to the ability of estrogen to increase the concentration of clotting factors in the blood (see estrogen and coagulation factors, page 37). The use of low-dose formulations would appear virtually to eradicate this complication.

In a 1984 study, doctors in Birmingham, England, reported in the *British Medical Journal* that oral contraceptives may predispose some susceptible women to colitis or inflammatory disease of the large intestine. Discontinuing the Pill improved symptoms in four of eight women studied who had the disease.

In another 1984 study, from Sweden, doctors compared the incidence and severity of appendicitis among Pill users and nonusers. Women not using oral contraceptives had a frequency of acute appendicitis that was twice as high during the second half of the menstrual cycle. Those on the Pill showed an incidence of appendicitis that was equally distributed throughout the month. One interesting and unexplained finding was that a significantly higher proportion of gangrenous and perforated appendices occurred in women using the Pill.

Can the Pill be used as a postcoital contraceptive?

A variety of estrogen compounds have been used as postcoital, or "morning-after," pills following unprotected intercourse at midcycle (see chapter 6). The combination of 0.050 milligrams of ethinyl estradiol and 0.5 milligrams of norgestrel, the components of Ovral, has been demonstrated to be a highly effective postcoital contraceptive. In a recent study, 608 women received two Ovral tablets within seventy-two hours of unprotected intercourse, followed by two tablets twelve hours later. The pregnancy rate was a remarkably low 0.16 percent. With this amount of estrogen and progestin ingested, it is not surprising that nausea and vomiting were the most frequent side effects observed. Use of birth-control pills in such high doses, while invaluable in emergencies, should never be made routinely by individuals who might be merely too forgetful to take the Pill in the prescribed manner.

Are headaches related to use of the Pill?

Headaches are occasionally a complication of oral contraceptive use and seem to occur more frequently during the week that the Pill is not being taken. Most investigators believe that it is the estrogen component of the Pill that is most responsible for these headaches. Headaches fall into either of two main categories: tension or migraine. It is vital that you and your doctor evaluate any Pill-related headache, since tension headaches are of little medical concern while migraine can have serious consequences.

Tension headaches are also called muscle contraction headaches because they are caused by the tightening of the muscles around the neck and the skull. They begin gradually and usually last one to four hours, often ending abruptly. Most sufferers of tension headaches describe the pain as a continuing ache or sensation of pressure that feels like a vise around the head. The pain sometimes moves down to the shoulders and the back and is often precipitated by anger, anxiety, depression, apprehension, or stress. The sudden drop in hormone levels during the week off the Pill seems to precipitate this type of headache for certain susceptible women.

For the more general type of tension headache that occurs during the withdrawal phase of each Pill cycle, some doctors recommend a daily progestin-only Minipill (see page 31). But the higher incidence of breakthrough bleeding and accidental pregnancy makes this a poor option for most women. More popular is a "tri-cycle" regimen of Pill use, in which a woman takes a low-dose combination pill every day without interruption until four packets are completed. A one-week break is taken every three months, during which time she menstruates. On the tri-cycle regimen, menstrual headache sufferers will have only four periods—and thus only four headaches—a year, instead of thirteen. Though these women will be taking sixteen rather than thirteen packs of pills each year, the increase in total hormonal dose does not appear to be harmful.

On rare occasions headaches may represent a symptom of a more serious condition, such as hypertension (see page 39) or an impending stroke (see page 36). Headaches that are severe, that occur frequently, and that begin or intensify after using the Pill require immediate attention and thorough evaluation by a physician, preferably a neurologist. If the cause of the headaches remains in doubt, it is best to discontinue the Pill permanently.

Should women who get migraine headaches use oral contraceptives?

Migraine is a special type of severe recurrent headache that, for some reason, appears to be more common in women than in men. It is considered a type of vascular headache because it involves the blood vessels of the scalp and brain. Many migraine sufferers experience early warning symptoms that precede the onset of the headache. This so-called aura is often characterized by exhaustion, irritability, loss of appetite, extreme sensitivity to light and sound, visual disturbances such as blind spots and double vision, numbness of the face, and weakness or even paralysis on one side of the body that may strongly resemble symptoms of a stroke. Some of these symptoms disappear with the onset of the headache, which may take the form of a throbbing sensation over one eye or be generalized over the entire head. Headaches may last anywhere from a few hours to four days and are almost always accompanied by nausea, vomiting, and intolerance to light. Migraine headaches among Pill users seem to occur most often during the week that the Pill is not taken.

Though the cause of migraines remains unknown, it is theorized that the symptoms associated with the aura are due to a disturbance in the circulation and blood flow within the smaller blood vessels of the brain. The headache is believed to be produced by a dilatation, or expansion, of the blood vessels outside the brain which causes pressure on surrounding nerves. Relief is often obtained with a popular drug called ergotomine which constricts the muscles in these dilated blood vessels, thereby reducing the diameter of the vessels and easing the pressure on the surrounding nerves. It is only in recent years that doctors have become aware that migraine may be a potentially dangerous condition. Ample evidence is now available to show that some migraine patients have a temporary decrease in blood flow to the brain as severe as that of a patient suffering from a stroke. Furthermore, permanent neurological damage following a migraine has been reported on rare occasions.

Since oral contraceptives may alter blood coagulation factors and produce circulatory changes, they are best avoided in individuals with a history of migraine headache. In one study, 50 percent of migraine sufferers found that their attacks worsened when they were on the Pill; 40 percent found that they were not affected; and 10 percent reported their migraine improved. Factors likely to characterize women whose migraine became worse while they were on the Pill were an age of thirty and higher, previous childbirth, a menstrual cycle longer than thirty-three days or shorter than twenty-seven days, and a tendency to experience headaches at the time of menstruation. There are also scattered reports of women with no previous history of migraine who developed it while on the Pill. Seventy percent of this group found that the frequency and intensity of their headaches improved significantly after they stopped using the Pill. While some doctors have noted less harmful effects with the Minipill, most women with migraines will fare better by using alternative methods of contraception.

Medically speaking, migraine is considered to be a "relative" rather than an "absolute" contraindication to use of birth-control pills. This means that doctors may cautiously prescribe the Pill under very specific circumstances, provided that the patient is fully aware of all potential complications and is monitored closely to be sure that there is no worsening of the intensity or frequency of the headaches. A relative contraindication becomes an absolute one—meaning that the Pill is forbidden and must be stopped immediately—when the migraine is severe enough to require ergotomine for pain relief or when the frequency of attacks increases. Other absolute contraindications include focal or isolated neurologic signs such as temporarily diminished vision in one eye, weakness of one arm or leg, speech difficulty at the time of the aura, and a "crescendo" migraine, one that becomes progressively worse over a couple of days.

Is the Pill effective in treating young women who experience menstrual cramps?

Primary dysmenorrhea is defined as pelvic pain occurring immediately prior to, or with the onset of, the period in a woman without any apparent gynecological disease. It is the most common gynecological disorder of teenagers and women in their early twenties, accounting for millions of hours lost from school and work each year. Primary dysmenorrhea occurs only in women who ovulate and it mysteriously disappears following childbirth.

While sufferers of primary dysmenorrhea appear perfectly normal on gynecological examination, it has been demonstrated that they experience uterine contractions during their periods that are of far greater intensity and duration than those of individuals who do not suffer from dysmenorrhea. In addition, the pain of their contractions is intensified because of a reduction in blood flow and oxygen to their uterine muscles.

Though psychiatrists have been telling us for years that severe dysmenorrhea represents a manifestation of deeper emotional disturbances, there is now unequivocal proof that women who suffer from it produce significantly greater amounts of prostaglandins in their menstrual fluid than do women with painless periods. Prostaglandins are chemical substances that can cause intense uterine contractions as well as headache, nausea, vomiting, and diarrhea if they enter the general circulation (see chapter 7). In one study, women with primary dysmenorrhea had prostaglandin levels that were seven times greater than those in other women. It is theorized that the thick, secretory endometrium, caused by the release of progesterone following ovulation, accumulates large amounts of prostaglandins in certain susceptible women (see chapter 1). With the onset of the period, this thick endometrium breaks down and a flood of prostaglandins is released.

Once scientists understood the mechanism behind primary dysmenorrhea, it was easy to eliminate the pain by developing medications that prevented the body from synthesizing prostaglandins. If taken just prior to, or at the onset of, the period, these so-called antiprostaglandins have proved to be godsends to 90 percent of women who suffer from primary dysmenorrhea. Drugs such as ibuprofen (Motrin, Advil, Nuprin), naproxen sodium (Anaprox, Naprosyn), suprofen (Suprol), and mefenamic acid (Ponstel) have become welcome and familiar additions to medicine cabinets throughout the world. Though not nearly as effective, aspirin is the oldest of the antiprostaglandins.

Combination birth-control pills are as effective as antiprostaglandins in relieving the symptoms of primary dysmenorrhea, because they prevent ovulation and suppress the formation of a thick, prostaglandin-filled secretory endometrium. Researchers have demonstrated that menstrual-fluid prostaglandin levels in Pill users are lower than those found in women with painless periods who are not on the Pill. Use of the Pill for a period of three to four months helps tremendously in breaking the miserable cycle of pain, and after the Pill is stopped, periods occasionally are permanently improved. More often than not, however, the pain will recur, necessitating restarting of the Pill for longer periods of time.

Some antiprostaglandins and oral contraceptives work equally well in relieving primary dysmenorrhea. The choice of one medication over the other will depend on a variety of factors, such as whether contraception as well as pain relief is desired and whether there is a medical reason for choosing one method over the other. For example, a history of a severe allergy to aspirin, previous gastrointestinal bleeding, or a diagnosis of a duodenal or gastric ulcer would preclude the use of an antiprostaglandin. The Pill, on the other hand, has been noted in one large study to decrease the incidence of ulcer disease. Regardless of which method is used, if pain relief is not achieved, the other medication should be added to the first (provided there are no medical reasons to withhold it). If menstruation still remains painful, you and your doctor should suspect secondary dysmenorrhea—pain caused by a gynecological disease such as PID (see page 49) or endometriosis.

What is endometriosis and how effective are birth-control pills in treating it?

Endometriosis is a fairly common, often painful, mysterious condition of young menstruating women caused by the presence of pieces of endometrium in areas other than its normal location within the uterus. The disease is most often diagnosed in women in their late twenties and thirties and is known as "the career woman's disease" because it occurs among those who delay childbearing to pursue other goals. Endometriosis is unlikely to occur in women who give birth to their first child before the age of twenty. But prior to the advent of newer diagnostic technology, it was believed that it was an unheard-of phenomenon in teenagers. We now know that this is untrue.

It is not known why certain individuals are susceptible to endometriosis and others aren't. Nor do we understand the method by which fragments of endometrium spread to other areas within the pelvis. The most popular theory is that of "retrograde menstruation," meaning that they are passed backward from the endometrial cavity into the fallopian tubes, and then out through the fimbriae (see chapter 1) into the abdomen at the time of menstruation. There, the endometrial tissue continues to function and respond to hormones as does normal endometrium. Unfortunately, when menstruation takes place, the blood passes into the pelvic organs that are involved, instead of out of the body.

Over a period of months and years, large cysts filled with old, dark blood and called "chocolate cysts" may form. The bursting of these cysts often requires emergency surgery. Scar tissue develops throughout the entire pelvis as the disease process continues. The ovary is most commonly involved, though other pelvic structures such as the ligaments supporting the uterus, the intestinal lining, and the urinary bladder may also become diseased. It is not uncommon for the back of the uterus to become firmly attached to the wall of the bowel, thereby assuming a retroflexed, or backward, tilt from which it can't be moved except through surgery. Infertility is very common in women suffering from endometriosis. Sometimes this is due to scarring around the tubes which prevents their normal movement and functioning. It is not unusual to encounter infertility associated with minimal amounts of endometriosis not involving the tubes or ovaries. In such cases, it is theorized that the endometriosis releases greater than normal amounts of prostaglandins (see prostaglandins, page 71) which adversely alter tubal and uterine transport of the egg.

Another enigma of the disease is that the symptoms are not often related to the amount of endometriosis that is present. I have seen patients in my own practice with chocolate cysts filling the entire pelvis, diagnosed only because they came in for a routine checkup. Others with severe pain have been noted to have only one or two tiny fragments of endometriosis in the pelvis. Again, the amount of pain may be related to abnormal prostaglandin synthesis in some fragments of endometriosis and not in others. The most common symptoms of endometriosis are severe dysmenorrhea (painful periods), lower abdominal soreness, and low back pain that persists throughout the month. Pain with intercourse is also very common.

Pregnancy appears to have a beneficial effect on most women suffering from endometriosis. Those who previously had severe pelvic pain often experience nine blissful months. This is believed to be a reaction created in the endometriosis sites by the high progesterone levels of pregnancy. Endometriosis fragments actually change in appearance and become smaller. Since no menstrual bleeding takes place during the nine months of pregnancy, no further bleeding is noted in the pelvis.

Dr. Robert Kistner suggested more than twenty years ago that progesterone given intramuscularly, or progestogens as birth-control pills, could create what he termed a "pseudopregnancy" in sufferers of endometriosis. By giving four Enovid tablets per day for at least nine months without stopping to allow a period, he claimed that 85 percent of his patients noted significant relief of symptoms. Subsequent reports by other doctors have not been nearly as optimistic. In a young woman with painful but minimal amounts of endometriosis, pseudopregnancy can be tried. Today's pseudopregnancy treatment consists of taking one tablet of a progestin-dominant birth-control pill every day for at least nine months. Enovid is no longer used to create pseudopregnancy because such high doses of this estrogen-dominant Pill could produce extremely serious complications. Though proof is lacking, many gynecologists believe that a low-dose birth-control pill taken in the usual cyclic manner will provide protection against the development and spread of endometriosis and the pain associated with it. The Pills create a much thinner endometrial lining and therefore less reflux of endometrial fragments and prostaglandins into the pelvis from the endometrial cavity.

In recent years, danazol (trade name Danocrine) has superseded the Pill as the primary hormonal method of treating endometriosis. Similar in chemical structure to the progestins in birth-control pills, danazol alters the abnormally located endometrial tissue so that it shrinks in size and becomes inactive. Significant relief from pain and rise in fertility rates often follow three to nine months of danazol therapy. For most women, these benefits are only short-lived, and symptoms recur months after the danazol is discontinued, but some fortunate individuals will experience permanent relief of symptoms. Research on the use of danazol as a contraceptive has also been conducted (see chapter 11, "The Future").

Most authorities agree that surgery is the one and only method of treating extensive endometriosis. When infertility is a problem, surgical removal of as much endometriosis as possible will allow a far greater chance of conception. Unfortunately, the only permanent cure for the pain and discomfort associated with the disease is hysterectomy, with removal of the ovaries if they are extensively affected. The chances of remaining endometriosis fragments growing again are enhanced if the ovaries are not removed. Rarely, after the ovaries have been removed, will the disease still flare up if replacement estrogen is given as a means of preventing menopausal symptoms created by removing the ovaries.

How would I know if I had dysmenorrhea due to a small amount of endometriosis or dysmenorrhea of unknown cause?

Often it is difficult, if not impossible, for your doctor to make this distinction. Certain clues in your history, such as pain throughout the month, are more likely to indicate endometriosis. If both birth-control pills and antiprostaglandin medication have failed to bring relief of symptoms, one's suspicions should be heightened. On a pelvic exam, it is sometimes possible for your doctor to feel the scarring and nodules of endometriosis in the ligaments supporting the uterus. An adherent, retroflexed, or backward, uterus also often suggests the condition. If birth-control pills are taken in the usual manner with one week of rest to allow menses, women with endometriosis may be more likely to experience pain at the time of bleeding than those with dysmenorrhea that is not caused by endometriosis. If your doctor is in doubt, viewing the pelvis with a laparoscope (see chapter 9) will clearly demonstrate the characteristic bluish or brown deposits of endometriosis on the ovary or other pelvic structures.

Is it true that some women experience loss of scalp hair after the birth-control pill is stopped?

Hair follicles go through various phases of growth in all individuals. Usually, 85 percent of scalp hairs are in an active growing phase, termed the *anagen* phase, and 15 percent are in the resting, or *telogen,* phase. Hair loss takes place during the telogen phase. For unknown hormonal reasons, some women note an alarming increase in scalp hair loss for two to three months following pregnancy or a discontinuation of birth-control pills. Microscopic study of hair follicles at this time indicates that 50 percent are in the telogen phase. The extra 35 percent of telogen phase hairs represents a total of millions of hairs lost during this time. This sometimes frightening condition corrects itself within three to six months, with 85 percent of the hairs returning to the anagen phase. Improvement might not be observed immediately, since it takes approximately one year for a strand of hair to achieve a noticeable length.

Are users of birth-control pills more susceptible than nonusers to infections?

Certain bacterial and viral infectious diseases have been found to be significantly more common among women using oral contraceptives: laryngitis, tracheitis (inflammation of the trachea, or windpipe), chronic nasopharyngitis (inflammation of the nose and throat), influenza, bronchitis (inflammation of the respiratory tubes into which the trachea divides), pleurisy (inflammation of the membrane surrounding the lung), and ulcers of the mouth.

In trying to find a scientific explanation for this higher rate of infection, researchers in California have studied levels of certain blood proteins called gamma globulins. These substances, because they provide immunity against infections and diseases, belong to a group of proteins known as immunoglobulins. Oral contraceptive users were found to have significantly lower levels of gamma globulins than nonusers. Furthermore, as the dose of estrogen in the Pill was increased, the gamma globulin concentration decreased even further. As a result, it was theorized that the decrease of gamma globulin may play a role in the increased prevalence of viral infections among Pill users. Further investigation will be needed to confirm or deny this relationship.

In a study presented at the Interscience Conference on Antimicrobial Agents and Chemotherapeutics in Chicago in 1981, researchers demonstrated that oral contraceptives may offer some protection against recurrence of one type of virus—the genital herpes simplex, or HSV-II, known to be sexually transmitted and responsible for causing painful blisters of the outer genitals which tend to recur over a period of months or even years. It was noted that the recurrence rate for HSV-II among women not using oral contraceptives was 1.6 times that of those using the Pill, with one recurrence every fifty-one days as opposed to a recurrence every eighty-one days among Pill users.

How do oral contraceptives alter the white-blood-cell count?

The white-blood-cell count (WBC) is one of the most commonly ordered tests in clinical medicine. An elevation of this count is often essential to your doctor's ability to diagnose common surgical and medical diseases, such as acute appendicitis. The normal range of a WBC count is usually between 4,000 and 10,000. In both pregnant women and women using the Pill, however, the count is often higher than 10,000. The degree of elevation appears to be related to the amount of estrogen in the Pill and the length of time that a woman has been using the Pill. The Pill user who is both obese and a heavy smoker may show a white-blood-cell count of over 14,000. (Reminding your surgeon of such facts may often save a normal appendix from extinction.)

Do oral contraceptives affect the urinary tract?

The ureters are two tubes that carry urine from the kidney to the urinary bladder. While several studies have demonstrated a dilatation, or widening, of the ureter in a small percentage of women using the older oral contraceptive formulations, this has not been noted with the newer low-dose Pills.

Conflicting results have been reported concerning the possible role of oral contraceptives in increasing bacterial growth in a woman's urine. While two studies found an association, two others did not. Most authorities consider the influence of oral contraceptives on the urinary tract to be minimal at best and possibly even nonexistent. Fear of urinary tract infections should certainly not deter a woman from using birth-control pills. This advice would apply even to those with a history of urinary tract infections. Diaphragm users are far more susceptible than Pill users to urinary tract infections (see chapter 4).

How soon after an abortion or childbirth should the Pill be started?

As illustrated in chapter 5, most women regain their fertility within a short time following a spontaneous or an induced abortion. When the terminated pregnancy is between eight and fifteen weeks, the average return of ovulation takes two to three weeks. If the pregnancy is between the sixteenth and twentieth week, ovulation will usually return four to six weeks later. For this reason one must conclude that birth-control pills should be instituted immediately following an abortion so that intercourse can be resumed after the required two-week period of abstinence without fear of pregnancy.

Most modern obstetricians allow their patients to resume intercourse three weeks postpartum. Statistically, 15 percent of non-nursing women will be ovulating by the sixth postpartum week, therefore pregnancy is more than a theoretical possibility if the Pill is not started by the third postpartum week. It is thus important that your doctor prescribe the Pill before you leave the hospital. Another good idea is for doctors to abandon the traditional six-week postpartum visit in favor of one at three or four weeks. Early and effective contraception could then be discussed and prescribed before ovulation becomes a concern.

Nursing women have less than a 5 percent chance of ovulating by their six-week postpartum visit. It has been demonstrated that women who nurse their babies at least every four hours, with no supplemental feedings, do not ovulate before the tenth postpartum week. Once supplementation is introduced, ovulation can occur at any time. Until recently, it was considered inappropriate to prescribe a combination oral contraceptive to nursing women because of its supposed capacity to decrease milk quantity and fat concentration. Another fear was that the estrogen in birth-control pills would pass to the baby via the milk. Recent studies with the new low-dose formulations, however, have shown that milk supply is not reduced if the Pills are started in the fourth to fifth postpartum week after nursing is well established. In addition, the weight gain of babies whose mothers use the Pill equals that of babies whose mothers employ other methods of contraception. The dosage of estrogen that reaches the infant through breast-feeding is less than 1 percent, not in excess of the natural estrogen levels received normally by nursing infants. Finally, researchers have noted no long-term adverse effects on the growth and development of children whose mothers use an estrogen-containing low-dose oral contraceptive. This positive information has prompted the Academy of Pediatrics to go on record as endorsing the use of low-dose oral contraceptives by women who have nursed successfully for the first six postpartum weeks. Despite these favorable reports, I am convinced that the majority of obstetricians in the United States will not prescribe the Pill to their patients who are nursing, preferring to await the results of larger and more convincing studies. The Minipill, a progestin-only formulation, has been more widely accepted than the combination Pill as a contraceptive for nursing women. While some research has shown that the quantity and quality of breast milk is not altered by the Minipill, other studies have shown the opposite. Based on all available data, I believe that the Minipill is a safe contraceptive option for the nursing woman.

Is there a law prohibiting doctors from prescribing contraception to sexually active teenagers without parental consent?

I hope you don't live in Utah, because it is the only state requiring written parental consent for contraceptive services to minors. In most states, the age at which an adolescent can receive prescription contraceptives without parental consent is the so-called age of majority, usually eighteen. Several states have a younger age of consent, whereas others, such as New York and California, have liberal statutes requiring that contraceptive services be provided to all persons in need of them, regardless of age or parental consent.

Several state laws have immunity provisions designated to protect physicians who provide contraception to minors. In these states, doctors can't be sued for caring for an adolescent patient without parental consent if he or she acted in good faith. To date, no physician in the United States has ever been successfully prosecuted for providing contraception to a minor without parental consent. The American Medical Association, the American Academy of Pediatrics, and the American College of Obstetricians and Gynecologists have all publicly supported the position that sexually active teenagers should be provided with contraception. In addition, the American College of Obstetricians and Gynecologists has stated that the confidentiality of the teenager in such matters must be respected and given precedence over the demands of angered and inquisitive parents attempting to breach it.

Studies have indicated that one of the major causes of delay by adolescents seeking contraception is fear of betrayal by the health care provider. Fortunately, the courts have repeatedly struck down as unconstitutional efforts by the Reagan administration to require minors at federally funded family planning clinics to secure parental approval before receiving contraception.

My advice to teenagers who fear that they will be reported to their parents is to call the doctor's office (use an alias if necessary) to determine his or her attitude about contraception. If the doctor appears hostile, uncooperative, or morally outraged, find a more sympathetic doctor or consult a local family planning clinic.

The incidence of teenage pregnancy is higher in the United States than in any other developed country. Today four out of every ten adolescent women are sexually active by the age of seventeen, and 14 percent of births in the United States are to teenage mothers. More shocking is the fact that half of all teenagers fail to use contraception during first intercourse. In light of these statistics, it is difficult to imagine any health care provider not enthusiastically supporting confidential contraceptive counseling to those most in need of it.

Aren't there new contraceptive methods on the horizon that are safer and equally as effective as the Pill?

Despite claims to the contrary, it is unlikely that any new method of contraception will be available for American men or women in the next five years that is equal in safety and efficacy to the birth-control pill. While everyone seems to be waiting for the perfect contraceptive suddenly to appear, the fact is that this is just not going to happen. It takes many years, extensive testing, and millions of dollars to bring a new contraceptive out on the market. Too often, the new contraceptive is merely a variation of an old, less-than-perfect method. In response to a 1986 article in *Family Planning Perspectives,* in which new and supposedly future methods of the "contraceptive revolution" were discussed, Dr. Carl Djerassi, one of the discoverers of the birth-control pill, chided the authors for "promising the public what we cannot possibly deliver." In his letter he warned of making impossible claims "or listing piddling variations of existing methods as 'new products.' "

As noted earlier, the hazards of the Pill have been grossly exaggerated. Sadly, negative misinformation continues to frighten women away from the Pill, evidenced by the 40 percent decline in Pill use over the past ten years. As a result, women are using less effective methods—or no method at all—and this is keeping the abortion rates in the United States at unacceptably high levels. The grim statistics speak for themselves: Of the 6 million pregnancies that occur in the United States each year, 3 million are unplanned and half of these end in abortion. Though there are innumerable reasons for this state of affairs, surveys clearly show that fear of complications is the most powerful deterrent to a woman's use of oral contraceptives. Sensational press coverage of each purported Pill side effect has historically been followed by an immediate and irreversible sharp decline in Pill use nationwide. The bare fact is that for the overwhelming majority of women under the age of thirty-five, oral contraceptives remain the safest and most effective means of preventing an unwanted pregnancy. There is no imminent contraceptive breakthrough to make us believe otherwise.

After a woman stops using the Pill, are there any lingering risks that may show up later in life?

Data from two large studies suggest that women who use the older and stronger oral contraceptive formulations may be at a higher risk of heart attack and stroke as late as ten years after they stop using them. In a 1981 article published in *The New England Journal of Medicine,* Denis Slone, M.D., and his associates at the Drug Epidemiology Unit of the Boston University School of Medicine interviewed 556 women between the ages of twenty-five and forty-nine with a proven diagnosis of myocardial infarction (heart attack). Compared to a control group of healthy women, those with myocardial infarction were far more likely to have used the Pill in the past. The women most at risk had used the Pill for at least five years; those who used it less than five years were at no greater risk than nonusers. In addition, the increased risk of heart attack among former Pill users was concentrated among obese heavy smokers and those who used the Pill in their thirties. The atherosclerotic changes in blood vessels caused by the high progestin dose in the old formulations is believed to be most responsible for causing them to narrow and eventually predispose to heart attack later in life.

Estrogen-induced changes in blood coagulation factors and hypertension caused by the progestogen in the Pill appear to be totally reversible as soon as it is discontinued.

3

IUDs

An intrauterine device, or IUD, is a device inserted into the uterine cavity and left there for varying periods of time for the purpose of contraception. Throughout the years, IUDs made of myriad materials and in a variety of sizes and shapes have been designed, manufactured, and used with differing degrees of success. All modern IUDs are made of polyethylene plastic and are coated in barium, making it possible for them to be seen on X ray. Most IUDs have a nylon "tail" which protrudes from the cervix into the vagina. While the merits and disadvantages of IUDs continue to be argued, the search for the ideal IUD remains an elusive goal of scientists.

Can you discuss the history of the IUD and its status as a contraceptive today?

According to one legend, the first IUDs were used by Arab camel drivers, who inserted stones into the endometrial cavities of their camels in order to prevent pregnancy on long desert crossings. The first twentieth-century IUD to be used by a woman was made of silkworm gut in the shape of a ring; it was introduced in Germany in 1909 by a doctor named Richter. In the 1920s and 1930s, rings of gut, silver, and gold were used in Germany, China, and Japan. They were soon discredited because of the high incidence of uterine infection associated with their use.

IUDs resurfaced in the early 1960s and peaked in popularity in the United States in the mid-1970s. It would appear that any gynecologist seeking immortality at that time was designing an IUD and naming it after himself: Margulies Spiral, Grafenberg Ring, Birnberg Bow, Majzlin Spring, Lippes Loop, Tatum-T—even the name of the infamous Dalkon Shield is derived from parts of the surnames of its discoverers. The more modest doctors in the East gave their IUDs exotic names such as Silent Protector, in Indonesia, and the Flower of Canton, in China. Over the past twenty-five years at least thirty-five IUDs of various sizes and shapes have been tested worldwide.

The optimism surrounding the use of IUDs ended abruptly in 1974 when the A. H. Robins Company, maker of the Dalkon Shield, revealed that its device was associated with a high incidence of pelvic infections as well as several deaths. Since then 14,000 lawsuits by ex–Dalkon users have led to worldwide condemnation of the device and a declaration of bankruptcy by its manufacturer in 1985. Lawsuits against other IUD manufacturers followed, and in September 1985 the Ortho Pharmaceutical Corporation discontinued the sale of its Lippes Loop, terming production "no longer economically feasible." The final blow came in January 1986 when G. D. Searle removed its widely used Copper-7 and Tatum-T from the American marketplace because of "unwarranted product litigation" and difficulties encountered in obtaining product liability insurance. Though both IUDs currently remain FDA-approved as safe and effective products, Searle has spent over $1.5 million successfully defending claims against these devices.

At the writing of this book, the Progestasert, manufactured by Alza Corporation, is the only IUD currently available in the United States. For a variety of reasons, this device has never gained great popularity here, accounting for only 1 to 3 percent of the IUD market while other devices were available. Epidemiologists forecast that the number of IUD users in the United States, estimated at 2.3 million in 1985, will decrease drastically over the next five years. The only women who will encounter no hardships from the absence of these devices in the United States are those who can make a trip to Canada or to a hundred other countries throughout the world where the Copper-7 and Tatum-T are still available. This so-called Canadian Connection has kept doctors across the border overwhelmed with requests by American visitors for the Copper-7 and Tatum-T. The majority of women in this country, however, now find themselves severely limited if their choice of contraception is an IUD. In addition, many vital questions remain about the safety of the IUDs they may presently have. Figure 3-1 shows some of the more famous (and infamous) IUDs.

Which is safer, the Pill or the IUD?

When epidemiologists calculate mortality (death) rates associated with any form of contraception, they include deaths attributed directly to the method itself as well as those that occur as a complication of an accidental pregnancy due to failure of the contraceptive. The following table shows that mortality rates associated with both the Pill and the IUD are very low.

Clearly, the death rates associated with IUD use do not vary greatly as a woman ages, and they compare favorably with those of a nonsmoker on the Pill who is younger than thirty-five. After that age, the risk of dying becomes much greater if you use the Pill rather than the IUD. Smoking only compounds this risk and subjects women in their twenties to higher death rates (see smoking and the Pill, chapter 2).

Figure 3–1. *Various types of IUDs.*

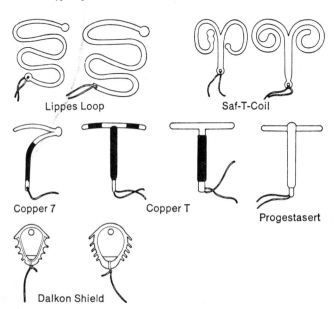

Lippes Loop

Saf-T-Coil

Copper 7

Copper T

Progestasert

Dalkon Shield

DEATHS ASSOCIATED WITH IUD AND PILL USE PER 100,000 WOMEN

METHOD	AGE					
	15–19	*20–24*	*25–29*	*30–34*	*35–39*	*40–44*
Pill/Nonsmoker	0.5	0.7	1.1	2.1	14.1	32
Pill/Smoker	2.4	3.6	6.8	13.7	51.4	117.6
IUD	1.3	1.1	1.3	1.3	1.9	2.1

SOURCE: *Compiled by the author.*

While mortality rates for IUD users compare favorably to those for women on the Pill, the same cannot be said of nonfatal complications and hospitalization rates. Several large studies have shown that the hospitalization rate for women using IUDs ranges between 3 and 7 of every 1,000 women per year, compared with only 1 per 1,000 for women on the Pill. In actual numbers, this translates to almost 10,000 hospitalizations annually among the more than 2 million IUD users in the United States, more than 90 percent of which are the result of fallopian tube infections and pelvic inflammatory disease (PID; see chapter 2). These serious infections are often associated with chronic pelvic pain, fever, and infertility resulting from tubal damage and scarring. In contrast, several studies have shown that the risk of PID is considerably lower for women using oral contraceptives than for IUD users. It is theorized that the progestin in the Pill alters the cervical mucus and makes it relatively impermeable to the ascent of PID-producing bacteria from the vagina and the cervix. IUD users who are most susceptible to the tragic consequences of PID, tubal damage, and infertility are those who are less than twenty-five, have never borne a full-term pregnancy, and have more than one sexual partner. Women fitting this profile have a PID risk of an astonishing 17 per 1,000. In contrast, IUD users more than thirty years old with one or more children and only one sexual partner have a PID risk of approximately 1 per 1,000. If one compares Pill and IUD complications with respect to a woman's age, it is interesting to note that the Pill favors the young and the restless while the IUD benefits older women who have children and who are less likely to change sexual partners. In 1985, two highly publicized, extensive studies emphatically confirmed these findings and reaffirmed the conclusions of past studies showing that the risk of PID, tubal damage, and infertility is greatly influenced by the type of IUD a woman uses.

In a 1984 report, published in the *Journal of the American Medical Association,* doctors at the University of Lund in Sweden looked through the laparoscope at the tubes of 546 women experiencing their first episodes of fallopian tube infection. They graded the infections as mild, moderate, or severe and found that Pill users had a significantly higher percentage of mild infections while IUD users were far more likely to experience severe infections.

Perforation of the uterus with an IUD is a serious complication of its use. It is estimated to occur in 40 out of every 100,000 IUD insertions (see IUD perforation) and is responsible for the hospitalization of almost 900 women each year in the United States.

Another serious IUD complication is septic, or infected, second-trimester spontaneous abortion, which may occur if a woman inadvertently becomes pregnant with the IUD in place. It is estimated that approximately 10 per 100,000 women with IUDs will be hospitalized annually with this complication and that 1 percent of these women will die from the infection. Figure 3-2 demonstrates these IUD hospitalization rates.

What is the purpose of an IUD's tail?

When you touch the tail or strings, or view them with a speculum as they protrude through the cervical os, you are assured that the IUD is in place. When it is inserted, a note should be made of the length of the tail, because an increase or decrease of the length on future examinations may mean that the IUD is not in its proper position. The strings also serve as a means by which the IUD can easily be removed.

Do the IUD tails differ from one device to another?

Unfortunately, many women are not told what type of IUD they have had inserted. This problem can easily be solved by doing a self-examination with a mirror, since the tail of each device has a characteristic appearance. Any knowledgeable doctor or family planning clinic should be able to examine you and answer this very important question. Descriptions of the appearance of the various IUD strings are listed in the following table.

How is an IUD inserted?

Prior to insertion of an IUD, a woman's cervix is grasped with an instrument called a *tenaculum.* Traction on the tenaculum holds the uterus in place and straightens the endometrial cavity to enable easier insertion of the device. A thin measuring rod, called a *sound,* is then placed through the cervix until it touches the top of the endometrial cavity. This is done to determine the maximum length of the cavity and to prevent insertion of the IUD beyond this limit.

All modern IUDs are elongated by being pulled into an inserter with a slightly larger diameter than the IUD itself. The inserter is then placed through the cervical os and the IUD is released into the endometrial cavity where it resumes its original shape. This is

Figure 3–2. *Estimated annual number of hospitalizations and rate per 100,000 IUD users. (Reprinted with permission from* Making Choices: Evaluating the Health Risks and Benefits of Birth Control Method, *The Alan Guttmacher Institute, 1983.)*

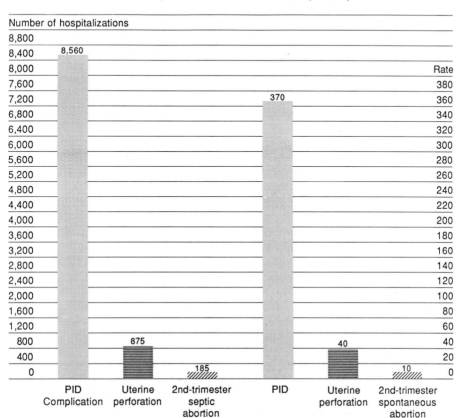

called "regaining its memory." When a T-shaped device is used, the two halves of the horizontal arm are folded downward against the vertical arm prior to insertion and the device is inserted in this I-shape. When the inserter is withdrawn from the top of the endometrial cavity, the two arms open outward again into their original T-shape.

It is vital that the IUD be placed at the top of the endometrial cavity if cramping and, more important, the risk of pregnancy are to be minimized. After the IUD is in its correct position, the tail is cut to a desired length, usually about 2 inches. Figure 3-3 shows how properly inserted IUDs will look.

When in the menstrual cycle should the IUD be inserted?

Until recently, it was universal practice to insert IUDs only during or immediately after menstruation. This precaution was taken because it verified to the physician that there was no possibility of an early, undiagnosed pregnancy. In addition, the cervical os is slightly more open at that point in the cycle, which may reduce the pain associated with insertion. Most doctors continue to adhere to this policy, but others now believe that it is safe to insert an IUD at any time during the menstrual cycle. In a 1980 study from the Centers for Disease Control, researchers analyzed the effects of inserting a Copper-T IUD at various times of the month in over 9,000 women. They found that during the first two months after IUD insertion the rates of expulsion or rejection of the device from the uterine cavity were lower when the IUD had been inserted later in the menstrual cycle. However, this benefit was offset by the fact that rates of IUD removal for pain, bleeding, and accidental pregnancy were higher when the IUD was inserted later in the cycle, especially after Day 17 of the typical 28-day cycle. Considering all the positive and negative aspects, the authors calculated that for every 1,000 insertions before Day 11 there would be only nine more discontinuations of IUD use due to expulsion, pain, bleeding, or accidental pregnancy than if the insertions had been done after Day 11. Based on these statistics they concluded that an IUD can be inserted with relative safety on the day it is requested if a woman's history indicates that she is unlikely to be pregnant at the time. In the absence of a period in a woman who menstruates only every few months, a negative pregnancy test is mandatory before insertion of an IUD. Though this sounds like a simple enough precaution, hundreds of women each year inadvertently have IUDs inserted while they are pregnant.

IDENTIFICATION OF IUD STRINGS

Type of IUD	Color of Strings	Number of Strings	Other Characteristics
Lippes Loop-A	Blue	1 or 2	1 thick; 2 thin
Lippes Loop-B	Black	1 or 2	1 thick; 2 thin
Lippes Loop-C	Yellow	1 or 2	1 thick; 2 thin
Lippes Loop-D	White	1 or 2	1 thick; 2 thin
Dalkon Shield	Black	1	Knot in thick string
Saf-T-Coil	Green	2	Thin strings
Copper-7	Older devices, black; newer devices, light blue	1	Thin strings
Copper-T	Light blue (variable)	2	Thin strings
Progestasert-T	Translucent	2	Thin strings

SOURCE: *Compiled by the author.*

Figure 3–3. *Proper insertion of IUD.*

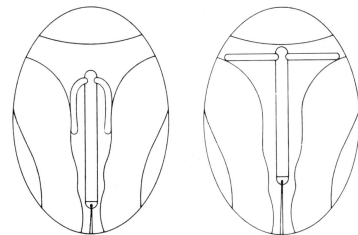

Should any other precautions be taken prior to having an IUD inserted?

It is vital that a pelvic exam be done immediately prior to inserting an IUD in order to determine the position, size, and shape of the uterus. Otherwise perforation of the uterus may occur. As mentioned earlier, "sounding" the uterus prior to inserting the IUD will also ensure against perforation. If there is even the slightest chance of a pelvic or tubal infection, the IUD must not be inserted until the diagnosis is confirmed and the infection adequately treated. The IUD insertion should be gentle, with no application of excessive pressure. All equipment must be sterilized in order to minimize the risk of infection.

How painful is an IUD insertion?

A gynecologist may tell a woman that insertion of an IUD is a simple, painless procedure. However, as most women with IUDs can attest, this is usually not true. The initial insult is the grasping of the cervix with a tenaculum, often described as feeling like a pinch or a tiny bee sting. For some women, a swarm of bumblebees would be a far more accurate description. The degree of pain associated with the insertion of the IUD is variable. There is usually little discomfort for women who have previously given birth, especially if the IUD is inserted within six weeks after a vaginal delivery. For others, especially women who have never given birth, the cramping may be excruciating, necessitating instant removal of the device. Certain individuals who have never had previous dilatation of the cervix, such as with an elective abortion, may experience "cervical shock syndrome" or vasovagal stimulation as the IUD inserter moves through the cervical canal, characterized by a dangerously slow pulse, heartbeat irregularities, fainting, seizures, or on rare occasions even cardiac arrest.

Use of a paracervical block is often helpful in relieving some, but certainly not all, of the pain associated with an IUD insertion. It is performed by injecting Xylocaine (lidocaine) or Nesacaine (chloroprocaine hydrochloride) or another similar drug into the cervix before the device is inserted (see chapter 7, "Abortion"). Some doctors have reported success with an anesthetic spray or gel applied to the cervix, while others recommend tranquilizers or an antiprostaglandin such as Motrin one hour before an IUD is inserted.

The diameter of the widest part of the inserter will determine to a great degree the amount of pain that an individual will experience. Theoretically, the Copper-7, with an inserter diameter of 3.07 mm., should cause less discomfort than the Tatum-T or Progestasert, which have diameters of 5.96 and 6.0, respectively.

How does an IUD prevent pregnancy?

This question has been a subject of great controversy among physicians as well as religious leaders. Certain religious groups claim that the IUD works solely by preventing implantation of an already fertilized egg, thereby causing an early abortion. Others have theorized that IUDs prevent pregnancy by increasing the speed at which an egg travels down the fallopian tube on its way to the uterus, thus reaching the endometrium at a time when it is too immature to implant. Another prevalent theory is that IUDs increase endometrial production of prostaglandins, which cause uterine contractions that inhibit implantation.

Although no conclusive medical evidence has come to light thus far, the prevailing opinion is that the presence of the IUD in the endometrial cavity stimulates an inflammatory reaction. As a result, large microscopic cells called *macrophages* are released, which are believed capable of destroying sperm before they can get into the tube to fertilize the egg, and the macrophages can undoubtedly destroy the fertilized egg as well. The addition of copper to some IUDs appears to enhance this inflammatory reaction. Copper may also react with certain enzymes in the endometrium to diminish sperm movement.

The Progestasert IUD releases small amounts of progesterone each day over a period of one year. This brings about subtle changes in the endometrial environment that impair implantation of the egg. In addition, it is believed that the progesterone alters the cervical mucus so that sperm are unable to penetrate it.

Are there certain women who should not use an IUD?

The IUD should not be used by women with abnormalities, irregularities, or tumors of the uterus, such as fibroids. Other contraindications are acute inflammation of the cervix, uterus, or fallopian tubes; undiagnosed vaginal bleeding; extremely heavy periods; anemia; extremely painful periods; and cancer of the cervix or uterus. If a woman's medical condition requires anticoagulants, such as coumadin or heparin, she should not be wearing an IUD. In addition, any woman who is concerned about her future fertility should probably avoid the IUD. This is especially true for those who have never given birth and who have more than one sex partner, since their risk of tubal infection is significantly higher than that of other women (see PID and IUD). Individuals with impaired blood coagulation caused by either a clotting factor or platelet abnormality or deficiency should not use the IUD. The same advice applies to women with heart disease, a history of rheumatic fever, or damaged heart valves. The use of the IUD with mitral valve prolapse remains controversial (see page 100).

How effective is the IUD as a contraceptive?

The most important factors in evaluating the efficacy of an IUD are the pregnancy rate; the expulsion rate; the removal rate for medical problems such as bleeding, cramps, and infection; and the patient continuation rate.

All reports about a particular device must be taken with a grain of salt, since the results are dependent on many factors and vary greatly from one study to another. Though the Progestasert is the only IUD currently available to American women, millions are still wearing other devices that were inserted before their production ceased. It is comforting for women to note that several IUDs voluntarily taken off the market by their manufacturers, such as the Copper-7, Copper-T, and Saf-T-Coil, have efficacy and safety rates comparable to those of the Progestasert (see table, page 86). Factors that may prevent meaningful comparisons between two different IUD studies include differences in the motivation of the patient group selected, the degree of experience among the individuals inserting the devices, and the attitude of medical personnel in encouraging or discouraging the use of a particular method of contraception. For these reasons it is extremely difficult for both the practicing doctor and the patient to obtain reliable data about a particular device. The table that follows is based on the most commonly quoted results from using some of the more popular IUDs. These results are expressed as events per 100 women using the device over the specific period of one year. This method of measuring success rates is referred to as events per 100 woman-years. For example, if 100 nulliparous women—women who have never given birth—were to use the Copper-7 for a period of one year, approximately 1.7 would become pregnant and 66.4 would continue to use it. The pregnancy rate in this case would be expressed as 1.7 per 100 woman-years.

Do the rates of effectiveness improve or worsen after the first year of IUD use?

Studies performed with most IUDs concur that effectiveness improves during the second and third years of use. In addition, rates of expulsion and medical removal diminish significantly. This obviously does not apply to the Progestasert device, which has to be changed yearly if it is to offer effective contraception.

The statistics for the Copper-7 among 100 parous users report 1.9 inadvertent pregnancies during the first year. In the second year, however, only an additional 1.1 would conceive, for a cumulative total of 3.0 per 100 woman-years. The third-year pregnancy rates for this device are even more impressive: 0.8 per 100, for a total three-year cumulative pregnancy rate of 3.8 per 100 woman-years. Similar favorable statistics with regard to pregnancy rates, expulsion rates, medical removals, and continuation rates during the second and third years are seen with the other devices as well.

How effective is a copper IUD that is left in place beyond the recommended three years?

This is an important question for the thousands of women in the United States who had Copper-7s and Copper-Ts inserted prior to their voluntary removal from the market by G. D. Searle in 1986. As the FDA deadline of three years for its removal approaches, scores of women in their thirties and forties who cannot take the Pill will be left with limited contraceptive options.

The prevailing opinion is that IUDs containing copper should be changed every three years, since much of the spermicidal and contraceptive action of the copper may be lost after this time, probably from the loss of the ionized copper from the surface of the device. Other research suggests that it isn't the loss of copper from the device that diminishes its contraceptive effect, but rather the formation of a microscopic crust over the copper which prevents its release and increases the risk of pregnancy. Some authors have described deterioration and fragmentation or breakage of the copper wire caused by exposure to endometrial secretions over a period of time. Fragmentation has been noted in some IUDs that have been in place for as little as six months; in others, no fragmentation has been detected after five or six years of use.

In contrast to these views is precise scientific research showing that the concentration of copper in the endometrial secretions remains at relatively the same level for up to four years after the insertion of a copper IUD. Even after six years, significant amounts of copper remain on the device and continue to be released into the endometrial cavity. Clinical experience suggests that the contraceptive effect of a copper-containing device may last as long as eight years. In a 1981 publication from Sweden, doctors studied a group of 278 women who used the Copper-7 for up to four years and a subgroup of 48 women who continued to use it beyond this time. Those

SUMMARY OF IUD EFFECTIVENESS DURING ONE YEAR OF USE

Device	Size	Pregnancy Rate Per 100 Woman-Years	Expulsion Rate Per 100 Woman-Years	Medical Removal Rates Per 100 Woman-Years	Continuation Rate Per 100 Woman-Years
Lippes Loop	A (small)	4.8–8.10	6.9	8.8–11.7	63.6
	B	2.0–5.8	6.5	9.0–21.1	59.2
	C	4.1	5.3	19.2	62.8
	D (large)	1.8–3.8	3.6	4.0–15.2	77.4
Saf-T-Coil		1.1–2.8	7.8–10	7.5–18.7	57–78.3
Copper-7		1.7 for nulliparous* 1.9 for parous	8.0 for nulliparous 5.7 for parous other studies: 3.3	13.6 for nulliparous 10.9 for parous other studies: 4.2	71.5 for nulliparous 66.4 for parous other studies: 88
Copper-T		2.1 for nulliparous 3.0 for parous	8.0 for nulliparous 7.8 for parous other studies: 5.3	13.9 for nulliparous 10.9 for parous other studies: 7.2	71.4 for nulliparous 73.4 for parous other studies: 81
Progestasert-7		2.6 for nulliparous 1.8 for parous	7.4 for nulliparous 3.1 for parous	15.1 for nulliparous 11.2 for parous other studies: 9.7	71.8 for nulliparous 79.8 for parous

*Parous describes a woman who has had a previous pregnancy, and nulliparous means a woman with no previous pregnancy.
SOURCE: Compiled by the author.

wearing the IUD for prolonged periods were satisfied with the device, experienced no adverse side effects, and had pregnancy rates that were about the same as women who had limited their use of the device to three years.

It is the impression of many experienced gynecologists that the contraceptive effectiveness of a copper device continues for many months and possibly years after the copper wire completely fragments and dissolves. The copper wire adds to contraceptive effectiveness during the first three to four years of use, but after the copper disappears, the plastic base continues to be highly effective in preventing pregnancy. Unfortunately, we do not know the pregnancy-preventing capability of the Ts and 7s stripped of their copper sleeves. Not enough data is presently available to endorse the use of copper-containing IUDs for five or more years by women who are now unable to get their devices replaced. However, it seems safe to say that they can be used effectively, regardless of FDA approval, for up to four years with extremely low pregnancy rates and few side effects. This extra year may provide valuable time for women to consider more carefully alternative contraceptive options.

How long can the standard plastic IUDs remain safely in place?

If you are currently wearing a nonmedicated polyethylene plastic IUD, such as the Lippes Loop or the Saf-T-Coil, there is little scientific evidence to guide you in making this decision. Opinions of authorities and results of various studies are often contradictory. For example, the vast majority of reports conclude that severe tubal infections and PID associated with IUD use are most likely to occur during the first six months following insertion and are not related to the number of years that the IUD is worn. But a 1984 report published in *Obstetrics and Gynecology* concluded that women using the IUD for five or more years were at greater risk of contracting a very rare but serious pelvic infection requiring hysterectomy or major tubal surgery. The authors of this study found that women who wore IUDs for shorter periods of time had many more tubal and pelvic infections but experienced less serious consequences. The unsolved dilemma was whether to chance an unlikely, though dangerous, infection by leaving the IUD in place or to change the device and stir up a far more common, though less serious, infection.

Some doctors suggest that plastic IUDs should be changed every three years because small calcification deposits may cover the surface of the device during that time and cause bleeding problems and loss of contraceptive efficacy. There are no scientific studies to support this contention, however. On the contrary, most people have noted a normalization of menstrual pattern and a lower pregnancy rate the longer a nonmedicated device is left in. Changing an IUD often initiates abnormal bleeding again, and therefore it has been my policy to leave these IUDs in place as long as my patient is free of complications. I have not regretted this decision, nor have several of my patients who have had the same IUD for ten or more years. The ideal time for many women to have their IUDs removed is when the diagnosis of menopause is confirmed.

What factors determine the expulsion rate of an IUD?

The expulsion rate is often determined by the skill of the person who has inserted the IUD. Many novices place the device too low in the endometrial cavity and even into the cervical canal. It must be placed in the upper part of the uterine cavity and conform to the shape of the cavity in order to prevent pregnancy and expulsion.

The expulsion rate is higher for nulliparous women (those who have never had children) than for parous women (those who have had children), probably because the muscles of the smaller, more rigid uterus of a nulliparous woman tends to contract and reject the device more readily. The highest expulsion rates occur with the smallest devices, and the lowest expulsion rates with the largest devices.

Time appears to be another important factor. Between 5 and 20 percent of women will expel their IUDs within the first year. Expulsion rates decrease with each month of IUD use, and the incidence of expulsion after the third year is extremely low. This is one of the great advantages that the older, plastic IUDs have over medicated devices such as the Progestasert, Copper-7, and Copper-T.

The symptoms of IUD expulsion may include severe cramping or pain, vaginal discharge, spotting between periods, spotting with intercourse, painful intercourse, lengthening of the IUD string, and the presence of the plastic part of the IUD at the cervical opening, discoverable during self-examination. It is not uncommon for an IUD to be unknowingly expelled into the toilet during a heavy and painful menstrual flow. If expulsion is not detected at that time, there may unfortunately be no indication that anything is wrong until symptoms of pregnancy begin to appear.

As you would expect, the risk of expulsion is higher after a previous expulsion has taken place. Only two out of five women who have had a previous expulsion will be able to retain a second device for a full two years. It is for this reason that women should examine themselves after each period to establish the tail length as well as the absence of plastic or copper protruding from the cervix or vagina. This is especially necessary during the first six months following insertion of the device. For women with a previous history of expulsion, an additional self-examination prior to and after intercourse will enhance safety. It is known that the uterine muscle contracts vigorously during orgasm, and it has been suggested that this action may help to expel an IUD at this time. However, no studies have been performed that show a higher expulsion rate following orgasm.

When and how can an IUD cause infection?

There are many studies clearly showing that women who wear IUDs are more likely to experience salpingitis (inflammation of the fallopian tubes), pelvic inflammatory disease (PID), and subsequent infertility. Infections associated with use of an IUD are caused by bacteria that find their way from the vagina and cervix into the endometrium and uterine cavity. While these infections may occur at any time, the incidence is highest during the first four months following insertion, leading investigators to surmise that the bacteria are initially introduced at the time the IUD is inserted. Even when sterile precautions are taken, some bacteria will always be transmitted from the cervix to the endometrium. The defense mechanisms of the vast majority of women are able to ward off these bacteria and prevent infection. Bacteria entering the endometrium after the first four months are probably aided in their ascent by the tail of the IUD, which serves as a conduit for infectious organisms entering the vagina and cervix. While many patients and their doctors erroneously believe that inert plastic IUDs, such as the Lippes Loop and Saf-T-Coil, should be changed every three to five years in order to prevent late infections from developing, the truth is that infection is less likely to occur with each year of IUD use. This view was reaffirmed by the Food and Drug Administration Advisory Committee, which concluded that evidence calling for IUD removal after a specific period of time was both "speculative" and "insufficient."

Once bacteria reach the endometrium they can travel directly to the fallopian tubes or pass through the muscle of the uterus and out into the lower pelvis, infecting the tubes, ovaries, and other pelvic structures. Occasionally the tube and ovary may become matted together in a ball of pus called a tubo-ovarian abscess. The rupture of such an abscess, though extremely rare, has a very high mortality rate. The bacteria might also enter the bloodstream and attack distant organs, producing an overwhelming reaction and drop in blood pressure called septic shock, which can also be fatal. If a woman survives such an infection, she may be left permanently sterile and in chronic pain due to destruction of her pelvic tissues. The incidence of pelvic infection in women using the IUD is approximately 2 to 3 percent, though only a small percentage of those infected suffer these severe complications.

Epidemiologists estimate that as many as 88,000 American women suffer infertility as a result of tubal damage associated with wearing IUDs. It is becoming increasingly clear that it is the woman and her lifestyle rather than the IUD itself that most determines whether or not these distressing complications will occur. Among nulliparous women, IUD users have at least double or triple the risk of infertility than women who have never used an IUD. This is especially true for nulliparous women less than twenty-five years of age. The most important factors in determining whether infection will occur appear to be the number of coital partners a woman has as well as her frequency of coitus. Several theories for this phenomenon have been proposed. One is that frequent coitus and orgasm produce uterine contractions that spread bacteria from the cervix to the endometrium. Other theories propose that the presence of an IUD somehow alters the cervical and endometrial immune responses to bacteria in certain susceptible women. In a 1986 report, published in *The American Journal of Obstetrics and Gynecology,* Finnish doctors compared the types of bacteria in the cervixes of women using barrier contraception with those using IUDs. They found more pathological (disease-causing) strains of bacteria among the IUD users.

The answer to the mystery of why pathological bacteria are more likely to enter the endometrium of women with multiple sexual partners was answered by Dr. Attilla Toth of New York Hospital–Cornell Medical Center. In her report, published in *The Journal of Reproductive Medicine,* Dr. Toth demonstrated that potentially dangerous bacteria are capable of attaching themselves to moving spermatozoa and traveling through the cervical mucus and into the endometrial cavity. Dr. Toth also noted that the number of attached bacteria was directly related to the sexual experience of the individual man—those with the greatest sexual experience had the highest number of bacteria attached to their spermatozoa. It would appear, therefore, that women with a greater number of coital partners are more likely to encounter a man with bacteria attached to his sperm. Of further interest was a 1986 report demonstrating that IUD users with PID were significantly more likely to have antibodies to chlamydia, the bacterial culprit most likely to cause PID and infertility (see chlamydia). Since antibodies to chlamydia indicate previous exposure to this bacterium, the authors of this article concluded that IUD users with more than one coital partner were more likely to encounter a chlamydia-carrying male than were less sexually active women. Doctors at Mount Sinai Hospital in Chicago provided further convincing proof that spermatozoa offer excellent transportation to chlamydia in need of a ride from the cervix to the fallopian tubes. In their 1987 study, they were able to detect the presence of the Chlamydia trachomatis bacterium attached to spermatozoa that they had recovered from the abdominal cavities of two women diagnosed as having salpingitis on laparoscopic examination (see laparoscopy).

Regardless of the mechanism by which IUD-associated infections and infertility occur, the vital lesson to be learned is that the IUD is the worst possible contraceptive device for a young, sexually active woman who has never given birth. In contrast, it is the perfect method for a woman in her thirties or forties who has completed her childbearing and is involved in a stable, monogamous sexual relationship.

What are some of the early signs of an IUD-related infection?

Occasionally a low-grade pelvic infection, tubal scarring, or infertility may occur without any warning symptoms. More often, however, there are clues that a problem exists. Symptoms that should alert a woman to the possibility of an early pelvic infection are: general pain in the lower abdomen, any temperature above 99°F, abnormal uterine bleeding, a foul-smelling yellowish discharge, chills, and pain with intercourse. Unfortunately, these infections sometimes become far advanced before a woman experiences any symptoms at all. Vague symptoms such as fatigue and flu-like aches and pains should also be cause for concern.

When in doubt about the cause of a low-grade fever or pelvic pain, your doctor should assume that the IUD is the culprit and immediately remove it while vigorously treating the infection with appropriate antibiotics. Placing the IUD in a sterile container and bringing it to a laboratory for bacterial analysis will help determine whether infection is present, what type of bacteria caused the infection, and what the sensitivity of the bacteria is to the antibiotic that has been prescribed. A culture for chlamydia and gonorrhea should also be obtained. The habit of some doctors of leaving the IUD in the uterus while treating the infection with antibiotics is to be deplored.

If a tubo-ovarian abscess has formed (a very rare occurrence) and it does not respond to antibiotic treatment, surgical removal of the infected tube and ovary is often necessary. When both ovaries are infected, removal of all structures involved in the infection, as well as a hysterectomy, is often necessary for cure. Several reports in the medical literature have described unilateral, or one-sided, tubo-ovarian abscess following IUD use. Removal of the infected tissue only on that side cured the disease. This one-sided involvement appears to be characteristic of IUD infections, whereas most infections produced by sexually transmitted diseases such as gonorrhea and chlamydia affect both tubes and ovaries. If your doctor, on pelvic examination, feels a slight enlargement of one side, the prudent move would be to determine immediately whether an IUD-related infection is present.

Is the risk of tubal infection and infertility related to the type of IUD that a woman wears?

There is no doubt that the infamous Dalkon Shield has been responsible for significantly higher rates of infection than any other IUD ever manufactured. Though this device was removed from the market in 1974, and a great deal of publicity urging women to have it removed has been disseminated, it is estimated that several thousand either uninformed or disinterested individuals continue to wear Dalkon Shields. An average of one woman each year appears in my office wearing a Dalkon and totally unaware of the device's history. The risk of salpingitis, or tubal infection, and PID has been estimated to be from five to eleven times greater for users of the Dalkon Shield compared to women without IUDs. And infertility resulting from tubal damage may occur three to seven times more frequently with this device.

While other IUDs have a far better safety record than the Dalkon Shield, they are not totally innocuous. The highest risk of tubal infection and infertility appears to be associated with the inert plastic devices such as the Lippes Loop and Saf-T-Coil. This finding was confirmed in two large 1985 studies published in the prestigious *New England Journal of Medicine.* In the first, from the University of Washington in Seattle, doctors interviewed 159 nulligravid women (women who have never been pregnant) with proven tubal damage as a cause of their infertility. Those who exclusively wore either a Lippes Loop or a Saf-T-Coil were 4.4 times more likely than women not using IUDs to experience tubal infertility. Women limiting their IUD use to copper devices had a minimal risk only 1.3 times greater than that of nonusers. The second study, based on data from seven different infertility centers and hospitals around the country, confirmed a greater risk with the inert devices than with the copper ones. These researchers also examined the relationship between IUD use and tubal infertility after a successful birth. Though there were only 69 women in this subgroup, it was found that there was no statistically significant risk of tubal infertility associated with use of copper IUDs once a woman had given birth. In contrast, those who gave birth and then used a Lippes Loop or Saf-T-Coil had a statistically significant, three-times-greater risk of sterility caused by tubal damage. Based on these studies, epidemiologists have calculated that 48 percent of the cases of tubal infertility among women who have had the Lippes Loop or Saf-T-Coil can be attributed to the IUD, giving a rate of 1,700 cases per 100,000 IUD users. For the copper devices, the statistics are a more favorable 23 percent and 600 cases per 100,000 users.

Laboratory studies have shown that the growth of the bacteria that cause gonorrhea is stopped in the area around the copper portion of the IUD. The plastic, however, affords no protection at all. The copper is not effective in preventing all bacteria from passing from the uterine cavity to the tubes and pelvis, and these IUDs should not be thought of as providing protection against sexually transmitted diseases or other infections. Unfortunately, none of the above reports analyzed the infection risk associated with use of the Progestasert, though the one report in the medical literature studying this relationship is very encouraging. In a 1983 publication in *The Journal of Reproductive Medicine,* Dr. Richard M. Soderstrom performed microscopic studies on the fallopian tubes of women using various IUDs. Evidence of salpingitis, or tubal inflammation, was found in 85 percent of the 175 women using either the Lippes Loop or the Saf-T-Coil but in none of the 22 women using the Progestasert. The reason for this excellent record with the Progestasert is unknown, but it is theorized that the release of progesterone somehow produces a quieting effect on the endometrium, which inhibits bacterial growth. Another theory is that menstrual blood is a good culture medium for bacterial reproduction, and since the Progestasert produces lighter periods than other IUDs (see Progestasert, page 92), it diminishes the ability of pathologic bacteria to grow and reproduce. Also contributing to a lower infection rate is the fact that the progesterone released from this device thickens the cervical mucus, thereby preventing bacterial penetration into the endometrium.

Some women may wish to resume use of an IUD after the resolution of an initial episode of salpingitis or PID. My practice is to encourage these women to use alternative contraceptive methods rather than risk a recurrence of a potentially serious infection.

Why are infection rates so much higher with the Dalkon Shield than with other IUDs?

In 1974, the A. H. Robins Company removed the Dalkon Shield from the market because of its association with salpingitis, PID, and septic (infected) accidental pregnancies. Dr. Howard Tatum, discoverer of the Tatum-T copper device, sought to discover why women using the Dalkon Shield were more prone to these infections. He studied the tails of all other IUDs under the microscope and noted that they consisted of a single or double segment of monofilament plastic thread. In contrast, the Dalkon tail is made of a bundle of filaments encased in a thin plastic sheath. When Dr. Tatum suspended the tails of various IUDs in a dye solution containing bacteria, he noted that the many filaments in the Dalkon allowed both the dye and the bacteria to move rapidly up the tail by capillary action. This did not happen with the other IUDs.

During accidental pregnancy with any IUD, the tail is often taken up into the endometrial cavity as the uterus enlarges. From the experimental model, Tatum theorized that infection with the Dalkon Shield is carried into the endometrial cavity from the infected tail, covered with bacteria from the vagina.

Ironically, isn't it true that the IUD has been used to enhance fertility?

In rare cases, scarring of the endometrium may occur when a D and C, or dilatation and curettage, is performed in the presence of an infected abortion or infected pregnancy tissue following childbirth. The scar tissue may prevent implantation of a fertilized egg when pregnancy is desired. This condition can be remedied if a doctor performs a repeat D and C and lyses (breaks down) the adhesions that are formed. If a large IUD, such as a Lippes D, is then inserted, the uterine cavity may be kept free of these adhesions. If the IUD is removed several months later, the adhesions will usually not return and pregnancy may then be possible.

What is the significance of finding actinomyces in the Pap smear of IUD wearers?

Actinomyces israelii is the official name of a bacterial organism detected in the Pap smears of 1 to 3 percent of IUD wearers. Using more sophisticated laboratory techniques, some research groups have found its frequency to be as high as 35 percent. Under normal circumstances, *Actinomyces israelii* is absent from the genital tract, but it is a common and harmless inhabitant of the mouth and lower intestine. An IUD acts as a foreign body that, in some unknown way, facilitates growth and reproduction of this organism inside the cervix and endometrial cavity. While some studies have shown that the incidence of actinomyces is heightened in plastic IUD wearers and lowest in women with copper-bearing IUDs, other research has shown equal distribution regardless of the type of IUD worn. In addition, most articles report a direct relationship between the likelihood of finding actinomyces and the duration of IUD use.

It has been theorized that *Actinomyces israelii* may be a sexually transmitted organism which is carried to the cervix through varied sexual activity. Oral sex is believed to play an important role since *Actinomyces israelii* is normally found in the mouth and not in the male genito-urinary tract. Furthermore, in a 1983 study from England, doctors found the organism in the genital tract of a significant number of women not wearing IUDs.

As many as 98 out of every 100 women with Pap smears that are positive for *Actinomyces israelii* will be totally asymptomatic. When the disease, called *actinomycosis*, is present, it is most often manifested by symptoms of pelvic inflammatory disease (see PID symptoms, this chapter and chapter 2). On rare occasions this organism will destroy pelvic structures, cause abscesses, and invade the abdominal cavity and the brain. Advanced widespread disease may prove life-threatening.

Medical opinions vary as to the management of the IUD wearer in whom *Actinomyces israelii* is found on a routine Pap smear. The prevailing strategy is to remove the IUD immediately and repeat the Pap smear four to six weeks later. If no evidence of *Actinomyces israelii* is present on the repeat Pap smear, the device can be safely reinserted. There is no evidence at this time to suggest that these women require antibiotic treatment. But a doctor who prescribes antibiotics can't be faulted, since PID and abscess formation have been reported on rare occasions as late as ten months after the IUD has been removed.

If there is even the slightest question of more extensive disease, as evidenced by symptoms of PID, antibiotics must be given. Fortunately, *Actinomyces israelii* is susceptible to antibiotics such as penicillin, erythromycin, tetracycline, cephalothin, and clindamycin. If antibiotic treatment is undertaken, it should be carried out for at least two weeks. It is probably best not to reinsert an IUD in these women. More severe cases need immediate and permanent IUD removal, prolonged antibiotic treatment, and, in some cases, extensive pelvic surgery.

What are the advantages and disadvantages of the Progestasert IUD?

The Progestasert is a T-shaped IUD that contains progesterone in its vertical arm. The progesterone is slowly released into the uterine cavity over a period of one year, which produces hormonal changes in the endometrium that prevent implantation of the egg. In addition it is believed that the progesterone alters the cervical mucus so that sperm are unable to penetrate it. It has been demonstrated that the small amount of progesterone released each day does not prevent ovulation.

The Progestasert is the only IUD currently manufactured in the United States, and while its efficacy, expulsion rates, and medical removal rates are impressive when compared to other previously manufactured devices (see table on page 86), it has failed to gain the popularity achieved with other IUDs. The most obvious reason for this is the distinct disadvantage of having to replace it every twelve months when it loses its progesterone contraceptive effect. It seems foolish to change an IUD so often, especially in light of the three-to-four month adjustment phase of higher expulsion and infection rates and heavier periods immediately following an IUD insertion. Having an IUD removed and inserted so often is likely to cause both inconvenience and discomfort in addition to the added expense of a doctor's fee for inserting a new device each year.

Another disadvantage of the Progestasert is that the diameter of its inserter is greater than that of other IUDs. While this will not be of any significance for the majority of women, it may be responsible for more pain on insertion for those with a small cervical opening. Earlier reports linking use of the Progestasert to a higher ectopic pregnancy rate have not been substantiated in more recent studies. One early concern about the Progestasert was that, in the event of an accidental pregnancy, the release of progesterone in close proximity to the developing fetus could cause an anomaly. However, studies to date of several newborn infants who were exposed to the Progestasert in utero have uncovered no anatomical or physiological defects. This is not surprising in view of the fact that the progesterone released from this device is identical to the hormone the body produces in great quantities during pregnancy.

In July 1986 the Alza Corporation, manufacturer of the Progestasert, raised the price of its device from $38.00 to $84.00. They cited the litigation-prone market as the reason for this increase. Since the doctor's fee for inserting the Progestasert is not included in this $84.00, many believe that cost will be a major deterrent to women using this device and replacing it each year.

On the positive side, the Progestasert does have certain distinct advantages over other IUDs. As previously mentioned, pregnancy rates, expulsion rates, and medical removal rates are as favorable and probably better than most other IUDs in the past. In addition, there may be a lesser likelihood of salpingitis, PID, and permanent sterility associated with use of the Progestasert, though more studies are required to confirm these findings (see previous discussion of PID and Progestasert). Several researchers have noted that this device may be more effective than other IUDs in relieving uterine cramps, partly because its T shape conforms to the shape of the endometrial cavity. In addition, the progesterone released by the device inhibits the endometrium's secretion of prostaglandins, which are responsible for causing severe menstrual pain (see prostaglandins). The progesterone in the device also suppresses endometrial growth, which in turn reduces the total amount of prostaglandins that are released each month. Since less endometrium is formed with the Progestasert, less tissue and blood is shed with each menstrual flow. In one study, measurable blood loss with periods decreased by 45 percent following insertion of a Progestasert. In another report, the Progestasert was found to lengthen the number of days between periods to more than thirty-two days in 8 percent of the women studied. In contrast, all other IUDs have been known to cause heavier and longer periods as well as occasional anemia secondary to blood loss.

Overall, one can only conclude that the advantages of the Progestasert far outweigh its disadvantages. It is certainly a logical contraceptive option for a woman in her thirties or forties who has completed her childbearing but does not want to be limited to choosing either permanent sterilization or less effective and less spontaneous methods of birth control.

How does an IUD perforate a uterus?

It is not the IUD but the person who inserts it who perforates the uterus. Perforation takes place at the time of insertion and is the sole responsibility of the individual inserting the IUD. A common misconception among women is that IUDs slowly work their way through the uterine wall over a period of time. While this may have been possible with older and more dangerous devices, such as the Majzlin IUD and Birnberg Bow, it does not occur with IUDs such as the Lippes Loop, Saf-T-Coil, Copper-7, Tatum-T, or the Progestasert.

The incidence of IUD perforation is listed as 1 in 2,500 insertions, but I am convinced that many cases go unreported. Perforation of an IUD into the tissues of the cervix or the uterine muscle wall is often "silent," meaning asymptomatic. In a partial perforation, at least part of the IUD has passed from the endometrial cavity and has embedded into the deeper tissues, while a complete perforation refers to passage of the device beyond the uterine wall and into the abdominal cavity.

When perforation rates are studied in terms of the individuals who inserted the IUD, investigators often find that one doctor is responsible for a great number of cases. If the person inserting the IUD is gentle, does not use excessive pressure, and performs a pelvic examination prior to insertion, perforation of the uterus should rarely happen. Approximately 20 percent of all healthy women have a retroflexed uterus—one that is tilted backward. If the person inserting the IUD omits the pelvic exam and assumes that the uterus is in an anterior position, as in figure 3-4, the procedure could perforate the cervix or the lower part of the body of the uterus. Under such circumstances the IUD could pass directly into the abdominal cavity.

As discussed earlier, before any IUD is inserted, a thin rod called a uterine sound should be passed gently through the cervix until the top of the corpus, or body, of the uterus is reached. In doing this, the position and length of the cavity can easily be determined (see figure 3-3, showing correct IUD insertion). This allows the person inserting the IUD to know the limits beyond which the inserter should not be passed. This simple maneuver prevents perforation through the top of the uterus.

How should your doctor diagnose and treat an IUD perforation?

Sadly, often the first clue that the IUD has perforated is when a woman becomes pregnant within a few months following its insertion. In the absence of a positive pregnancy test, perforation may be suspected when neither you nor your doctor can locate the IUD strings. Since the tail or strings may be taken up into the endometrial cavity when the IUD is in its proper location, the mystery of a lost IUD may be solved simply by passing the uterine sound into the cavity and feeling for the IUD. If the IUD can be touched with the sound, rest assured that all is well. If the IUD can't be palpated, an ultrasound examination can demonstrate its location with great precision. If ultrasound is unavailable, an X ray taken with a probe in the uterus will confirm the presence of the IUD as well as its relationship to the endometrial cavity. An alternative method is to insert a second IUD and take an X ray. If both IUDs are in

Figure 3–4. *Perforation while inserting the IUD.*

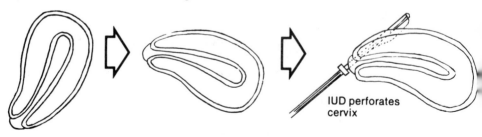

IUD perforates cervix

Doctor assumes uterus is anterior (side view)

Uterus is posterior

close contact, they are probably in the right place and the one with the visible string can then be removed. A third technique is to fill the endometrial cavity with an X-ray dye solution and then take a picture, called a *hysterogram*. If the IUD is seen outside the area of the dye, it means perforation has occurred.

Hysteroscopy is another technique for visualizing and retrieving lost and embedded IUDs from the endometrial cavity and uterine wall. In this procedure, local anesthesia is applied to the cervix, and a small viewing instrument is passed through the cervical os and into the endometrial cavity. If the IUD is present, a variety of special forceps may be used to grasp and remove it.

If diagnostic tests reveal that the IUD is in its correct position in the endometrial cavity, there is no need to bring the string out through the cervix. Attempts to do so may dislodge the IUD. Furthermore, infection rates may be lower when the string doesn't pass into the vagina (see chapter 11, "The Future").

When it has been determined that an IUD is located in the abdominal cavity, it can be removed through the laparoscope (see chapter 9). The IUD must not be left in the abdominal cavity because it may be responsible for an inflammatory reaction of the surrounding intestine, or a blockage of a loop of intestine that may adhere to it. IUDs containing copper are the most difficult to remove because they cause the greatest inflammatory reaction. The Dalkon Shield also produces a marked inflammatory reaction in the abdomen, due to the little-known fact, first revealed in the August 1974 investigations, that each Dalkon Shield actually contained 2 milligrams of copper.

How soon after an abortion or a full-term pregnancy can an IUD be safely inserted?

Most gynecologists prefer not to insert an IUD for at least two weeks following an elective abortion for fear that it will increase a woman's risk of infection, heavy bleeding, expulsion of the device, and perforation of the softer, more stretchable uterine musculature associated with pregnancy. Much of this policy, however, is based on outdated and inaccurate information from the late 1960s and early 1970s. Recent studies are far more optimistic. In fact, several publications have shown that immediate insertion of an IUD at the time of an abortion is associated with a slightly lower incidence of expulsion and perforation than at other times. In addition, cramping is minimized since the cervix is already dilated. Since ovulation may occur as soon as eight to ten days following an induced abortion, early IUD insertion also offers the advantage of immediate contraceptive protection.

In the past, a variety of IUDs were designed specifically for the purpose of insertion at the time of a full-term birth. Despite these efforts, expulsion rates for all IUDs remain significantly higher at this time. Opinions differ as to whether uterine perforation is more likely to occur when IUDs are inserted during the immediate postpartum period. In one study of almost 1,700 postpartum women who had IUDs inserted prior to discharge from the hospital, the author reported no uterine perforations. Other reports have not been as favorable. However, all studies agree that expulsion rates can be minimized if the person inserting the device is skilled, gentle, and able to place it in as high a position as possible in the endometrial cavity (see figure 3-3). In a 1984 report studying data on 2,595 IUD insertions, doctors found a significantly higher probability of expelling the device when it was inserted between ten minutes and thirty-six hours following delivery of the placenta. In contrast, expulsion rates were lowest for IUDs inserted within the first ten minutes. Other studies have found that the best time for postpartum IUD insertion is between the fourth and eighth week.

According to a 1983 article, published in *Obstetrics and Gynecology,* a woman who nurses her baby is at greater risk than a non-nursing woman of experiencing uterine perforation with an IUD. This report studied 32 women admitted to the hospital for IUD removal due to complete perforation into the abdominal cavity and 106 women admitted for removal of devices embedded in the muscle of their uteri (plural for *uterus*). They concluded that complete perforation was 10 times more likely and embedding 2.7 times more likely among women nursing at the time the IUD was inserted. In trying to explain their findings, the authors pointed out that nursing women have very low estrogen levels. This in turn causes a temporary atrophy or thinning and reduction in uterine size, thereby predisposing to perforation. It should be pointed out, however, that a 1982 study on this subject concluded that lactation had no effect on IUD perforation rates.

If I can't feel the strings, should I assume that my IUD has perforated?

In view of the fact that perforation occurs at a rate of only 1 in 2,500 insertions and that one out of every three women is unable to feel the strings even when they are in place, perforation should not be a major concern. Nevertheless, the location of your IUD must be determined. If you have been able to feel your strings in the past and suddenly are unable to do so, the odds are undoubtedly in your favor that all is well but that the string has been taken up inside your cervix. The strings will usually disappear soon after insertion if perforation has occurred. An exam by your doctor, in which the IUD is palpated with a uterine sound, will prove reassuring to both of you.

Some doctors prefer to cut the IUD strings very short, but may not explain this to their patients. This increases your difficulties in palpating the strings and the likelihood of their disappearing inside your cervix. I recommend that a woman take the time to learn to palpate her cervix and check for the IUD tail. This process should be repeated after each period, especially for the first six months, to help reassure you that the device is indeed in place.

As previously stated, if you are unable to feel your IUD strings the possibility of an accidental pregnancy must be acknowledged.

What are the dangers of becoming pregnant while using an IUD?

If the strings are visible in your cervix and you decide to continue with the pregnancy, the device should be removed immediately, regardless of the type of IUD. The risk of miscarriage will then be approximately 25 percent, compared with 50 percent if the IUD is left in place. The risk of miscarriage is normally 10 to 15 percent. The likelihood of losing a pregnancy when removing an IUD is often determined by its position in relation to the pregnancy, or gestational, sac. IUDs located below the sac can usually be safely removed, while those above will often precipitate a miscarriage. The position of the IUD in relation to the gestational sac can be accurately determined on ultrasound examination.

If the IUD strings cannot be seen, you can assume that it has been expelled without your knowledge, has been taken up into the uterus with the pregnancy, or has perforated the uterus earlier and is now in either the *myometrium* (tissues of the cervix) or the abdominal cavity. Locating the IUD without radiation exposure to the fetus may be easily accomplished with use of ultrasound. Since even a single X ray taken early in pregnancy to locate an IUD causes undue radiation exposure to the fetus, it is not recommended unless ultrasound is unavailable.

Women must understand the potentially great risk of infection while carrying a pregnancy with an IUD. For this reason early elective abortion should be considered. If you decide against terminating your pregnancy, maintain great vigilance and have the pregnancy terminated at the first evidence of infection. Symptoms of infection include cramping, low-grade fever, and abnormal bleeding or discharge. The risk of a second-trimester spontaneous abortion is increased twenty-six-fold among women carrying pregnancies in the presence of an IUD. Even more frightening is the fifty-fold increase in the maternal death rate.

At the time of delivery, the IUD will often be found attached to the placenta or in the endometrial cavity. If the IUD is not located at that time, either an ultrasound or X ray should be taken.

Women often express fears that an IUD may harm or cause deformity of the fetus by entangling a limb or other parts of the body. Fortunately, this does not happen since the IUD always lies outside the gestational sac of the baby. However, a 1979 study demonstrated that pregnancies that progressed to term with an IUD in place resulted in babies of slightly lower than normal birth weight. Concern has been expressed about whether chemicals, such as progesterone and copper, lying in close proximity to the developing fetus can cause damage. From what is known about the relationship between hormones and the fetus from research on birth-control pills (see chapter 2), this concern is certainly understandable. It is incorrect, however, to compare the fetal effects of progesterone released from the Progestasert with those of the synthetic progestins contained in birth-control pills. While the latter have the potential to cause anomalies, natural progesterone is a hormone found in abundance throughout all pregnancies. To date, there have been no malformations reported among infants following exposure to the Progestasert in utero.

Is ectopic pregnancy more common in women using an IUD?

Since the IUD prevents pregnancy in the uterus and not in the tube, any woman wearing an IUD who is found to have a positive pregnancy test should strongly suspect an ectopic pregnancy. In fact, about 3 to 4 percent of all pregnancies conceived among IUD wearers are ectopic, meaning outside the normal location in the endometrial cavity. While the fallopian tube is overwhelmingly the most common site for an ectopic pregnancy, for reasons unknown there is a significant increase among IUD users in the number of ectopics located in the ovary.

Several articles over the years have concluded that present and former IUD use increases a woman's risk of an ectopic pregnancy. Tubal infection and scarring—appearently greater with the IUD than other forms of contraception—hinder the fertilized egg from passing down the tube to its normal intrauterine location. As a result, it was theorized that the fertilized egg became trapped in the tube and grew in this abnormal location. More recent data suggest that the IUD does not increase a woman's risk of an ectopic pregnancy, but only appears to do so since it is so effective in preventing a normal pregnancy from occurring. In other words, it is a relative rather than an absolute increase in the percentage of ectopic pregnancies that we see among IUD users who accidentally conceive. Other recent research suggested that women with IUDs had only a 40 percent greater risk of an ectopic pregnancy compared to women not using contraception.

One reason for the conflicting and confusing findings in many of these studies is that, with or without the IUD, the incidence of ectopic pregnancy has almost tripled in the last ten to fifteen years. In 1970, the incidence was 4.8 ectopics per 1,000 births, compared to 1983 statistics of 14 per 1,000 births.

In a study published in the April 1977 issue of *Fertility and Sterility,* researchers reported that the percentage of ectopics among pregnant Progestasert patients was 16 percent, compared to 3 percent for women who inadvertently conceived while using a variety of other IUDs. At the time it was theorized that the release of progesterone from this device prevented the egg from moving down the tube as fast as it usually does (see Progestasert). An inadvertent pregnancy with the Progestasert was thus believed more likely to grow in the lining of the tube instead of in the endometrium of the uterus. Subsequent research by the Alza Corporation over the past few years has failed to confirm the greater risk of ectopic pregnancy with their device.

Certainly, if you conceive while using the Progestasert or any other IUD, your doctor should strongly consider the diagnosis of ectopic pregnancy. Symptoms of pregnancy accompanied by lower abdominal discomfort and a slight amount of dark vaginal bleeding should further arouse suspicion. Occasionally, it is possible for a doctor to feel an enlargement in the tube that contains the ectopic pregnancy. Movement of the cervix either through intercourse or pelvic examination will usually elicit extreme pain in the lower abdomen.

If only a minimal amount of tissue along with the IUD is removed during an abortion on an IUD user with a positive pregnancy test, ectopic pregnancy should again be strongly suspected.

It is vital that an ectopic pregnancy be diagnosed before it ruptures, since this can cause massive intra-abdominal hemorrhage and even death. Diagnosis prior to rupture is easy with the newer, highly sensitive quantitative determinations of the beta-subunit of the pregnancy hormone human chorionic gonadotropin, known as B-HCG. Combined with the use of ultrasound and laparoscopy, this test has significantly increased the number of ectopic pregnancies diagnosed prior to rupture. The benefits of this new technology are reflected in a fourfold decline in death rates from ectopic pregnancy over the last decade.

Isn't ultrasound dangerous if a woman has a copper IUD?

Ultrasound use in medicine may be either diagnostic or therapeutic. One of the many uses of diagnostic ultrasound is to locate the position of IUDs. There is a common misconception that using ultrasound in this manner could "heat" an IUD and cause damage to surrounding tissues. Based on laboratory and clinical experience, it is safe to say that these fears are unfounded. Despite the increased heat conductivity of metals, metallic objects within the body actually reflect a much higher percentage of incoming ultrasound energy and absorb it poorly, thus lessening any anticipated heating effect.

Therapeutic ultrasound is used for the treatment of a variety of medical problems such as low back pain and muscle aches and pains. The exposure to this form of energy is far greater than with diagnostic ultrasound, but there is no proof that it is harmful to a woman wearing a metallic IUD.

Is it safe for a diabetic woman to wear an IUD?

Since diabetic women are more prone than other women to a variety of bacterial infections, some gynecologists are hesitant to insert an IUD in these individuals. At present, however, there is no evidence that diabetic women are more likely than other women to contract salpingitis or PID while wearing an IUD.

Of greater concern than infection are the findings of a 1982 article in the British medical journal *Lancet*, in which a team of doctors from the Royal Infirmary in Edinburgh noted an incredible 36 percent pregnancy rate among diabetic IUD wearers, compared with 4 percent among nondiabetics. Electron microscopy of the copper-bearing IUDs removed from these women showed that 40 percent of those worn by diabetics were encrusted with sulphur and chloride deposits, compared with 15 percent of those removed from nondiabetic women. In addition, diabetic women were more likely to show erosion of the copper in their devices and less likely to have calcium deposits on them. These facts prompted the Scottish physicians to suggest that the high risk of pregnancy in diabetic women with IUDs may be linked in some way to a difference in their endometrial metabolism.

Another interesting association between diabetes and the IUD was reported by Dr. William N. Spellacy and his associates at the University of Florida College of Medicine in 1979. They evaluated carbohydrate and lipid metabolism in thirty-one women before and after one year's use of the Progestasert. There were no changes in lipid tests, though one of the blood glucose values and all of the blood insulin values were elevated. The authors concluded that the increased insulin secretion needed to maintain the blood glucose at normal levels was caused by the progesterone being released from the IUD and absorbed into the bloodstream. These changes were mild enough to encourage the authors to confirm the safety of the Progestasert, however, even in women with borderline abnormalities in their glucose metabolism prior to insertion of the device.

Do women using the IUD have a higher incidence of vaginal discharge?

The characteristic discharge associated with use of the IUD is watery, mucuslike, clear, and odorless. It does not cause itching or irritation of the vulva, and is believed to result from stimulation of the glands of the inner cervix by the presence of the IUD tail or strings. This discharge will be most noticeable near or at the time of ovulation. Cutting off the tail completely will help relieve the discharge somewhat, but it is not advisable since locating and removing the IUD will then become more difficult.

Can the tail of the IUD cause discomfort for my partner during intercourse?

Discomfort with intercourse is a rather common complaint from male partners in the days immediately following a woman's IUD insertion. This is due to the firmness of the strings of the tail, but they soften after having been bathed in the vaginal secretions for a few weeks. If your partner continues to complain of penile irritation, your doctor can cut the strings so that they barely protrude through the cervical os.

Does intercourse or orgasm cause IUDs to move?

If the IUD is in its proper location, having intercourse should not jostle it. Intercourse may cause movement of the uterus, and orgasm is known to be associated with uterine contractions, but neither should cause displacement of an IUD.

If I suddenly experience abnormal bleeding after several years with the same IUD, should I have it replaced?

The presence of bleeding in a woman using the IUD does not necessarily mean that the IUD is responsible for the bleeding. In this particular case, removing one IUD and immediately inserting another will only delay diagnosing the true cause of the bleeding. The more logical treatment in such situations is to remove the IUD and observe the menstrual pattern while another method of contraception is used. If the menstrual pattern reverts to normal, another IUD may be tried. If it doesn't, either an office sampling of the endometrium or a diagnostic D and C should be performed.

What is the relationship between IUD use and cancer of the cervix and endometrium?

I have often heard this question from my patients. There is no evidence thus far to indicate that any relationship exists between use of the IUD and cancer of any type.

How can the heavy and prolonged periods that are associated with IUD use be prevented?

The Progestasert is currently the only IUD available for insertion in the United States and is the only IUD that actually may reduce rather than increase menstrual flow. If you are currently wearing another IUD, keep in mind that the heaviest amount of bleeding is associated with insert devices such as the Lippes Loop and Saf-T-Coil, while the copper IUDs exert an intermediate effect on menstruation.

While heavy and prolonged periods as well as bleeding between periods can occur at any time after an IUD is inserted, it is most likely to happen during the first three to six months. This complication has been reported in as many as 15 to 20 percent of all IUD users and remains the main reason why women stop using the IUD. In a 1986 report from Finland, 20 percent of women wearing a copper IUD demonstrated laboratory evidence of iron deficiency secondary to heavy periods, and half of this group were overtly anemic. For this reason, many gynecologists obtain a hemoglobin blood test on all women before inserting an IUD and repeat the test at six- to twelve-month intervals in order to detect the first sign of a borderline or low hemoglobin. To prevent anemia, IUD wearers with heavy periods should take iron supplements daily.

Many remedies to decrease blood loss associated with IUD use have been tried. Vitamins C and K, cortisone, and ergotrate, a drug used to contract uterine muscles following pregnancy or abortion, have all been unsuccessful. In a 1983 study from India, doctors gave vitamin E to fifty-one women with heavy periods caused by their IUDs. Though all noted a significant decrease in blood loss, further studies on a far greater number of women must be carried out before this form of treatment can be endorsed.

Hormonal treatment in the form of birth-control pills and other hormones does control the bleeding, but most women have chosen the IUD specifically to avoid the hazards and discomfort of these medications.

It is theorized that the presence of an IUD increases the concentration of prostaglandins released from the endometrium (see prostaglandins). Prostaglandins increase vascularity and decrease blood platelet activity, and this mechanism is believed responsible for causing heavy bleeding associated with IUDs. Several articles over the last few years have impressively demonstrated that drugs classified as prostaglandin inhibitors significantly reduce menstrual pain and blood loss in 60 to 80 percent of all IUD wearers (see prostaglandin inhibitors). If taken immediately with the onset of the period, these medications can reduce menstrual blood loss by as much as one-third. Interestingly, one study noted that the greatest percentage of reduction in menstrual blood loss was among IUD wearers who had the heaviest periods and those who used the Lippes Loop and Saf-T-Coil. Examples of prostaglandin inhibitors include ibuprofen (trade name Motrin), naproxen (trade name Naprosyn and Anaprox), and mefenamic acid (trade name Ponstel). Though aspirin is another antiprostaglandin medication, it increases menstrual bleeding if ingested within five days before the period. In addition, women who take aspirin and aspirin-containing products may increase their chances of becoming pregnant. In a study from the University of Wisconsin Medical School, seventy-eight women who became pregnant while wearing IUDs took an average of seven times more aspirin a month compared to a control group. To prevent inadvertent pregnancy, the doctors conducting this research suggested that women wearing IUDs take aspirin only during the menstrual period and at doses below those normally recommended.

Is it safe for women with heart disease to wear an IUD?

All doctors should carefully question and examine women for evidence of heart disease before inserting an IUD. Those with a history of congenital heart disease or a murmur secondary to rheumatic fever are at risk of contracting a life-threatening bacterial infection of their heart valves, called *endocarditis*. Though this condition is extremely rare, it may occur when bacteria are introduced into the endometrial cavity at the time that the IUD is inserted. From the endometrium, the bacteria can enter the bloodstream and travel to the heart valves and infect them. In order to destroy the main strains of bacteria that cause endocarditis, cardiologists recommend prophylactic antibiotics starting on the day before and continuing until the day after the IUD is inserted. The antibiotics should be a combination of penicillin or ampicillin, or another antibiotic class known as cephalosporins, combined with either gentamycin or streptomycin. There are many cardiologists and gynecologists who believe that the risk of IUD infection in the months and years following the initial insertion of an IUD is just too great for women with heart disease.

Mitral valve prolapse is a mild, usually harmless heart condition that has received much publicity in the 1980s (see discussion of birth-control pills and mitral valve prolapse in chapter 2). It has been estimated that 10 to 17 percent of women have some degree of mitral valve prolapse. Women with this condition usually show no symptoms and require no medication or limitation of their activities. Since IUD insertion carries a low risk of endocarditis, and since endocarditis develops only rarely in women with mitral valve prolapse, most doctors do not prescribe antibiotics under these circumstances. Occasionally, prophylactic antibiotics are used for more serious cases of mitral valve prolapse in which there is a significant murmur or ultrasound evidence of marked mitral valve ballooning, or prolapse.

Can an IUD be removed at the same time that a tubal sterilization is performed?

The most commonly used method of sterilization in the United States is the burning or coagulation of the fallopian tubes with a laparoscope, a viewing instrument inserted into the abdominal cavity through the umbilicus (see chapter 9, "Tubal Ligation"). While some gynecologists will remove an IUD at the same time that they perform laparoscopic sterilization, others hesitate because they believe it increases a woman's chances of postoperative salpingitis and pelvic inflammatory disease (PID). There are no scientific studies to substantiate such a fear, but a relevant report was published in 1986 in *The Journal of Reproductive Medicine* on forty-nine women who underwent laparoscopic sterilization combined with removal of their IUDs. The doctors found it a safe procedure that was not associated with an increased risk of postoperative infection. They concluded that cauterization, or burning, of the tubes completely destroyed the tubal segments and any bacteria living in them. It is not known at the present time whether removal of an IUD combined with tubal sterilization methods other than cauterization, such as banding and clips, results in an increased risk of postoperative salpingitis and PID.

What is a reasonable fee for inserting an IUD?

Fees vary. They may range from $25.00 in a family planning clinic to more than $200 in certain exclusive practices. As previously stated (see Progestasert), as of July 1986 the price of a Progestasert to doctors and others who insert them rose from $38.00 to $84.00. Bear in mind that this fee does not usually include the doctor's charge for inserting the device and that a Progestasert must be replaced yearly. Though the total cost is probably comparable to that of a year's supply of birth-control pills, for many women it is less of a financial burden to pay small amounts for pills every few months than to receive one large bill for an IUD insertion.

Since the Copper-7 and Tatum-T are available in Canada at a total insertion cost of 40 to 75 Canadian dollars, many American women are combining long weekend vacations with visits to Canadian doctors and clinics for one of these IUDs. It could be well worth the trip in view of the fact that these devices do not have to be changed for three or possibly four years after insertion.

What safeguards should be made available to women before the Progestasert is inserted?

Physicians should obtain either oral or written consent before inserting an IUD. Women should have adequate time, well in advance of the date scheduled for actual insertion, to read the labeling and to study the list of all potential IUD complications. The Alza Corporation, manufacturer of the Progestasert, has published an excellent patient information bulletin containing all of the important facts one should know before having this device inserted.

I have noted in my own practice that a considerable number of women opt for safer alternatives when given time to reflect on the potential hazards of this form of contraception. In the following chapter I will discuss some of these safer, though somewhat less effective, methods.

4

BARRIER CONTRACEPTION

With the removal of most IUDs from the U.S. market and the widespread though unsubstantiated fear that many women have of oral contraceptives, there has been a sudden and well-deserved awakening of interest in barrier contraception. While diaphragms, condoms, spermicidal jellies and creams, and aerosol foams have been available for many years, it is the newer methods such as the TODAY brand vaginal contraceptive sponge, contraceptive suppositories and tablets, and cervical caps that are most responsible for the rise in popularity of barrier devices. In addition, the fear of contracting newer and more devastating forms of sexually transmitted diseases has served as a stimulus for the use of these so-called old-fashioned methods. From 1973 to 1982 oral contraceptive and IUD use declined significantly, while from 1982 to 1987 the drop has been precipitous. In contrast, barrier method popularity has demonstrated a dramatic rise over the past fourteen years. It is estimated that approximately 23 percent of women currently practicing contraception use some type of barrier method. The wisdom of this trend is supported by large epidemiological studies that have repeatedly confirmed that barrier contraception backed up by early induced abortion of unwanted pregnancies is the safest method of birth control.

DIAPHRAGM

What is a diaphram?

A diaphragm is a flexible metal ring covered with latex rubber in the shape of a shallow dome (see figure 4-1). It is placed in the vagina so as to completely encircle the cervix, thereby preventing sperm from entering the uterus (see figure 4-2). When used with a spermicidal (sperm-killing) jelly or cream applied to the side of the dome facing the cervix, it can be a very effective contraceptive.

How long has the diaphragm been used as a contraceptive?

Believe it or not, an early description of three different types of primitive diaphragms appears in Egyptian writings and drawings dating back to 1850 B.C. These devices consisted of honey adhering to crocodile dung to form a potent barrier to sperm, and probably to romance as well. Later, more sophisticated discs of oiled silk paper were introduced in China and Japan, while Europeans employed linen cloths and wafers of molded wax. During the eighteenth century, some women inserted a ball of gold into the vagina in order to prevent pregnancy. Though today's diaphragms resemble those first used in Germany at the end of the nineteenth century, it was Casanova who first

Diaphragm

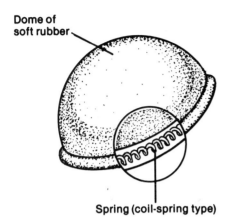

Dome of
soft rubber

Figure 4–1. *Coil-spring diaphragm.*

Spring (coil-spring type)

envisioned one of the more original diaphragms around 1750: the rind of half a lemon placed against the cervix. The rind served as a mechanical barrier against sperm while the citric acid of the juice proved a strong spermicidal agent. For centuries prior to this discovery, less effective mechanical barriers had been used, such as leaves, plugs of wool soaked in oil, fig pulp, and sea sponges. Sponges had the advantage of being relatively clean and were reusable. In recent years there has been a resurgence in the use of these simple sea sponges in many areas of the world.

It was illegal in the United States in the early 1900s to provide contraceptive services to women. In defiance of this law, Margaret Sanger devoted her life to this cause. In 1916, her sister was imprisoned for distributing diaphragms, which had been illegally imported from Germany.

Modern diaphragms are used by approximately 6 to 8 percent of all women practicing contraception in the United States today.

Where do I get a diaphragm and how do I learn to use it properly?

You must be measured or fitted for your correct diaphragm size in a doctor's office or in a family planning clinic. The doctor may supply the diaphragm himself or a prescription for the specific type and size can be filled by a pharmacist. Spermicidal creams and jellies are available without a prescription. It takes only a few minutes to be measured for a diaphragm, but once the size is determined it is the obligation of the person fitting it to take the time to explain the simple anatomy involved as well as the proper insertion technique. You should practice inserting the diaphragm without assistance and then have its proper position checked by the person instructing you. Regardless of how many attempts may end in failure, you shouldn't leave the office or clinic until you are satisfied that you fully understand the insertion technique.

Occasionally when a woman has become discouraged after several unsuccessful insertion attempts, I will tell her to practice in the privacy of her home and then return to the office on another day wearing the diaphragm so that we can be sure it is inserted correctly. Obviously, it is important to use alternative contraception during this learning period. Once the insertion technique is learned, the diaphragm is extremely simple to use.

What determines the diaphragm size?

The diaphragm size is dependent on the size and shape of the vagina, which in turn is determined by body size, body build, body structure, previous intercourse, and previous childbearing. With childbearing, the vaginal walls and supporting muscles often undergo stretch and become weaker. A woman usually needs a larger size diaphragm after giving birth. In addition, the type of diaphragm prescribed will depend on the firmness or laxity of your vaginal tissues. The diameter of the rim determines the diaphragm size, and sizes are measured from 60 to 105 millimeters.

What is the proper way to insert a diaphragm?

For greatest effectiveness the diaphragm should be inserted within the six hours prior to coitus, since the spermicidal cream or jelly will lose its potency after this time. Inserting the diaphragm several hours earlier and then injecting cream into the vagina

Figure 4–2. *Correctly placed diaphragm.*

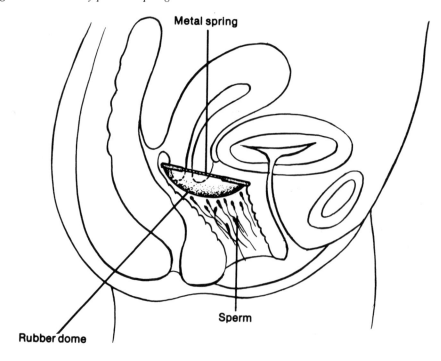

Figure 4–3. *Proper insertion of diaphragm.*

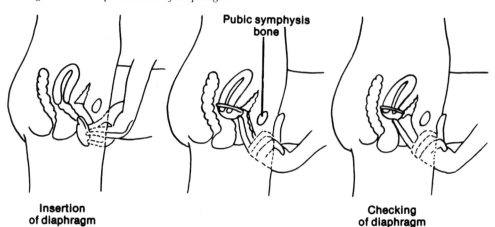

immediately before intercourse isn't enough, since these substances must first be applied to the side of the dome facing the cervix. When applying the cream or jelly to the diaphragm, put a very thin film on the rim to prevent the sperm from passing between the rim and vaginal wall. Applying too much to the rim will make the diaphragm more likely to slip during intercourse. A teaspoonful of cream or jelly in the cup is usually adequate.

The diaphragm can be inserted while you are in any position you find comfortable; probably the most commonly used position is standing with one foot resting on a stool or toilet seat. First squeeze the diaphragm in half by pressing the rim between the thumb and middle finger, and then insert it (figure 4-3). The diaphragm may be inserted by hand or by using a small plastic or metal inserter (figure 4-4), available wherever diaphragms are sold. Insertion is easier if you push the rim against the back wall of the vagina as far as possible, ensuring that the back of the rim has passed beyond the cervix. Then release the diaphragm from its bent position. Feel the dome with your finger to be sure that the cervix is in its center and that the rim completely encircles it. The front rim of the diaphragm should fit snugly under the pubic symphysis bone (see figure 4-3).

What are the different types of diaphragms?

There are three basic diaphragm types. The coil-spring type is made of a cadmium-plated coil spring encased in latex (see figure 4-1), and is compressible when bent in any plane. The two most popular brands of this type are the Ortho Diaphragm and the Koromex Coil Spring. The coil-spring diaphragm is especially suited to women with strong vaginal muscle tone and a deep arch behind the pubic symphysis bone.

The flat-spring, or Mensinga, diaphragm is also covered with latex but it contains a flat, watch-type spring that allows it to be compressed in one plane only, rather than at any point of the rim as are the more flexible coil-spring types. This feature often allows for easier, less slippery insertions. The Ortho-White Diaphragm is an example of a flat-spring diaphragm, which works best for the nulliparous woman with strong vaginal muscles and the woman whose vagina is of normal length but somewhat narrowed. It is more applicable to those with a shallow, rather than a deep, arch behind the symphysis bone as determined by vaginal examination at the time the diaphragm is fitted. The flat-spring diaphragm is also preferable in situations where the uterus is tilted forward, or anteflexed, and the cervix is long and facing backward, or posteriorly.

If you are unable to place the diaphragm behind your cervix, an arcing-spring diaphragm is probably best. When compressed, this diaphragm assumes a half-moon, or arc, shape that makes it easier to pass along the vaginal floor and beyond the cervix. Women with poor vaginal muscle tone, mild cystocele, rectocele, or uterine prolapse (see chapter 10, "Hysterectomy") will benefit most from this type of diaphragm. Other indications include marked anteflexion or retroflexion of the uterus and a shallow pubic arch, which makes it difficult to secure the front rim of the diaphragm behind the pubic symphysis bone. Examples of arcing diaphragms are the Ortho All Flex and the Koro-Flex Arcing Spring Diaphragm.

Comparative studies of failure rates among the three diaphragm types have never been conducted.

Another type of diaphragm, called a Matrisalus, is rarely, if ever, used today. Its rim is in the shape of a special pessary named Smith-Hodge. *Pessaries* are devices made of plastic or rubber that come in a variety of sizes and shapes. When inserted into the vagina they are helpful in supporting sagging vaginal tissues found with cystocele, rectocele, and severe uterine prolapse. This type of diaphragm has been used for both contraception and for support of these tissues. However, it is extremely difficult to fit.

Figure 4–4. A–D *Proper use of the diaphragm inserter.*

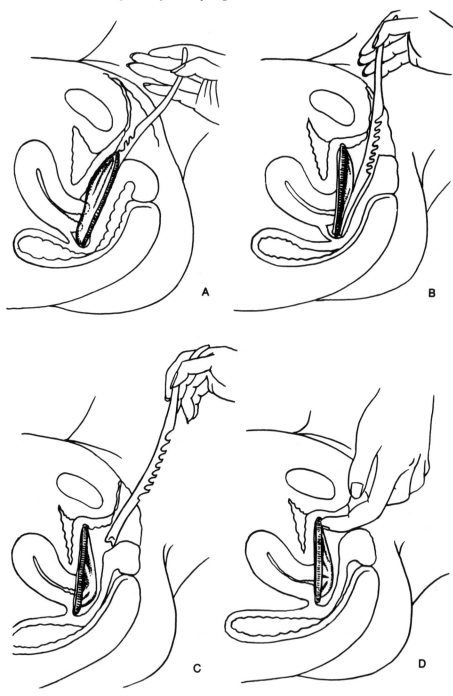

How is a diaphragm inserter used?

Diaphragm inserters, or introducers, are intended for use only with the coil- and flat-spring diaphragms. Inserters cannot be used with an arcing-spring diaphragm because the arcing spring is too flexible and becomes dislodged soon after it is placed on the inserter. By far the most popular inserters are the Ortho Universal Introducer and the Koromex Introducer, plastic devices that are designed for use with any coil- or flat-spring diaphragm brand.

One end of the inserter has a smooth, round hook for use in removing the diaphragm, simply by grasping it under the front rim. To insert the diaphragm (refer to figure 4-4), one end of its rim is placed in the notch at the end of the inserter without the hook. Each of the little notches located in the middle of the inserter has a number corresponding to each diaphragm size. Place the diaphragm on the inserter by squeezing it and slipping one end of the rim in the end notch and the other end in the notch corresponding to your diaphragm size. It is best to apply spermicidal jelly or cream after the diaphragm is on the inserter. Otherwise, stretching the slippery, lubricated diaphragm onto the inserter may prove difficult and messy.

After you have inserted the diaphragm as far as possible, release it by giving the inserter a slight twist. After the inserter is removed, use your index finger to push the front of the diaphragm securely under the pubic symphysis bone.

How successfully does the diaphragm prevent pregnancy?

Until recently, most studies have demonstrated pregnancy rates to be significantly higher with a diaphragm than with an IUD or birth-control pills. Even in highly motivated women, the lowest pregnancy rates achieved were usually no better than 6 per 100 woman-years. In the medical literature, the most commonly quoted pregnancy rates attributed to diaphragm use vary between 13 and 20 per 100 woman-years, though failure rates have been reported in some studies to be as low as 2.2 and as high as 23 pregnancies per 100 woman-years. In one study from Oxford, England, involving 4,000 diaphragm users, researchers demonstrated a remarkably low pregnancy rate of only 2.4 per 100 woman-years. Furthermore, these rates fell sharply as a woman's age increased and with each month that the diaphragm was used. It is also of interest to note that the pregnancy rate was lower for women who already had as many children as they wanted than for those who desired more children or who were uncertain about their intentions in this respect. These findings demonstrate the importance of motivation in the success of this method of contraception.

Unfortunately, there have been no recent studies dealing with diaphragm efficacy, but in 1976 the Margaret Sanger Research Bureau published the results of the largest contemporary diaphragm study ever conducted in the United States. Of 2,168 women using this method of contraception, accidental pregnancies in the first twelve months of use ranged from a low of 1.9 per 100 women less than eighteen years of age to a high of 3 per 100 women aged thirty to thirty-four. At the end of one year, approximately 84 women out of every 100 elected to continue using the diaphragm. The Margaret Sanger Research team attributed the success to patients' motivaton as well as to the motivation, skill, and patience of the instructors teaching the proper use of the diaphragm. They also noted that once a patient chose the diaphragm method, she used it successfully regardless of her age, ethnic background, marital status, or number of children.

It is interesting that the pregnancy rates cited in these reports are so much lower than those quoted in several other large studies conducted in the United States and Europe. It is obvious from these discrepancies that the success of the diaphragm depends to a great degree on skillful explanation given by an enthusiastic instructor to a motivated woman. With that combination, the pregnancy rate for diaphragm users should approach that of the IUD.

Figure 4–5. *Pregnancy rates by method of contraception and motivation of user. (Courtesy of* Contemporary OB/GYN, *Medical Economics Company.)*

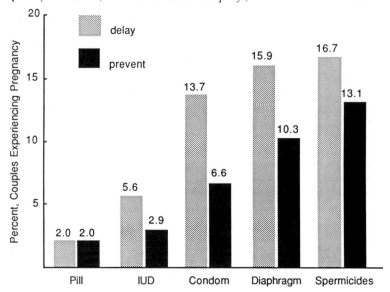

How does diaphragm use compare in effectiveness to other contraceptive methods?

Since the range of effectiveness varies dramatically between individuals and from one study to another, accurate comparisons are difficult if not impossible. Further complicating meaningful interpretation is the fact that different investigators use different statistical methods and definitions of effectiveness. Figure 4-5 shows the results of a study comparing the accidental pregnancy rates for different methods of contraception during the first twelve months of use per 100 married American women from fifteen to forty-four years of age. Though no single study can determine the true effectiveness of a particular contraceptive, figure 4-5 does give us a good general idea of the relative pregnancy risk associated with each method during the first twelve months of use.

It is especially interesting to note in the figure that the success of any method is directly related to the motivation of the individual to use it carefully and consistently. When the intention is to prevent rather than to delay pregnancy, failure rates will be significantly lower with all methods except the Pill.

How can pregnancy rates for diaphragm users be reduced?

Improper placement, because of either poor instructions by medical personnel or excessive haste by the woman using the diaphragm, is the main cause of pregnancy. No more than six hours should elapse from the time the diaphragm with spermicide is inserted until coitus takes place. To minimize pregnancy risk, two hours or less is preferred. In addition, the diaphragm must be left in for at least six hours after intercourse to ensure that all sperm in the vagina are dead. If you remove a diaphragm before that time, living sperm can enter the cervix. A second intercourse within six hours should be preceded by insertion of more spermicidal cream or jelly into the vagina, offering additional protection against the influx of new sperm. It is important that great care be taken at this time not to disturb the diaphragm from its secure position. If multiple acts of coitus takes place, the diaphragm should not be removed until at least six hours have elapsed after the last encounter. Though it is possible that repeated acts of intercourse could necessitate use of the diaphragm for more than twenty-four hours, its use beyond this length of time is not recommended due to the greater risk of toxic shock syndrome, or TSS (see toxic shock syndrome, page 118). Never douche while a diaphragm is in place, because the solution dilutes the spermicide and increases the risk of pregnancy.

If the diaphragm appears to move during intercourse, the size should be rechecked. It is better to have a diaphragm that is too large than one that is too small, but if bleeding or discomfort follows coitus it may mean that the diaphragm is too large and is irritating the vaginal walls. Sizes should also be rechecked following full-term pregnancy, second-trimester abortion, or a weight gain or loss greater than fifteen pounds.

Examine your diaphragm frequently for defects or holes by running water over the dome and observing for leaks. Another method is to hold the diaphragm up to the light and stretch the rubber gently between your fingers. When removing the diaphragm from the vagina, hook your index finger under the front rim as it is pulled out, taking care to avoid puncturing the dome with your fingernail. Then wash the diaphragm with soap and water, dry it, and dust it with cornstarch. A diaphragm lasts longer if it is stored in its container when not in use. Eventually the latex rubber of the diaphragm will deteriorate, so it is a good practice to replace it routinely every two to three years. Often, the rubber around the rim will pucker before cracks appear. At the first sign of puckering, the device should be replaced.

Perhaps the greatest obstacle against reducing pregnancy rates is the maturity and motivation of the couple using the diaphragm. Although all methods of contraception require a certain degree of motivation, it is especially true of the diaphragm. Too often a "diaphragm failure" really means that it was never used. The best diaphragm success rates are in those women who insert the diaphragm every night before going to bed, and remove it the following morning. When intercourse is spontaneous at other times during the day, a mature man patiently waits while his partner inserts the diaphragm. The woman does not have to be the one who inserts the diaphragm; active participation by her partner in this act can represent both a sensual and a mature expression of his feelings.

If all these precautions are followed, why does the pregnancy rate with diaphragm use remain so high?

Unfortunately, other factors prevail. The vagina expands naturally during sexual excitation and intercourse, which can cause even a properly fitted diaphragm to become loose. Frequent penile thrusts and woman-above coital positions can also loosen the diaphragm and increase the risk of pregnancy.

Aren't there some authorities who believe that fitting a diaphragm is unnecessary and that one size can fit all women?

In 1980 Edward M. Stim, M.D., claimed that all women can use a 60 millimeter arcing-spring diaphragm and achieve pregnancy rates of only 1 per 100 woman-years. In addition, based on his research of over 1,200 women, Dr. Stim claimed that spermicides were unimportant in reducing the pregnancy rate and only served to discourage diaphragm use because of their messiness.

Following presentation of his data at the annual meeting of the Association of Planned Parenthood Physicians, Dr. Stim's theories were soundly denounced by several authorities in the field of contraceptive research. Based on currently available data, one would be ill-advised not to use a properly fitted diaphragm in combination with a spermicidal jelly or cream.

Are there any medical problems associated with use of the diaphragm?

There is no doubt that diaphragm users are more susceptible to urinary tract infections than women using other forms of contraception. In a 1985 report, published in the *Journal of the American Medical Association,* Dr. Stephen D. Fihn and his associates at the University of Washington in Seattle found the incidence of urinary tract infections to be 27 per 1,000 patient-months for women using the diaphragm, compared with 8.9 per 1,000 patient-months for those on oral contraceptives. These differences could not be attributed to differences in age, number of children, sexual activity, or previous urinary tract infections. Other researchers have repeatedly confirmed these findings. The most likely reason for the association between diaphragm use and urinary tract infections is that the front rim of the diaphragm impinges on the urethra and partially obstructs it. As a result, some women are unable to empty the urinary bladder completely after intercourse. The stagnant urine remaining in the bladder becomes a perfect site for bacterial contamination, reproduction, and infection. Replacing an ill-fitting diaphragm with a slightly smaller size will often relieve the problem without incurring an increased risk of pregnancy. In one study conducted by urologists, women with recurrent urinary tract infections were refitted with smaller diaphragms and instructed to void immediately after intercourse. Follow-up one year later showed that almost 100 percent of the women who used this regimen were infection-free.

It has been suggested that the mere presence of the diaphragm in the vagina alters its bacterial flora and predisposes to a variety of urinary and vaginal infections. One bacterial organism, named *Escherichia coli,* is a common cause of urinary tract infections. Doctors have been able to culture *Escherichia coli* from the vaginas of diaphragm users with significantly greater frequency than from those of other women, suggesting a greater likelihood of bacterial passage of this organism from the vagina to the urethra. The alteration of the vaginal flora by the diaphragm also helps explain why women who choose this method of contraception seem to be more susceptible to vaginitis caused by bacteria and yeast. Recurrent yeast or monilial infections may occasionally result in the presence of microscopic spores of the organism surviving on the latex rubber of the diaphragm for prolonged periods of time. Reusing the diaphragm can then recontaminate the vagina. To rid your diaphragm of monilial spores would require boiling it, which would destroy its shape and reduce its effectiveness. It is probably a better idea to treat the vaginitis pharmaceutically and then purchase a new diaphragm.

A small percentage of men and women experience allergic reactions to the latex rubber or to the spermicide. Symptoms may include a rash, severe burning, and itching. If this occurs, alternative methods of contraception are recommended.

One of the most ominous, and fortunately one of the rarest, complications of diaphragm use is toxic shock syndrome, or TSS (see TSS question in this chapter). This potentially deadly disease is caused by a bacterial organism named *Staphylococcus aureas* and is far more likely to occur with use of tampons at the time of the period. Researchers have theorized that this organism can enter the circulation via abrasions of the vaginal wall caused by pressure of the diaphragm. Though toxic shock syndrome has been reported to occur with diaphragms left in place for as little as seven to nine hours, in the majority of instances the time has exceeded twenty-four hours. Removal of the diaphragm six to eight hours after intercourse will almost completely eliminate the risk of TSS.

It has recently been suggested in the medical literature that the sexually transmitted hepatitis B virus and perhaps the deadly AIDS virus could be transmitted via reusable diaphragm fitting rings which are used in clinics and doctors' offices. This should never occur if the disinfection procedure recommended by the ring manufacture is carefully carried out. To inactivate these viruses, the rings must be washed with soap and water followed by immersion in a 70 percent alcohol solution for fifteen minutes. Diaphragm fitting rings should be routinely checked for deep cracks or scratches that could make adequate cleaning and disinfecting difficult.

Which women can benefit most from using the diaphragm?

The diaphragm is an ideal contraceptive for women for whom accidental pregnancy would not be a physically, emotionally, or religiously devastating experience.

Women more than forty years old and those approaching menopause are well advised to use the diaphragm since the chances of conception are lower at this age, while the dangers and side effects of the Pill are greater. The diaphragm is also an ideal contraceptive for a woman having infrequent intercourse. Taking birth control pills every day in anticipation of only an occasional sexual encounter appears to impose too high a risk on a woman. If you normally abstain from intercourse during the menstrual period because it would be too messy, inserting the diaphragm over the cervix at that time solves the problem. Since the risk of pregnancy is minimal during the menstrual period, the diaphragm may be removed at your leisure over the next one to two hours following coitus. Once again, leaving the diaphragm in for longer periods of time during the menses may make one more susceptible to TSS.

Are there women who should not use the diaphragm?

Occasionally, anatomical factors, such as a severely anteflexed or retroflexed uterus (see chapter 1), prevent proper diaphragm encirclement of the cervix. Complete uterine prolapse and severe cystocele and rectocele may also deter you from using the diaphragm (see chapter 7). Also, women who have not been accustomed to having intercourse may find the diaphragm uncomfortable, at least for the first few encounters.

If you feel uneasy about touching your genitals, chances are you will not be comfortable using a diaphragm. Some women find inserting the diaphragm and jelly to be repugnant and messy. To avoid getting excessive amounts of jelly or cream on your hands, you can use an inserter instead. Many men find the presence of spermicide at the entroitus, or opening to the vagina, a distinct source of displeasure during oral-genital sex. Still other couples believe that the spontaneity of precoital lovemaking is lost when time is taken to insert a diaphragm.

As previously mentioned, the diaphragm is not the best choice of contraception for women needing 100 percent protection, or those with recurrent bacterial urinary tract infections or vaginitis caused by monilia. In addition, in situations where there is a sensitivity to either the latex rubber of the diaphragm or the spermicidal preparations, other measures would be preferable. Finally, if you or your sexual partner are not motivated to use this method enthusiastically, it will undoubtedly fail.

Is there anything else I should know about contraceptive jellies and creams used with a diaphragm?

If you experience burning, irritation, or a rash in the genital area from the ingredients of a spermicide, switch to a brand with a different active ingredient. At the present time, your choices are limited to nonoxynol-9, octoxynol-9, glyceryl ricinoleate, methoxypolyethoxy ethylene glycol, p-diisobutylphenoxypolyethoxyethanol, dodeco-ethylene-glycol monolaurate, and ricinoleic acid hexylresorcinol. Until recently, several contraceptive jellies and creams contained phenylmercuric acetate, which is an organic mercury compound. This dangerous chemical is no longer found in any vaginal contraceptive preparations currently manufactured in the United States.

The majority of women using a diaphragm prefer contraceptive jelly to the cream because it provides better lubrication during intercourse. The brand of contraceptive agent does not have to be the same as that of the diaphragm, and you should sample a variety of brands to determine which you prefer. The table that follows lists the most commonly used vaginal spermicidal (sperm-killing) agents. Aerosols or foam should not be used with a diaphragm because they cannot adhere to the latex rubber to form a seal between the cervix and the diaphragm membrane. But if intercourse is repeated within six hours of the initial coitus, with the diaphragm already in place with cream or jelly, an applicator full of foam may be inserted. Some women mistakenly use petroleum jelly with a diaphragm. This substance not only has little if any spermicidal effect, but can also cause deterioration of the latex rubber.

Though the manufacturers of the various creams and jellies always specify whether a product is to be used alone or only with a diaphragm, my conversations with various drug representatives have convinced me that all the creams and jellies listed in this table can be used with the diaphragm. But not all creams and jellies designed for use with the diaphragm are safe enough to be used alone. The pregnancy rate achieved under such circumstances may range from a not-so-low 11 to a high of 38 per 100 woman-years.

COMMONLY USED VAGINAL SPERMICIDAL AGENTS

PRODUCT

Creams	Spermicidal Agent	Percentage of Spermicidal Agent	Manufacturer
Conceptrol	nonoxynol-9	5 %	Ortho
Delfen	nonoxynol-9	5	Ortho
Koromex	octoxynol	3	Schmid
Foams			
Because	nonoxynol-9	8	Schering
Delfen	nonoxynol-9	12.5	Ortho
Emko and Emko Pre-Fill	nonoxynol-9	8	Schering
Koromex	nonoxynol-9	12.5	Schmid
Jellies			
Conceptrol	nonoxynol-9	4	Ortho
Koromex	octoxynol	1	Schmid
Ramses	nonoxynol-9	5	Schmid
Suppositories			
Encare	nonoxynol-9	2.5	Norwich-Eaton
Intercept	nonoxynol-9	5.6	Ortho
Ortho-forms	nonoxynol-9	2	Ortho
Semicid	nonoxynol-9	5	Whitehall
S Positive	nonoxynol-9	10	Jordan-Simner
Sponge			
Today	nonoxynol-9	—	VLI
Film			
VCF	nonoxynol-9	28	Apothecus

SOURCE: *Compiled by the author.*.

It is not clear why the stronger preparations are not promoted for use both alone and with the diaphragm. Company representatives have given me several answers, including fear of deterioration of the rubber with prolonged use, and fewer packaging problems by enclosing one jelly or cream with each diaphragm rather than four or five possible choices. The most logical reason given to me is that the contraceptive action of the less concentrated spermicides is more than adequate when they are used with a properly fitting diaphragm. Pregnancies that result from diaphragm use are rarely due to insufficient concentration of the spermicide.

How much does a diaphragm cost?

The cost of a diaphragm at a retail pharmacy ranges between $14.00 and $16.00. Arcing-spring diaphragms, such as the Ortho All-Flex, are sometimes more expensive because of their unique construction. The discount pharmacies I sampled sold diaphragms for $12.00 to $15.00. If you take good care of your diaphragm it should last for several years. As soon as it becomes puckered or cracked, or loses its shape, it is best to get a new one immediately. Diaphragms may become discolored with time, but they can still be used. To check for small defects, hold the diaphragm up to the light and stretch the rubber between your fingers. Defects can also be detected by filling the dome with a small amount of water and checking for leaks.

Contraceptive jelly and cream costs about $7.00 to $8.00 per tube at a retail pharmacy and slightly less at a discount pharmacy. The best buy is a large tube since it contains enough spermicide for approximately ten applications. The premeasured and preloaded single dose applicators, such as Conceptrol Disposable Contraceptive Gel, are proportionately far more expensive than the larger do-it-yourself products.

Does a diaphragm help prevent sexually transmitted diseases?

By forming a seal with the cervical os, the diaphragm plays a very important role in preventing the ascent of sexually transmitted bacteria, such as chlamydia and gonorrhea, into the uterus and fallopian tubes. Type 2 herpes simplex virus is known to be transmitted via sexual intercourse. Though the diaphragm can't prevent herpes of the outer genital area or lower vagina, it does help stop its spread to the upper vagina and cervix.

Cancer of the cervix is also thought to be a sexually transmitted disease. Evidence shows that it is most prevalent in women who engage in intercourse both at an early age and with numerous sexual partners (see chapter 2). Until recently, it was believed that the herpes virus was most responsible for the development of precancerous changes of the cervix—known as dysplasia, pre-invasive cancer, or carcinoma-in-situ—as well as for the more dangerous invasive form of the disease. There is now considerable evidence to suggest that the human papilloma virus, or HPV, is probably the cause of precancerous and cancerous cervical disease. This is the same organism responsible for venereal warts of the vulva and vagina, though only a few specific strains of the virus have been implicated in inciting cellular abnormalities in the cervix. Several medical publications have suggested that the diaphragm offers a mechanical barrier against HPV or whatever agent is responsible for causing cervical cancer. In a 1978 article from Oxford University in England, doctors compared rates of dysplasia and carcinoma-in-situ among 17,000 women using the diaphragm, IUD, or birth control pills for contraception. Their findings, charted in per 1,000 woman-years, are a convincing endorsement of the diaphragm's protective effect:

	Oral Contraceptives	IUDs	Diaphragm
Dysplasia	31	28	0
Carcinoma in-situ	45	43	0

Based on these statistics, the authors hypothesized that the diaphragm protected the cervix from direct contact with seminal fluid and its cancer-causing agent.

It should be pointed out, however, that these two studies do not prove convincingly that the diaphragm is protective against cancer of the cervix. Certainly other factors such as the personality, sexual habits, and lifestyle of a woman choosing one form of contraception over another would have to be more intensively studied before definite conclusions could be drawn.

In addition to studying the effects of diaphragm use in preventing sexually transmitted diseases, researchers have attempted to learn more about the role played by spermicides. Laboratory studies have demonstrated that nonoxynol-9, the spermicide found in most contraceptive foams, jellies, and creams, has the ability either to kill or to inactivate the organisms responsible for causing gonorrhea, syphilis, chlamydia, herpes, trichomoniasis, and venereal warts. Even the deadly AIDS virus, HTLV-III, can be inactivated with nonoxynol-9.

Unfortunately, what occurs in the laboratory may not take place in the human body. This was demonstrated in a 1984 study by doctors at the University of Alabama at Birmingham who compared 735 women with gonorrhea and about 1,000 controls without gonorrhea. While the women using spermicides had a 33 percent reduction in their gonorrhea risk, closer examination of these statistics revealed that this only occurred when it was combined with either a diaphragm or a condom. Use of the spermicide alone played no significant role in preventing gonorrhea. In a similar 1982 study evaluating 645 women hospitalized for pelvic inflammatory disease (PID), epidemiologists at the Centers for Disease Control concluded that hospitalization rates for PID could be reduced by 40 percent if spermicides were used with either a diaphragm or a condom. When used alone, they offered no PID protection. Interestingly, the diaphragm fared better than the condom as a barrier to PID. Based on their statistics, these epidemiologists estimated that the six million barrier-method users in the United States are spared 20,000 episodes of PID and 5,000 hospitalizations for this disease each year.

THE TODAY SPONGE

What is the TODAY Vaginal Contraceptive Sponge and how does it prevent pregnancy?

While natural sea sponges have been used for contraception since the days of antiquity, the modern version of this idea was approved by the FDA in 1983. Since then, the TODAY Vaginal Contraceptive Sponge has gained great popularity in the United States, with an estimated 1.5 million users annually.

The TODAY Vaginal Contraceptive Sponge, manufactured by the V.L.I. Corporation of Irvine, California, is best described as a small, round, disposable, soft, squeezable polyurethane sponge that contains one gram of the spermicide nonoxynol-9. The sponge has a concave dimple on one side which is intended to fit over the cervix and decrease the chance of dislodgement during intercourse (see figure 4-6). The other side of the sponge has a woven polyester loop or retrieval string used to facilitate its removal. Unlike the diaphragm, the TODAY sponge is available in only one size and does not require a prescription.

To activate the spermicide in the sponge, you must moisten it in tap water immediately before inserting it deep in the vagina. Once it is in place, the sponge releases nonoxynol-9 at a steady rate for up to thirty hours, providing immediate and continuous contraception. Though it must never be left in the vagina for longer than twenty-four hours (see TSS, page 118), it has the unique advantage of not requiring any additional applications of spermicide for as long as it is left in place. To ensure the

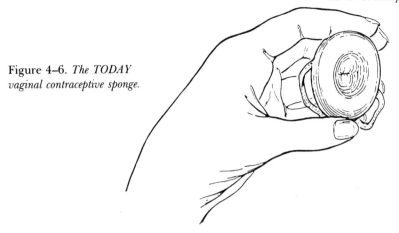

Figure 4–6. *The TODAY*
vaginal contraceptive sponge.

greatest sperm-killing effect, it is best not to remove the TODAY sponge until at least eight hours after the last coital act. After removal, the sponge should be discarded.

While many women express concern that the sponge's small size will prevent it from adequately covering the cervix and blocking the ascent of sperm, the fact is that this is its least important mechanism of contraceptive action. Far more effective is the dispersion of nonoxynol-9 over the cervix and upper vagina. In addition, laboratory research has shown that the TODAY sponge has the capacity to absorb sperm for up to twenty-four hours.

Isn't it true that the TODAY sponge contains carcinogenic agents?

When the TODAY sponge was first introduced in 1983, detractors claimed that it contained three compounds known to be carcinogenic: dioxane, ethylene oxide, and toluenediisocyanate (TDA). Careful analysis by the FDA, however, has demonstrated that there is no risk of cancer associated with the TODAY sponge.

Dioxane should not be confused with dioxin, a highly toxic compound. Dioxane is found in all nonoxynol-9 spermicides, and practically 100 percent of it evaporates and disappears in the process of manufacturing the sponge. Ethylene oxide is used in the process of synthesizing nonoxynol-9. When mixed with water, it forms a harmless compound with the nonoxynol-9 and the polyurethane in the sponge. And the TDA is rendered harmless in the sponge's manufacturing process. Any remaining traces of it would be present only in inactive, infinitesimal amounts.

Several laboratory studies have demonstrated that, regardless of the barrier method used, a small amount of the spermicide placed in the vagina will be absorbed into the bloodstream. Though it has been theorized that this may have a cumulative effect and eventually produce organ damage and cancer, at the present time there is no evidence to support this hypothesis.

How do pregnancy rates associated with use of the TODAY sponge compare to those of the diaphragm?

Data accumulated from several medical centers in the United States and the United Kingdom clearly show that the diaphragm is more effective than the TODAY sponge in preventing pregnancy. In a 1985 U.S. study, doctors reported an overall pregnancy rate of 17 per 100 woman-years among 723 TODAY users, compared with 13 per 100 woman-years for 717 women using the diaphragm. Further breakdown of these statistics revealed that parous women, those who have had children, had far less success with the TODAY sponge than with the diaphragm. For these women, pregnancy rates were an astounding 28 per 100 woman-years with the sponge, and 13 per 100 woman-years with the diaphragm. In contrast, nulliparous women fared much better with the sponge. They experienced pregnancy rates of only 14 per 100 woman-years, versus 13 per 100 woman-years with the diaphragm.

As a possible explanation for the higher pregnancy rates seen among parous sponge users, it has been suggested that its small diameter may be insufficient to fit snugly over the larger cervix of a woman who has given birth. A possible solution to this problem might be to manufacture a larger sponge for parous women. The laxity, or loss of tone, of a woman's vaginal muscles following childbirth may contribute to the shifting of the sponge's position during coitus from its preferred location in the upper vagina.

In 1985, researchers in the United Kingdom also compared pregnancy rates between TODAY and diaphragm users and found overall pregnancy rates of 25 and 11 per 100 woman-years, respectively. In the case of parous women, the British investigators confirmed the greater success of the diaphragm, with only 17 pregnancies per 100 woman-years versus an unacceptable 28 per 100 woman-years with the TODAY sponge. In contrast to the American studies, however, they reported higher pregnancy rates for nulliparous sponge users (23 per 100 woman-years) and lower rates for nulliparous diaphragm users (10 per 100 woman-years).

All researchers to date have agreed that accidental pregnancy rates for both the diaphragm and the TODAY sponge dropped by as much as one-third during the years of use beyond the first year. This is probably due to greater familiarity and expertise acquired over a period of time with either method chosen.

What are some of the advantages of the TODAY sponge over the diaphragm?

The strongest selling point for the TODAY sponge is its simplicity—one size fits all, and it can be purchased over the counter at any pharmacy. In contrast, the diaphragm has to be accurately fitted for size and requires a prescription, and its user must have some degree of expertise which can only be obtained via instruction by a trained professional. A further inconvenience for a woman using a diaphragm is that its size must be rechecked following a midtrimester (second-trimester) abortion, childbirth, and changes in weight (see page 103).

Though the TODAY sponge and the diaphragm are both inserted prior to intercourse, the sponge has the distinct advantage of interfering less with sexual spontaneity because it can be inserted rapidly and with less precision and messiness. Furthermore, additional applications of spermicide are not required for repeated coital acts, as they are with a diaphragm. Because of its larger size and firm rim, the diaphragm is more likely to impinge on the urethra and predispose to urinary tract infections. To reduce this risk, it is best for a diaphragm user to empty her bladder immediately before and as soon after coitus as possible. This, too, often interferes with sexual spontaneity. In contrast, the small, soft sponge poses little if any risk of urinary tract infections.

While each TODAY sponge is discarded following use, the diaphragm must be cleaned, dried, powdered, and checked frequently for defects and leaks. In addition, spores of vaginitis-producing yeast may reside on the diaphragm for prolonged periods of time.

Neither the sponge nor the diaphragm should be worn during the immediate postpartum period. After this time, the sponge is found to be far more comfortable, especially for the nursing woman. This is because nursing causes an estrogen deficiency which is manifested in a marked thinning and tenderness of the vaginal tissues; the firm rim of the diaphragm only serves to aggravate this condition.

Aside from a lower pregnancy rate, does the diaphragm offer any other advantages over the TODAY sponge?

From a purely financial point of view, the diaphragm is a far better investment than the TODAY sponge. While the initial fee for fitting and purchasing the diaphragm may run as high as $75.00, the only other costs incurred over the next few years are those of the spermicide. A large tube of spermicide can cost between $7.50 and $11.50, depending on the pharmacy. Assuming a coital frequency of three times a week, this size tube should last at least one month. Using $9.50 as the average cost of spermicide, one year's supply will cost $114.00, and three years of diaphragm use will cost $342.00 + $75.00 = $417.00.

The TODAY sponge is sold in packages of three, six, and twelve. In my survey of local pharmacies, the average price quoted for each was $5.00, $9.25, and $16.00. Assuming one purchases the largest and least expensive package and uses three sponges weekly, the cost over three years will total an astronomical $624.00.

While insertion of the TODAY sponge is far easier than the diaphragm, many women find that it is more difficult to remove. In the American study previously mentioned, 6 percent of sponge wearers discontinued its use either because of inability to locate the retrieval string or because of tearing and fragmenting of the device. In some cases, removal of the TODAY sponge required medical assistance. Statistically, 33 percent of all complaints registered against the TODAY sponge relate to difficulties encountered in removing it.

In the above-mentioned study, 4 percent of sponge wearers stopped using it because of allergic reactions to either the spermicide or the polyurethane, compared to 1 percent of the women wearing the diaphragm. Discontinuation rates due to "discomfort" in using the method were 6 percent in the TODAY group and 3 percent for the diaphragm users. Discomfort was usually manifested by vaginal itching.

Of all the statistics comparing the TODAY sponge with the diaphragm, one of the most frightening is that 17 percent of sponge wearers reported displacement or expulsion of the device during or after intercourse, compared to only 2 percent for women using the diaphragm. As previously mentioned, this phenomenon is more apt to occur in parous individuals and probably accounts for their higher pregnancy rates when compared to nulliparous sponge wearers.

Some women have rejected the TODAY sponge because they find that it causes excessive vaginal dryness as a result of its ability to absorb vaginal secretions and the male ejaculate. Other women have considered this a beneficial effect.

Though never proven scientifically, it is probable that the diaphragm, by virtue of its tighter fit, offers greater protection than the sponge against the passage of chlamydia and gonorrhea bacteria into the cervix. In addition, the diaphragm is probably more effective in protecting the cervix against the human papilloma virus (HPV) and the herpes virus (see sexually transmitted diseases).

This belief, however, does not negate the fact that the TODAY sponge does offer a significant degree of protection against sexually transmitted diseases. Doctor Michael J. Rosenberg and his associates at Family Health International compared the incidence of chlamydia and gonorrhea among more than 400 TODAY users and an equal number of women using other methods of contraception. In their 1987 report, published in the *Journal of the American Medical Association,* they concluded that the TODAY sponge offered a significant degree of protection against these two diseases. On the negative side, women using the TODAY sponge had a higher incidence of candida or yeast vaginitis, a harmless and easily treated condition (see yeast and birth-control pills, chapter 2).

What is toxic shock syndrome and how is it related to the use of the TODAY sponge and the diaphragm?

Toxic shock syndrome, or TSS, is a potentially fatal condition caused by the endotoxin (poison) released by certain strains of the *Staphylococcus aureus* bacterium. When TSS was first recognized, in 1978, it was believed to occur only among menstruating women who used superabsorbent tampons, such as the brand Rely. Since then, however, TSS has been known to strike nonmenstruating women as well as men, and individuals undergoing nasal surgery involving the insertion of nasal packing are especially prone to TSS, since this is a favorite site of the organism. Infected skin abscesses, burns, insect bites, lacerations, and postoperative incision infections have all been reported to initiate TSS. For reasons that remain obscure, a strong association appears to exist between the development of TSS in women who have had a tubal ligation at least one year earlier. While women on birth control pills appear less likely to contract TSS, users of barrier contraception are at greater risk. As of 1987, the Centers for Disease Control have confirmed nineteen cases of TSS associated with the use of the TODAY sponge and twenty-seven cases with the diaphragm.

It is curious to note that while *Staphylococcus aureus* is a ubiquitous bacterium, TSS is an extremely rare condition. In fact, the organism can be cultured from the vaginas of 5 to 9 percent of healthy women at midcycle and of as many as 17 percent at the time of menstruation. It remains a mystery why the immune system of only a small percentage of women is unable to fight the endotoxin.

The portal of entry for the endotoxin into the bloodstream is through tiny ulcerations on either the skin surface or body membranes. Laboratory studies have clearly demonstrated that pressure on the vaginal walls from a diaphragm, sponge, or tampon over a period of several hours can cause these microscopic defects.

As a result of the great amount of publicity surrounding TSS, it is understandable why so many women suspect this condition at the first sign of illness. In fact, it is extremely rare and the overwhelming majority of gynecologists have never seen a patient with TSS. The likelihood of developing TSS from a tampon during a period is approximately 1 in 20,000 to 40,000, while the risk for the TODAY sponge is only 1 for every 2 million sponges used. Rates for the diaphragm are believed to be approximately equal to those of the sponge. In a 1987 report, funded by the V.L.I. Corporation and published in *Obstetrics and Gynecology,* researchers found that the TODAY sponge actually inhibited the growth of the *Staphylococcus aureus* organism and lowered its endotoxin levels in a variety of bacterial culture tubes. Most authorities therefore agree that the use of the diaphragm or the TODAY sponge does not represent a significant TSS health risk.

Nevertheless, when TSS does occur, it is a dire medical emergency. The first symptom is usually a sudden temperature elevation to greater than 101°F (38.9°C). This is often accompanied by diarrhea, vomiting, muscle aches, and a diffuse, red, sunburnlike rash. Any of these symptoms should warn you to call your doctor immediately. Hypotension, or a drop in blood pressure, often accompanies TSS as does disorientation and altered consciousness. Laboratory studies frequently show an abnormally low platelet count as well as abnormal liver and kidney function tests. A characteristic finding noted one to two weeks after the onset of symptoms is a peeling of the skin on the palms and soles.

Treatment of TSS demands immediate hospitalization, correction of hypotension with intravenous fluids and a variety of other medications, the taking of cultures to identify the bacteria, and administration of specific antibiotics to which the *Staphylococcus aureus* organism is sensitive. With immediate and expert medical care, complete recovery can be expected. Of the forty-five cases of toxic shock syndrome reported with diaphragm and Today use, there were no deaths. But the overall death rate from TSS has been quoted in the medical literature as 3 percent.

What can a woman do to reduce her risk of TSS?

In 1986, the Centers for Disease Control analyzed the reported cases of TSS associated with use of the TODAY sponge. They concluded that a woman is more likely to contract the disease if she has worn the sponge during menstruation or in the weeks immediately following childbirth; if she has left it in for longer than thirty hours; or if she experienced difficulties or fragmenting of the sponge when removing it from the vagina. Review of the TSS cases occurring with use of the diaphragm also confirmed the dangers of leaving it in beyond twenty-four hours. It was surprising to find, though, that TSS developed in less than nine hours in two young women using the diaphragm for the first time. Possibly the tightness of the new diaphragm rim in these two cases caused pressure and micro-ulcerations of the vaginal walls.

For aesthetic rather than contraceptive purposes, some women wear their diaphragm or TODAY sponge during coitus at the time of the menstrual period. Others wear it during the first three postpartum weeks in order to control bleeding. While this practice is probably harmless if the device is removed in less than one hour, leaving it in beyond an hour should be discouraged since secretions can accumulate and provide a site for infection. Some researchers have theorized that blood that is blocked from flowing out of the vagina may back up and pass through the fallopian tube into the abdominal cavity. From there, the *Staphylococcus aureus* endotoxin may get absorbed into the bloodstream.

To minimize risk, it is a good idea to remove the sponge or the diaphragm as soon as possible after six hours have elapsed following the last coital encounter. Never leave either device in place for more than twenty-four hours—preferably fewer than twelve hours. After removing the sponge, inspect it carefully to be certain there are no missing fragments.

Finally, any woman with a previous vaginal culture that is positive for *Staphylococcus aureus* should not use the sponge or the diaphragm. Oral contraceptives are a far better choice, since it is believed that they decrease the risk of TSS by reducing the amount of menstrual flow.

It is best not to use tampons exclusively during the menstrual period. Instead, you should alternate tampons with sanitary napkins. At night it is safer to use napkins instead of leaving a tampon in during the long hours of sleep. Ideally, tampons should be changed at intervals of no longer than four hours.

If you believe that you have a problem related to the use of the TODAY sponge, call its manufacturerer, the V.L.I. Corporation of Irvine, California, on its twenty-four-hour toll-free hotline: 1-800-223-2329. If you have symptoms suggestive of TSS, forget the hotline and call your doctor immediately.

CERVICAL CAPS

What is a cervical cap and how long has it been in existence?

A cervical cap is a device that is much smaller than a diaphragm, designed to fit snugly over the cervix rather than against the vaginal walls (figure 4-7). While cervical caps have been created from many different materials and fashioned into a variety of inventive shapes, all are held in place and exert their contraceptive effect by adhering to the cervix and preventing the entry of sperm from the vagina.

The cervical cap is often considered to be a new and promising contraceptive device, but it has actually been in existence in Europe since the nineteenth century. The first description of the cervical cap in the medical literature is by a German gynecologist named Friedrick Adolphe Wielde in 1838. He created wax impressions of women's cervixes and then had small rubber caps custom-made to the exact size of the impressions. Since then, cervical caps have been made from various strengths

Figure 4–7. *Varieties of cervical caps.*

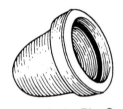

Prentif Cavity Rim Cervical Cap

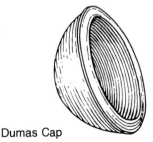

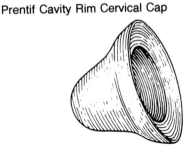

Dumas Cap   Vimule Cap

of rubber, silver, copper, and other metals, as well as Lucite and Silastic plastic. Despite claims to the contrary, many authorities are convinced that cervical cap technology has not progressed much beyond Dr. Wielde's original work.

Why are some American women wearing cervical caps while others are denied access to them by their gynecologists?

The manufacture and sale of contraceptive devices such as the cervical cap are under the authority of the FDA. To date, the FDA has refused to endorse the use of any brand of cervical cap until extensive testing of its safety and efficacy have been completed. An American woman who is currently using a cervical cap for contraception has probably obtained it from one of a small number of FDA-approved medical protocols testing various caps on an "investigational" basis. Another source is various women's health clinics or doctors' offices that have imported cervical caps from England. It is estimated that as many as 20,000 Prentif Cavity-Rim Cervical Caps, manufactured by Lamberts, a London-based company, have been imported into the United States since the early 1980s.

Many feminist groups have voiced anger at the "information blackout" surrounding the cervical cap, assailing the Food and Drug Administration (FDA) and the male-dominated medical establishment for denying women this "ideal" contraceptive. Recent studies have clearly demonstrated that the cervical cap may be far less than perfect. In fact, prolonged use of one type of cap, known as the Vimule, was found to cause redness, abrasions, cervical and vaginal lacerations, and overgrowth of the vaginal tissues. Fortunately, these problems were detected by doctors conducting investigational studies under FDA supervision. As a result of these important revelations, the Vimule Cap was removed from further investigational studies in 1983. The clinical trials of another highly publicized cervical cap, known as the Contracap, were abruptly halted in 1981 following reports of an excessive number of cap dislodgements and pregnancies attributed to the unpredictable consistency of the alginate used in the caps. New FDA-approved trials using Silastic Contracaps were begun again in 1983. Had it not been for these clinical trials, the deficiencies in the original Contracap would not have been detected until a large number of American women had experienced dislodgement of the device and inadvertent pregnancy.

There is no conspiracy by the FDA or the AMA to prevent distribution of an effective and safe cervical cap. When and if such a device proves to offer real advantages as a contraceptive, it will undoubtedly pass the necessary scrutiny imposed by the FDA.

How does the cervical cap compare to other barrier methods in terms of preventing pregnancy?

As new statistical data become available, it is more and more obvious that the cervical cap is a less than ideal method of preventing pregnancy. In one 1986 study of 217 women fitted with a cervical cap, doctors noted a disappointing pregnancy rate of 23 per 100 woman-years. Upon closer analysis of these findings, it was found that the highest rates were among younger women having more frequent coitus, those who were less educated, and individuals who had had a previous abortion or a full-term birth. Neither the total length of time that a woman wore the cap nor the number of hours that it had been left in place following intercourse had any bearing on the pregnancy risk. Five recent studies evaluating a variety of cervical caps showed pregnancy rates of 7.6, 13, 16.9, 21, and 44 per 100 woman-years. These numbers are hardly reassuring for the woman seeking an efficient method of contraception.

With the exception of the Contracap, most cap manufacturers have stressed the importance of placing a small amount of spermicidal jelly or cream inside the cap before fitting it on the cervix, but statistical analysis has failed to demonstrate that this precaution has any effect on lowering the pregnancy rate. One report actually showed that the lowest pregnancy rates were among former diaphragm users who did not use spermicides in their cervical caps. This would suggest that previous diaphragm use affords a woman a greater degree of familiarity with her anatomy and helps her to master the correct placement of the cap over the cervix. Since taking the time to insert spermicide further delays the spontaneity of lovemaking, women who use a spermicide are more likely to discontinue cap use than those who bypass this step. If you prefer to apply spermicides to your cervical cap, your risk of pregnancy will probably be less if you use a jelly rather than a cream. This is because the accumulation of cervical secretions in the cap forms a water-soluble layer over the oil-based cream, which is more likely to provide a safe passage for those few sperm that have circumvented the rim of the cap. In contrast, the more water-soluble jellies readily dissolve in the cervical secretions and render them spermicidal.

Studies of the cervix show that it is far more mobile and changeable in size and shape than previously believed. It is now known that a woman's cervical size fluctuates not only during the monthly cycle, but during sexual excitation and orgasm as well. This helps explain the high pregnancy rate associated with use of the cap and the frequency of caps becoming dislodged or falling off the cervix during intercourse and activities requiring intense straining and bearing down. In a 1983 study, cap dislodgement was reported in 31 percent of the women studied, tripling their risk of accidental pregnancy. Current researchers now know that as many as 10 percent of women wearing cervical caps need at least two different sizes to accommodate the changes in their cervixes each month. Obviously, this necessity will increase the cost of using the cap.

Because insertion and removal of the cervical cap is difficult, many women simply lose interest in the method. Researchers use the term "noncompliance" and "inconsistent use" to explain why pregnancy rates are so high in women supposedly using the cervical cap. In one recent study, an incredible 70 percent of those fitted with a cervical cap stopped using it after only twelve months.

One can conclude from these dismal statistics that use of the cervical cap should not be encouraged as a primary means of contraception. Even if you have access to a professional or a clinic that fits cervical caps, you should explore all other contraceptive options first. Cap use should be reserved only for women who are extremely motivated or those who are unable to use alternative contraception.

In what other ways does the cervical cap compare to the diaphragm or the TODAY sponge?

Originally the main argument in favor of the cervical cap was that, unlike the diaphragm and the TODAY sponge, it could be left in place for several days at a time. However, the chief complaint against the cap has been malodor, especially when it is worn for two or more days. In two separate studies, 27 percent and 33 percent of all cap wearers reported this problem. In addition, as many as 15 percent have noted a greater incidence of vaginitis associated with use of the cap. Leaving the cap on the cervix for prolonged periods of time may also cause the surrounding tissues to grow over the cap rim. Contusions, lacerations, and small ulcerations of the cervix and vagina are also more likely with the cervical cap. In a 1984 report from California, doctors studied 600 women wearing the cap and found that 6 percent of them converted from normal to abnormal Pap smears during this period of time. To date, no other studies have demonstrated such a relationship.

Promoters of the Contracap device have stated that its unique one-way valve alleviates the problem of malodor because it allows the escape of blood and cervical secretions while preventing the entry of sperm. Further extensive testing of this device is necessary before we can substantiate these claims.

Although there have been no cases of toxic shock syndrome (TSS) associated with use of the cervical cap, most epidemiologists believe this is only because not enough women have used it yet. Given the knowledge that abrasions and ulcerations do occur with the cap, it is undoubtedly just a matter of time before cases of TSS will be reported in the medical literature. To minimize this risk, cap wearers should not wear the device for any longer than is absolutely necessary.

Some of the newer caps are made of softer and more flexible synthetic plastics, which may offer the advantage of somewhat greater comfort than the diaphragm for both partners during coitus. In addition, the caps' smaller sizes may lessen the chances of a urinary tract infection. However, the TODAY sponge is equal to the cap in both regards and is much easier to insert and remove.

The durability of the cervical cap is probably less than that of the diaphragm, but unlike the latter the cap is more difficult to replace because of the limited availability of caps to only a select group of doctors and clinics. Over time, most caps lose their elasticity and are best replaced every twelve to eighteen months. In a 1984 report, doctors examined cervical caps under the microscope and found marked deterioration in most of those that had been worn for more than one year. Many of the caps that had been worn for longer periods of time also appeared damaged. One interesting observation was that deterioration of the cap was related more to how many hours at a time it had been worn rather than to the total accumulated hours of use.

It is more difficult to clean a cervical cap than to clean the flatter diaphragm. The disposable TODAY sponge wins the cleanliness award since it is discarded immediately after each use.

In summary, there is little reason to believe that the cervical cap, even in its most modern designs, will ever become an overwhelmingly popular form of barrier contraception.

VAGINAL SPERMICIDES

While one of the most recent over-the-counter vaginal spermicide products is the TODAY Vaginal Contraceptive Sponge (see "The TODAY Sponge"), other, fairly reliable preparations in the form of creams, jellies, aerosol foam, tablets, and suppositories have been available for years.

All spermicidal preparations consist of two components: an inert base that holds the spermicidal agent in the vagina against the cervix; and a spermicidal agent, such as nonoxynol-9 or octoxynol. Some creams and jellies are designed for use with the diaphragm, while others may be used alone or in conjunction with a condom or an IUD for added pregnancy protection at the time of ovulation. Vaginal contraceptive products intended for use with the diaphragm are formulated to cling to the diaphragm and cervix and usually contain a lower concentration of spermicide. The products intended to be used alone, in addition to a higher spermicide content, are formulated to spread over the cervical opening and form a protective barrier. Foam does not form an adequate seal between the diaphragm and cervix, and therefore it should not be used with the diaphragm.

When any of these products are used as the sole contraceptive agent, it is very important that they be inserted far up into the vagina, as close to the cervix as possible, if they are to achieve maximum effectiveness.

How does the contraceptive aerosol foam compare to the jellies, creams, tablets, and suppositories in preventing pregnancy?

Contraceptive aerosol foam is probably the most effective of these methods. Skepticism about foam is based on studies demonstrating pregnancy rates as high as 29 per 100 woman-years. Other investigators, however, have claimed pregnancy rates as low as 1.55 and 1.80 per 100 woman-years. These rates are lower than those for the IUD and diaphragm. The most commonly quoted pregnancy rates for the foam, creams, and jellies is 15 per 100 woman-years. The critical factor in the success or failure of contraceptive foams seems to be whether users are motivated and diligent enough to use the method correctly with each coital encounter.

How can I achieve the lowest possible pregnancy rates with foam?

Since most of the spermicidal effect of foam is lost after thirty minutes, be sure to insert it within that time period before intercourse. It is important to insert a fresh applicator of foam if more than thirty minutes elapses as well as immediately before repeated acts of intercourse.

Foam is sold in large cans containing enough spermicide for several coital acts, and in more expensive prefilled applicators designed to be used only once. When you buy your first large can of foam, you will need to purchase an applicator with it. These applicators may be used repeatedly and should be washed with soap and lukewarm water to remove any remaining foam. Refill cans of foam are usually less expensive because they do not contain the plastic applicators. The proper use of the applicator and its plunger is demonstrated in figure 4-8. It is a good idea always to keep an extra container of foam on hand. With the large cans, there is often no way of knowing when the supply is about to run out. Using a single, premeasured applicator, such as Emko Pre-Fil, may be more helpful. Foam and all other spermicides should be stored at room temperature, since excessive heat can reduce their efficacy. Storage for periods of time longer than two years is ill-advised. Most products have an expiration date stamped on the package.

Shake the can or prefilled applicator vigorously about twenty times just prior to using it to ensure that the foam will have the consistency of shaving cream and that the spermicide will be evenly dispersed into the base. It is also important not to douche for at least eight hours after intercourse. To prevent foam from running out of the vagina, insert a tampon after intercourse.

The amount of foam an applicator holds may vary from one product to another and may often be a source of confusion. The volume, or number of cubic centimeters (cc's), of foam per applicator for some of the more popular brands is as follows: Delfen: 5 cc; Koromex: 5 cc; Emko Pre-Fil: 10 cc; Emko: 17 cc; and Emko Because: 17 cc. The smaller volume of the Delfen and Koromex products prompts many authorities to recommend that two full applicators be used prior to coitus.

Figure 4–8. *Proper method of inserting vaginal cream, jellies, or foam.*

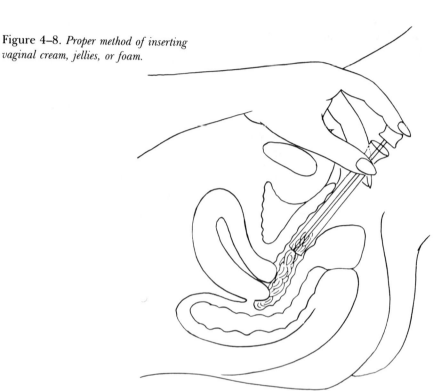

Delfen foam is considered to have the best spermicidal effect. Though Emko would appear to be equally potent, to date no scientific studies have compared these two agents. Since they contain different spermicides, if you experience burning or irritation with one you can try switching to another brand.

Are there any other advantages to foam contraception?

Theoretically, foam should offer faster protection than any other agents because it is more rapidly distributed throughout the vagina and quickly forms a barrier over the cervix. This advantage applies to contraceptive creams and jellies as well, though the barrier may be more complete with foam. Intercourse and ejaculation can immediately follow insertion of these products, in contrast to suppositories and tablets which usually require a wait of ten to fifteen minutes before completely liquifying and becoming effective. Since intravaginal distribution of tablets and suppositories is partially dependent on penile thrusting, there is a greater chance of pregnancy if the male ejaculates quickly after penetration.

Another advantage of foam is that it is not nearly as messy to use as the other vaginal spermicides. It is less likely to drain out of the vagina after use, and less likely to leak out of the vagina during intercourse.

As previously mentioned, all spermicides have been observed in laboratory tests to retard the growth of viruses and bacteria responsible for causing herpes, AIDS, gonorrhea, syphilis, and chlamydia. In actual practice, however, there is no convincing data confirming the effectiveness of these agents in preventing the spread of venereal disease. Certainly they are less effective than either the condom or the diaphragm in that respect.

What are the disadvantages of using vaginal spermicides?

In addition to higher pregnancy rates than other contraceptive measures, vaginal spermicides can interfere with sexual spontaneity. These preparations are somewhat messy to use, they tend to drip out of the vagina, and they have a rather unpleasant taste. To correct this last problem, the Nova Corporation of America has introduced Flavo-Cept Contraceptive Jelly and Cream, containing nonoxynol-9 in a raspberry-flavored cream and a cherry-flavored jelly.

As previously mentioned, some men and women have allergic reactions to the spermicide or base in many of these products. It is often helpful for such individuals to try a different preparation. Vaginal and penile irritation is especially prevalent with the stronger spermicidal preparations.

What is the cost of these products?

A can of foam, which contains approximately twenty applications, costs between $9.00 and $9.50 at most pharmacies. The individual premeasured applicator of Conceptrol costs approximately $1.00 and is sold in packets of six and ten for $6.80 and $9.60, respectively. The brand Because is not premeasured but has to be drawn up into an applicator. It is therefore less expensive, at six for $5.50. Contraceptive creams and jellies are about equally priced, at approximately $8.00 for a $2\frac{1}{2}$ ounce tube and $10.00 for $4\frac{1}{2}$ ounces.

What are the advantages and disadvantages of using vaginal spermicidal suppositories?

The three most popular spermicidal suppositories sold in the United States are Encare (Eaton-Merz), Intercept (Ortho Pharmaceutical), and Semicid (Whitehall Laboratories). Though each manufacturer has spent millions of dollars trying to prove its product superior to all others, the fact is that they all contain the spermicide nonoxynol-9. A major disadvantage of all three products is that they must dissolve over a period of ten to thirty minutes after placement in the vagina prior to sexual intercourse. It is important that a new suppository be inserted if intercourse does not take place within one hour after insertion, and immediately prior to subsequent coital acts. On rare occasions, a suppository will take even longer to dissolve. Not only can this cause increased friction and penile and vaginal irritation, it may also increase a woman's risk of pregnancy. There is some evidence to suggest that with intercourse in the female-superior position, it is best not to rely on vaginal suppositories for contraception.

While some couples find suppositories less cumbersome than foams, jellies, and creams, others complain that they are sometimes difficult to remove from their surrounding foil. Several of my patients have complained of intense vaginal burning soon after inserting a suppository. This seems to occur most often with Encare.

The pregnancy rate associated with vaginal contraceptive suppositories has been reported to range from a low of 0.3 to a high of 42 per 100 woman-years. The most commonly quoted rate is 15 per 100 woman-years. When Eaton-Merz Laboratories first introduced Encare, they promoted it by referring to a West German survey showing a pregnancy rate of only 1 per 100 woman-years. They proclaimed "a new era in nonhormonal contraception" and implied in their advertising that the efficacy of their suppository was equal to that of the Pill and the IUD. Other suppository manufacturers followed the Eaton-Merz lead and used misleading advertising as well. Fortunately, in 1980, the Federal Trade Commission ordered all suppository manufacturers to cease using the words *highly, extremely,* and *very* in combination with the words *effective* or *reliable* in advertising their products. In addition, they were instructed not to claim that their product was more effective than other spermicides.

One clear advantage of the suppositories is that they come in small packages that can be easily carried in a pocket or a purse. The price is also reasonable. A box of twelve Encare Ovals or Intercept suppositories costs between $5.50 and $6.00, while a box of ten Semicid suppositories costs slightly less. This averages out to 50 cents per suppository, a reasonable price when compared to other methods.

If used by a woman before she is aware that she is pregnant, can contraceptive spermicides harm the fetus?

Within the past six years, at least four separate reports have noted a higher incidence of chromosomal abnormalities, spontaneous abortions, and birth defects among women using spermicidal contraception. The theory is that because spermicides damage, but don't necessarily kill, sperm cells, they may allow an abnormal sperm to fertilize an egg.

Many knowledgeable scientists and epidemiologists have questioned the validity of these findings, and the preponderance of subsequent information has totally exonerated all currently used spermicides. One investigation, conducted by doctors at the Centers for Disease Control in Atlanta in 1983, compared two groups of mothers who gave birth to infants with birth defects; one group had used spermicides at the time of conception and the other had not. They found no specific anomaly patterns in the spermicide group and concluded that there was no evidence of a link between spermicides and chromosomal abnormalities or birth defects. In the most recent study addressing this question, Dr. James L. Mills and his associates at the National Institute of Child Health and Human Development studied the outcome of pregnancies in women who had used spermicide either before or after their last menstrual period. Their research, published in *Fertility and Sterility* in 1985, evaluated the incidence of malformation, low birth weight, premature delivery, and spontaneous abortion among these women. They compared their results with those obtained from pregnancies among women who had been using other methods of contraception either immediately before or soon after they conceived. The malformation rates were actually found to be slightly higher in the women who had not been exposed to spermicide.

Based on a thorough review of all available data, medical experts have concluded that there is no relationship between use of a spermicide at the time of conception and an adverse pregnancy outcome. The FDA has decided not to require changes in the product labeling on spermicide packages. Pregnancy termination is not warranted if pregnancy follows spermicide failure.

CONTRACEPTIVE FILM

What is VCF and how does it compare with other vaginal contraceptives?

VCF or Vaginal Contraceptive Film is the newest vaginal spermicidal agent on the market. It is a paper-thin, two-inch square vaginal insert containing the spermicide nonoxyol-9, polyvinyl alcohol, and glycerine. When placed high in the vagina, five minutes to two hours prior to intercourse, VCF dissolves into a sperm-killing gel and achieves contraceptive efficacy equal to any of the vaginal spermicides currently being manufactured. VCF is less messy and more comfortable to insert than other vaginal contraceptives, and it cannot be felt by either partner during intercourse. Its main advantage over the TODAY sponge is that it does not have to be removed after intercourse since it completely dissolves in the vaginal secretions.

VCF was first introduced in England more than ten years ago, and it has been tested extensively throughout Europe under the trade name C-film. Apothecus, Inc. of Great Neck, New York, has FDA approval for marketing VCF at many pharmacies in a discreetly packaged matchbook-size box of twelve. Its retail price ranges from $5.00 to $7.00.

CONDOMS

A condom is a thin sheath, made of either latex rubber or lamb intestinal membrane, which fits over the penis and prevents sperm from escaping. (see figure 4-9) Other names for condoms are safes, prophylactics, rubbers, bags, sheaths, skins, balloons, French letters, and Trojans. (The latter is actually the name of one of the more popular brands.)

The condom is an excellent method of birth control and is probably the oldest, having been described by Fallopius in 1564. Though the linen bag he fashioned for the prevention of syphilis was not an instant success, he did eventually achieve immortality by having the fallopian tubes named after him because of his research on them.

Not until two centuries later was the penile sheath given the name *condom,* after a British physician named Condon who first described it. The condom's dual purpose of "protection from venereal disease and numerous bastard offspring" helped it gain worldwide popularity. As with the diaphragm, Casanova was one of the first to popularize its use, in eighteenth-century Italy. Today the condom is the most frequently used method of birth control worldwide, and in the United States it ranks third, behind the Pill and sterilization. It is estimated that the condom is favored by 10 to 15 percent of all contraceptive users, with more than 300 million purchased each year. In recent years, condom sales have increased at a yearly rate of 10 percent.

The prime reason for the sudden increase in condom sales has been the realization that it is the most effective means of preventing the many potentially devastating sexually transmitted diseases, such as chlamydia, herpes, gonorrhea, syphilis, and AIDS. In addition, advertising in popular magazines has recently stressed the fact that women, as well as men, must assume the responsibility for purchasing condoms, as much for protection against disease as for contraception. Newer and more innovative designs have further helped the condom to gain popularity.

After all the problems that women have experienced with birth-control pills, IUDs, abortions, and sterilization techniques, it is a sad commentary that this 400-year-old device is still the primary male contraceptive.

How effective is the condom?

Several studies have demonstrated that if a couple uses the condom consistently with each act of intercourse, pregnancy rates should be no greater than 2 per 100 woman-years. Recent studies from the United Kingdom actually reported rates of less than 1 per 100 woman-years for conscientious users, and only 3.3 per 100 woman-years for those who were less diligent. If foam, creams, or jellies are used in conjunction

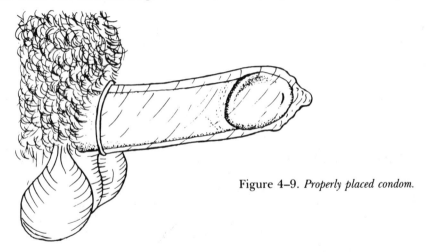

Figure 4–9. *Properly placed condom.*

with the condom, failure rates should be even lower. These statistics are in sharp contrast to earlier studies that showed pregnancy rates ranging between 9 and 15 per 100 woman-years.

The most exciting news in condom contraception is the introduction of Ramses-Extra and Ansell Prime Super-Thin Condoms. These two unique products contain nonoxynol-9 on their inner and outer surfaces. Researchers have demonstrated that sperm motility, or movement, was reduced to 10 percent within 30 seconds of ejaculation into one of these condoms. This percentage was lowered to 4.3 and 1.5 percent, respectively, after 60 and 120 seconds. In contrast, motility rates remained greater than 50 percent for up to 20 minutes after using conventional condoms. These figures convincingly demonstrate that the spermicidal condom is highly effective in immobilizing and killing sperm. Though as yet unproven, these two new products should significantly decrease pregnancy rates associated with a condom's slipping or falling loose immediately after intercourse.

It is reassuring to note that the risk of pregnancy from a defective condom is extremely small, probably no greater than 0.3 percent. The chance of rupture or tearing of the high-quality latex produced in the United States is less than 1 in 300, and condoms made of lamb intestinal membrane are equally durable. Even a pinpoint defect in a condom is unlikely to allow enough sperm to exit from the condom to result in a pregnancy. It is best to ignore the standard advice of testing a condom for leaks by filling it with water or blowing it up with air like a balloon. These maneuvers only increase the risk of creating a defect in the latex.

When and how does a man put on a condom?

Latex condoms are unrolled onto the erect penis. Some models of sheep intestine condoms are also put on this way, while others are pulled on like a glove. Many, but not all, latex condoms have a rubber receptacle in the tip to hold the sperm. The man using a condom without a receptable should leave a little space between the end of the condom and the penis for this purpose (refer to figure 4-9). It is a common misconception that this practice prevents rapid ejaculation from bursting the rubber. The real reason for the space at the end of the condom is that it prevents sperm from being forced down the penile shaft and out the lower part of the condom. Air should be squeezed out of that space, called the receptacle tip, with the fingers prior to intercourse. The condom should be unrolled the full length of the erect penis, and uncircumcised men should retract the foreskin underlying the end of the penis.

Though men should be cautioned to put on the condom before intercourse rather than immediately before ejaculation, the reason usually given for this is incorrect. It is often stated that the first few drops of a man's discharge, which are present during erection and before ejaculation, contain enough sperm for pregnancy to occur. Most knowledgeable urologists dispute this notion, claiming instead that pregnancy is nearly impossible from this small amount of pre-ejaculatory discharge. The wise reason for putting on the condom before penetration is that a man may forget the condom along with his conscience once intercourse is begun.

How can a man determine his condom size?

Men need not be "fitted" by a urologist for a condom. Condoms come in one standard size and are sold in drugstores in packages of three or twelve. Inexperienced men must remember that the words *large* and *small* on condom packages denote the number of condoms and not anatomical dimensions.

Which is the best condom?

The best condom is the one that a couple is most likely to use consistently. No one condom is best for everyone, and couples are advised to experiment with a variety of types and brands to find one that is mutually satisfying (see table that follows).

CONDOM PRODUCTS AND THEIR DESCRIPTION

Brand Name and Manufacturer	Type	Approximate Cost
Conture (Warner-Lambert)	rubber, shaped, packaged with lubricant	
Excita Sensitol (Schmid)	rubber, shaped and/or ribbed, packaged with lubricant	3/$2.00
Fetherlite (Schmid)	rubber, plain end, packaged dry rubber, plain end, packaged with lubricant	12/$6.00
Fiesta Sensi-Color (Schmid)	rubber, reservoir end, packaged with lubricant	
Fourex (Schmid)	lamb cecum, regular end, packaged with lubricant	3/$6.30–6.50
Guardian (Youngs)	rubber, reservoir end, packaged with lubricant	12/$20.00–26.00
Hugger (Ansell)	rubber, reservoir end, packaged with lubricant	
Mentor (Mentor)	rubber, reservoir end, packaged with lubricant, adhesive at base to prevent slippage	
Naturalamb (Youngs)	lamb cecum, regular end, packaged with lubricant	

CONDOM PRODUCTS AND THEIR DESCRIPTION *(Continued)*

Brand Name and Manufacturer	Type	Approximate Cost	
Nuda (Warner-Lambert)	rubber, shaped/thin, packaged with lubricant		
Nuform Sensi-Shape, Lubricated (Schmid)	rubber, shaped and/or ribbed, packaged with lubricant		
Nuform Sensi-Shape, nonlubricated (Schmid)	rubber, shaped and/or ribbed, packaged dry		
Prime (Ansell)	rubber, reservoir end, packaged with lubricant		
Prime Super-Thin (Ansell)	rubber, reservoir end, packaged with spermicide and lubricant		
Prime, nonlubricated (Ansell)	rubber, reservoir end, packaged dry	3/$2.50–3.00	12/$6.00–7.40
Ramses (Schmid)	rubber, plain end, packaged dry		
Ramses Sensitol (Schmid)	rubber, plain end, packaged with lubricant	3/$2.50–3.50	12/$6.00–8.00
Rough Rider (Ansell)	rubber, studded, packaged with lubricant		

Product	Description	Price (3)	Price (12)
Sheik Plain End (Schmid)	rubber, plain end, packaged dry		
Sheik Reservoir End, Lubricated (Schmid)	rubber, reservoir end, packaged with lubricant	3/$2.30–2.50	12/$5.50–6.60
Sheik Reservoir End, nonlubricated (Schmid)	rubber, reservoir end, packaged dry	3/$2.00	12/$5.30
Stimula (Warner-Lambert)	rubber, ribbed, packaged with lubricant		
Sultan (Ansell)	rubber, ribbed, packaged with lubricant		
Tahiti (Ansell)	rubber, colored, packaged with lubricant		
Trojan-Enz, nonlubricated (Youngs)	rubber, reservoir end, packaged dry	3/$1.50	12/$4.00
Trojans (Youngs)	rubber, plain end, packaged dry	3/$1.35	12/4.00
Trojans Plus (Youngs)	rubber, shaped and/or ribbed, packaged with lubricant		
Trojans Ribbed (Youngs)	rubber, shaped and/or ribbed, packaged with lubricant	3/$2.00	12/$5.50–6.00

SOURCE: *Compiled by the author.*

As previously noted, condoms containing the spermicide nonoxynol-9 have been marketed in the United States since 1982. Such condoms were available in Great Britain several years earlier and presently account for over 40 percent of all condom sales. If the British experience is at all predictive, brands such as Ramses Extra and Prime Super-Thin should have a successful future in the United States.

Fourex and Naturalamb are "skin" condoms made of a thin, though very strong, lamb intestinal membrane, and are thoroughly lubricated. Though they make up less than 5 percent of all condom sales in the United States, many couples prefer them because of their special feel. Although skins are actually thicker than latex condoms, the greater sensation some men report with skin condoms is due to increased heat transmission from the vagina. This sensation is significantly inhibited with the latex products. A couple who avoids latex condoms because of decreased sensation should try skin condoms before abandoning this method of birth control. The two major disadvantages of skin condoms are their tendency to slip, because of the degree of lubrication, and their high cost. Skin condoms are usually two to three times more expensive than latex products.

Several companies produce condoms of excellent quality latex rubber that may be purchased with or without lubricant and a receptacle at the tip. Regardless of the brand, lubricated condoms are always more expensive than the nonlubricated variety. The lubricant most commonly used consists of a nonirritating surgical jelly, though the newest development in lubricated condoms is the special silicone lubricant, found in condoms such as Trojan Plus and Ramses Sensitol. Many couples now prefer this so-called dry lubricant, since it is not as messy.

Contouring and texturing are additional features of some condoms. There are two types of contouring: One involves flaring of the condom from its base to allow greater movement of the penis within the condom (Nuform, Excita); the other is a constriction just in front of the glans, or head, of the penis, helping the condom fit more snugly over the glans (Conture, Hugger). Condom texturing may be in the form of ribbing, dots, or small projections from the condom to increase sensation. Ribbing consists of several very thin horizontal notches in the latex. Sultan and Stimula are examples of ribbed condoms; Nuform, Excita Sensitol, Trojans Plus, and Trojans Ribbed may be purchased with or without ribbing. Advertisers are quick to point out that ribbing is a great sexual stimulant to women during intercourse. If you believe this, you're being ribbed. Based on the evaluation of these condoms by several of my patients and their husbands or partners, I am convinced that the enhanced sexual benefits of these condoms are strictly in the imagination of their manufacturers.

For the couple seeking the ultimate, Ansell Corporation offers a rubber-studded condom appropriately named Rough Rider. And for those who enjoy dressing up before intercourse, Ansell offers Tahiti condoms in a variety of bright colors. Nuform is also available in different colors. Those who are financially secure may favor the gold Trojan Plus condom. The latest addition to the condom competition is Mentor, which contains a thin adhesive substance at its base to prevent slippage.

All rubber condoms produced in the United States undergo very precise quality control testing of their tensile strength by the various manufacturers. In addition, the FDA has established standards for testing a condom's minimal thickness, and pressures below which it should not burst or tear. Foreign brands of condoms are not uniformly subjected to the testing given American condoms and are more likely to be defective. Condoms made in the United States of lamb membrane are also subjected to testing by their manufacturers as well as by the FDA. But, because these condoms are made of an animal membrane, rather than a uniformly manufactured substance such as latex rubber, the tests they undergo tend to be less specific and less standardized.

Is it true that condoms are actually used by couples who are trying to conceive?

On rare occasions, a couple will be infertile because a woman forms antibodies against the sperm of her partner. When the antibody level is high, sperm deposited in the vagina and cervix may be immediately destroyed or inactivated by these antibodies. For such couples, the antibody level of the woman will diminish if her partner wears a condom during coitus for periods of six months or more. Then attempting conception without a condom exactly at the time of ovulation often proves successful.

How can pregnancy rates with a condom be reduced?

Precise laboratory studies have shown that even a properly packaged condom can demonstrate microscopic defects when exposed to temperatures equivalent to those of a car's glove compartment on a hot day. The common practice of many boys of obtaining a condom at the onset of puberty and hiding it in their wallets while waiting for an opportunity to use it is not a good idea. The waiting period may last a couple of years, and when the moment finally arrives the condom is usually in less-than-perfect condition. It is therefore important not to store condoms for prolonged periods of time or to keep them in places subject to high temperatures.

A nonlubricated condom should never be lubricated with petroleum jelly, Vaseline, or cold cream, which can cause rubber to deteriorate. K-Y Jelly or Lubrin tablets are suggested instead. Both may be purchased without a prescription at any pharmacy. Adequate lubrication helps decrease the condom's risk of breaking when the vagina is dry.

Though a condom holds firmly to the erect penis, after ejaculation it may easily slip off the flaccid penis. Because of this danger, it is best to withdraw the penis soon after intercourse, before it is completely soft. In addition, the base of the condom should be secured firmly against the penis to prevent the condom from slipping off. Penile thrusting can also loosen a condom, especially one with an abundance of lubricant inside and outside, like the Fourex and Naturalamb products. The new Mentor condom, with its adhesive at the base, is reportedly less likely than other condoms to slip off.

Using foam, jellies, or contraceptive creams in addition to the condom will add tremendously to its effectiveness. When spermicides and condoms are used together by a conscientious couple, the pregnancy rates should approach that of the birth-control pill. Even if not always used, it is good to keep a spermicide nearby in the event a condom slips off or tears following ejaculation. If this happens, immediate injection of foam deep into the vagina may help thwart a potential pregnancy. The new spermicide-containing condoms, such as Ramses Extra and Prime Super-Thin, would appear to be an even safer option.

Each condom should be used only once. Finally, one must not forget the ten most important letters in condom contraception: M-O-T-I-V-A-T-I-O-N!

How effective is the condom in preventing sexually transmitted diseases?

The condom is superior to all other contraceptive methods in preventing the spread of sexually transmitted diseases. Laboratory studies suggest that the addition of the spermicide nonoxynol-9 to some condoms may further add to their efficacy in this matter. No clinical studies have demonstrated that nonoxynol-9 kills disease organisms in actual practice as well as it does in the laboratory, however. Provided the condom doesn't slip off or tear, a woman or a man will have 100 percent protection against transmission of chlamydia and gonorrhea from an infected partner. Trichomoniasis ("trich") and nonspecific vaginitis (NSV) are two types of sexually transmitted vaginitis caused, respectively, by a microscopic protozoan and a bacterium. Though harmless, both organisms produce a profuse, foul-smelling, vaginal discharge. Men are almost always asymptomatic though capable of transmitting these organisms. Metronidazole (trade names: Flagyl, Protostat) is the prescription drug of choice for both conditions, but it must be given to both symptomatic and asymptomatic partners if a cure is to be permanent. Condom use effectively prevents the spread of trichomoniasis and nonspecific vaginitis.

Condom protection against syphilis and herpes is less effective than it is against other sexually transmitted diseases, since these organisms are capable of being introduced through the exposed skin of the labia or the scrotum. Similarly, venereal warts caused by the human papilloma virus (HPV) can probably spread via contact of skin surfaces. There is no doubt, however, that the condom offers a great deal of protection, especially for a woman whose partner's virus is inside the urethra or on areas of the penis that are completely covered by the condom. Only very specific strains of the HPV virus cause precancerous and cancerous changes of the cervix. One might theorize that the strains of HPV that reach the cervix are either at the tip of the penis or in the ejaculate, a supposition reinforced by a 1981 article in the *American Journal of Obstetrics and Gynecology*. The authors of this report, Dr. A. Cullen Richardson and Dr. James B. Lyon, instructed 139 women with a biopsy-proven diagnosis of cervical precancer to have their mates wear a condom with each act of coitus. After periods of observation of no less than six months, 136 women showed complete regression of their disease as evidenced by normal Pap smears and examinations. Could it be that interruption of the constant HPV inoculations on the cervix reversed the cervical abnormality? We are anxiously awaiting the results of other large studies to confirm or refute the findings of Drs. Richardson and Lyon.

Dr. Franklyn H. Judson and his associates at the University of Colorado Health Services Center in Denver, Colorado, tested the permeability of several brands of nonlubricated latex condoms to chlamydia and herpes organisms. In a laboratory simulation of intercourse using a mechanical dildo device reminiscent of a Rube Goldberg experiment, they created 50 to 100 thrusts over a period of ten minutes. They found that neither organism passed through the condom's wall. In a 1984 report, doctors using a similar device found that the herpes virus was unable to penetrate either the latex or the lamb membrane condoms.

No factor has contributed more to the resurgent interest in the condom than the fear and concern surrounding the epidemic of AIDS, the fatal disease caused by the HTLV-III virus (also known as HIV and LAV). It is now only too clear that heterosexuals as well as homosexuals and bisexuals are at risk of contracting AIDS. There is strong epidemiologic evidence to show that nothing will slow the spread of AIDS more efficiently than conscientious condom use. In a 1986 study, researchers at the University of California in San Francisco tested the permeability of latex and lamb membrane condoms to the AIDS virus. Each condom studied prevented the passage of the virus through its wall. An observation made by several researchers, though not yet statistically proven, is that condom breakage is more likely to occur with anal than with vaginal intercourse.

In summary, laboratory and clinical experience suggests that conscientious use of condoms will provide protection from a wide variety of sexually transmitted diseases. The condom's role as a contraceptive may eventually become secondary to its function as a disease preventative.

Why don't more people use the condom?

As with the diaphragm and vaginal spermicides, many couples complain that the spontaneity of sex is lost by stopping to put on a condom immediately before intercourse. For other couples it is a tolerable delay—even pleasurable, if the woman places the condom on her partner's erect penis.

Men often complain that the condom diminishes the sensation of the penis being in direct contact with the vaginal walls. Some men find, however, that the newer lubricated condoms actually enhance their penile sensitivity and enjoyment of coitus. Latex condoms do not allow heat to be transmitted from the vagina to the penis, and many men refuse to use them for this reason. Skin condoms, made of lamb intestinal membrane, often correct this problem.

"Rubber condom" dermatitis is a rare skin condition characterized by itching and swelling at the end of the penis due to an allergic reaction to a latex condom. A rash may begin at the tip of the penis and spread up the entire shaft to involve the scrotum, as well as other areas of the body. The same reaction in a latex-rubber-sensitive woman is usually milder, producing a rash on the vulva and inner thighs. Individuals with rubber sensitivity will experience no further difficulty if they switch to a condom made of lamb intestinal membrane, such as Fourex and Naturalamb.

Newer condoms containing the spermicide nonoxynol-9 may also be responsible for allergic skin reactions among sensitive individuals. If there is a history of such an allergy, Ramses Extra and Prime Super-Thin should not be used.

What do condoms cost?

The table on pages 129 to 131 lists the average price for a variety of condoms. As expected, the cost is slightly less when they are purchased in larger quantities.

There is no doubt that the condom will continue its resurgence as a reliable and safe method of preventing pregnancy and of controlling a large number of sexually transmitted diseases that are prevalent throughout our society.

5

COITUS INTERRUPTUS
AND RHYTHM

These methods of contraception are far less effective than barrier methods.

COITUS INTERRUPTUS

What is coitus interruptus?

Coitus interruptus is intercourse in which the male partner withdraws his penis from the vagina before ejaculation. Emission of sperm then takes place away from the vagina and external genitalia of the woman. It is an ancient technique, mentioned in the Bible where Onan "spilled his seed upon the ground." Other, more modern synonyms are withdrawal, pulling out, and the French method. Worldwide (and among teenagers in this country), it is probably the most used form of contraception. Coitus interruptus has a failure rate resulting in somewhere between 15 and 25 pregnancies per 100 woman-years of use.

Why is withdrawal such an unreliable method?

As discussed in chapter 4, it is doubtful that the first few drops of a man's discharge, which are present during erection but before ejaculation, can be responsible for pregnancy. In contrast, it is known that the first few drops of the "true" ejaculate, released at the time of orgasm, contain the greatest concentration of sperm. Depositing even a small amount of this fluid in the outer part of the vagina, or even on the labia, may result in sperm migration to and through the cervical os. For this reason, withdrawal should never be depended on for contraception by men with poor ejaculatory control or by those who experience premature ejaculation. Even when the method is practiced faithfully by a man with good control, the split-second timing required makes it inherently too dangerous for real reliability.

Women often object to coitus interruptus because it places the man in total control of both coitus and contraception. In addition, it is difficult for a woman to relax completely and achieve a full sexual response when she must worry whether or not he will "pull out" in time. A woman's orgasm may not be achieved or may be blunted with early withdrawal. Too often coitus is terminated abruptly, without any warning. Finally, for some women the postorgasmic warmth and closeness is spoiled by the presence of the external ejaculate.

Is there any way to improve coitus interruptus?

Many highly motivated couples have used withdrawal successfully for prolonged periods of time. When excellent communication and mutual respect exist between a couple, coitus interruptus is most likely to be successful. Frank discussion of coital

136

techniques may be helpful in determining which position will give the greatest degree of ejaculatory control. The "spoon position"—in which the couple curls side by side in a semifetal pose—is often very satisfactory both physically and emotionally. In this position the male partner is unable to thrust very deeply because he is behind the woman and has little leverage (see figure 5-1).

In the spoon position, a woman's legs are together, which helps to close the labia so that if ejaculation does take place on the labia there is less chance for sperm migration. This position also allows the woman to enjoy breast and clitoral stimulation during intercourse.

Another valuable aid for withdrawal users is the "squeeze technique." First introduced by J. H. Semans in 1956 and later popularized by Masters and Johnson, this method is also used as a treatment for premature ejaculation. In the squeeze method, the woman takes the superior position and stimulates the man to the point of imminent ejaculation. He must learn to signal her when he reaches this stage. She then temporarily withdraws the penis from the vagina and places her thumb on the undersurface of the penile glans at the frenulum, while placing her first and second fingers next to each other on either side of the coronal ridge (see figure 5-2). Strong pressure should be applied by squeezing the thumb and first two fingers together for approximately three to four seconds. When this technique is used on an uncircumcised male the coronal ridge should be felt through the skin covering, and the frenulum position should be estimated, since they will not be visible.

When the penis is erect, squeezing causes little if any discomfort, and considerable pressure with both hands may be necessary for adequate results. The desired effect is for the man to lose his urge to ejaculate immediately, though his erection will maintain 70 to 90 percent of its fullness. The penis is then reinserted and pelvic movements are resumed thirty to forty-five seconds after the squeeze. Following this technique there is little fear of imminent ejaculation for some time, occasionally for as long as twenty minutes. The squeeze technique may be repeated throughout coitus whenever the man lets his partner know that he is aroused and that orgasm may be imminent. With close communication, eventual ejaculation outside the vagina can easily be accomplished. It must be remembered that this technique will not work successfully if employed at the last moment before ejaculation.

The "stop-and-go" or "stop-start" technique can be used along with the squeeze technique to improve ejaculatory control during coitus interruptus. The stop-and-go method involves total cessation of all sexual stimulation, caressing, and thrusting just as ejaculation becomes imminent. The moment a man reaches that level of arousal,

Figure 5–1. *Spoon position.*

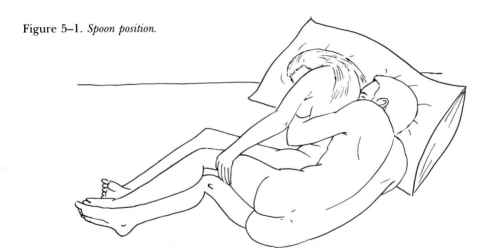

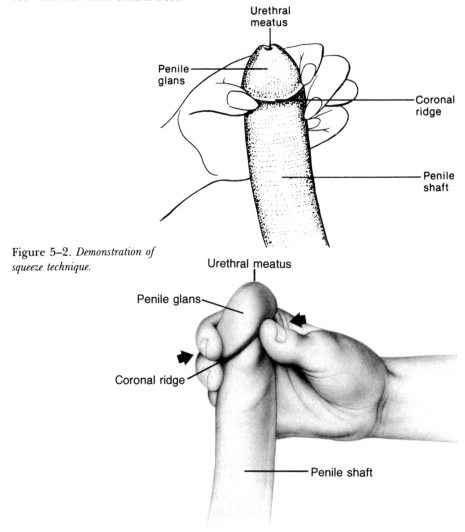

Figure 5–2. *Demonstration of squeeze technique.*

he communicates this to his partner, and everything stops as abruptly as the movement in an E. F. Hutton television commercial. After thirty seconds of complete inactivity, the intense desire to ejaculate will recede and stimulation can then be resumed.

Though research into the relative efficacy of these two techniques has been inconclusive, it is generally believed that the stop-and-go method is probably less effective than the squeeze technique in interrupting a man's ejaculatory cycle. In actual practice, however, many couples prefer the former method.

RHYTHM METHOD

What is the rhythm method?

The rhythm method is a birth-control technique based on limiting intercourse only to those times of the month thought to be free from the threat of pregnancy. It is the only contraceptive technique sanctioned by the Catholic Church. Many proponents of the rhythm method consider its name to be obsolete, and believe that the terms "natural family planning," and "fertility awareness" best describe the various techniques encompassed by this form of contraception. Since 1980, the U.S. government has increased the funds allotted to programs promoting natural family planning from a low of $400,000 in 1980 to its present level of almost $20,000,000 annually. In 1986, the Georgetown University School of Medicine received a $15 million grant from the Agency for International Development for a five-year study of the effectiveness, availability, and acceptability of natural family planning. These funding changes took place as the result of a congressional directive stating that these programs be strongly supported. Congress in turn was pressured by anti-abortion and pro-life lobbying groups opposed to "artificial" contraceptive methods. Despite the large sums of money devoted to the promotion and development of natural family methods, no significant inroads have been made in gaining new advocates or in drastically reducing the relatively high failure rates associated with their use.

It should be emphasized that most people who either practice or teach natural methods of family planning are morally and religiously opposed to the use of other means of birth prevention during the fertile days of the menstrual cycle. Strict adherents of "pure" natural family planning stress the importance of abstinence and self-control during these days in order to preserve the "naturalness" of the method and to strengthen the bond of shared responsibility, dedication, and faithfulness between couples. Many natural family planning supporters are adamant about the importance of coitus only within the marriage and the acceptance of a child should a pregnancy occur. While I appreciate and respect this position, I am also aware of the realities and frailties of our society in the 1980s. Since this book is intended for the majority of individuals seeking practical contraceptive advice, I recommend alternative methods of contraception during the fertile days of the month, when pregnancy is most likely to occur.

The rhythm method has been and will probably continue to be used widely throughout the world despite its decline in popularity in the United States. The results of a study released in 1977 showed that in 1965, 31.8 percent of white Catholics in the United States practiced rhythm but that by 1970 that figure had declined to 17.8, and by 1975 to 5.9 percent, while use of rhythm among non-Catholics went from 4.2 to 3.6 to 1.7 percent in the same years. Therefore, the importance of achieving maximum success with it is readily apparent.

The rhythm method may be divided into three categories: the calculation of the "safe" period, based on the length of previous menstrual cycles, known as the calendar technique; the charting of the daily basal body temperature; and the daily self-examination of the cervical mucus. These are all methods of determining ovulation in order to avoid coitus at that time. The sympto-thermal method of contraception is a combination of the temperature and cervical mucus methods. In addition, other signs of impending ovulation can be observed: breast tenderness, abdominal cramps, a change in position and firmness of the cervix, and for some women a slight amount of vaginal spotting. Though pregnancy rates for the rhythm method have been quoted in some studies to be as high as 30 per 100 woman-years, in the hands of a conscientious couple a more accurate rate is probably 10 to 19 per 100 woman-years.

Knowledge and use of all rhythm techniques should lower these failure rates to a more acceptable level.

How do I calculate the safe period based on the length of previous menstrual cycles?

The success of the calendar technique in determining the safe time for intercourse is based on three biological phenomena. The first is that ovulation will occur 14 days, plus or minus 2 days, prior to the onset of menses regardless of the length of the cycle. A woman with a 37-day cycle, measured from the first day before the next period, usually ovulates between Days 21 and 25. It is a misconception that ovulation occurs on the 14th day of the cycle, unless of course one has the textbook 28-day cycle, which is true of only 8 percent of women of childbearing age. The second and third phenomena crucial to the success of this technique are that an unfertilized egg survives no longer than twenty-four hours, and that most sperm remain viable no longer than forty-eight hours.

Chart the length of your cycle for a period of at least six months, then calculate your fertile days by subtracting 18 from the number of days of the shortest cycle over those months. That number represents the first fertile, or unsafe, day. Subtract 11 from the number of days of the longest cycle in order to determine the last fertile day, or the day on which the unsafe time ends. The following table demonstrates the method of calculating the unsafe days.

CALCULATING THE UNSAFE DAYS OF THE MENSTRUAL CYCLE

Length of Shortest Cycle in Days	First Unsafe Day after Start of Period	Length of Longest Cycle in Days	Last Unsafe Day after Start of Period
21	3	21	10
22	4	22	11
23	5	23	12
24	6	24	13
25	7	25	14
26	8	26	15
27	9	27	16
28	10	28	17
29	11	29	18
30	12	30	19
31	13	31	20
32	14	32	21
33	15	33	22
34	16	34	23
35	17	35	24

SOURCE: *Compiled by the author.*

For example, if you note that your shortest cycle is 25 days and your longest is 28 days, your first fertile, or unsafe, day will be Day 7, and your last fertile day will be Day 17. You must therefore avoid unprotected intercourse from Day 7 through Day 17 of future menstrual cycles.

If you are a sexually active woman with irregular menses, you obviously will not enjoy these restrictions on your sexual life. Furthermore, when the calendar technique of rhythm is used as the sole form of contraception, the best pregnancy rate achieved is an unsatisfactory 14 per 100 woman-years. The more often quoted figure, however, is 20 per 100 woman-years.

How is the daily temperature used in determining the unsafe days?

Following ovulation, progesterone is produced by the corpus luteum and is responsible for the elevation of a woman's temperature for approximately 14 days, until the onset of menstruation. The basal body temperature—the oral temperature taken immediately after waking each morning, before getting out of bed—will rise between 0.4° and 0.8°F. during those 14 days. Charting an accurate daily record of your temperature will enable you to determine your safe and unsafe times of the month.

Some women show a definite dip in temperature at the exact time of ovulation (see figure 5-3). By definition, the dip should be at least 0.1°F. below the previous six daily temperatures and occur within three days of the subsequent temperature rise. While many natural family planning enthusiasts have emphasized the importance of the temperature dip, recent studies have questioned its reliability in pinpointing the time of ovulation. In one report, published in 1980, researchers found that only ten of sixty-six normal cycles showed the classic body temperature dip. In other studies, in which the time of ovulation was accurately ascertained with blood tests, the temperature dip agreed with the laboratory results no more than 34 to 55 percent of the time. Based on these statistics, one would have to seriously question the predictive value of this factor.

The temperature rise usually takes place within twenty-four hours after ovulation. In actual practice, not all temperature charts are as easily interpreted as that demonstrated in figure 5-3. Occasionally the temperature rises gradually each day by less than 0.4°F., and at other times it may have a steplike appearance, with a 0.2°F. rise every two or three days. This may lead to inaccuracies in interpreting the safe days. Most confusing of all is the fact that 3 percent of women with hormonally proven ovulatory cycles show no temperature elevation at all.

You should take your basal temperature with a basal body thermometer, which has large, easy-to-read numbers and a temperature range of 96°F. to 100°F. These thermometers may be purchased at any pharmacy under the trade name of Ovulindex, and they usually cost $9.50 at a regular pharmacy and $8.50 at a discount pharmacy.

For greatest accuracy, rectal or vaginal temperatures are preferred to oral, but whatever method you choose, you should stick with it from one day to the next.

Since the egg is usually incapable of being fertilized twenty-four hours or more following ovulation, a temperature rise for three or more days should begin the period of safety from pregnancy. For the woman with predictable menstrual cycles, intercourse prior to ovulation should be safe until 7 days before the earliest recorded day of temperature rise based on the cycles over the preceding six months. Though sperm have been known to live for longer than forty-eight to seventy-two hours, they usually do not.

Figure 5-4 shows one woman's earliest recorded day of temperature rise to be on Day 15. Deducting 6 days will tell her that coitus should be safe for the first 8 days of the cycle. In addition, the 3rd day of temperature elevation, on Day 17, marks the first day that coitus can be resumed without fear of pregnancy. When the temperature

Figure 5–3. *Temperature method of rhythm contraception.*

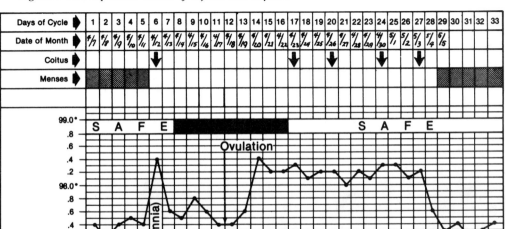

Figure 5–4. *Combined form of the temperature method.*

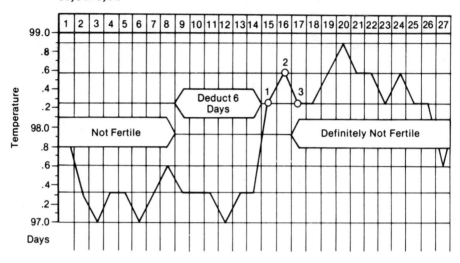

chart is used in this manner to determine safe coital days both before and after ovulation, it is referred to as the "combined form" of the temperature method.

What are the chances of conception with the temperature method?

Three early studies demonstrated pregnancy rates to fall between 14 and 24 per 100 woman-years. The only fairly recent report was conducted in 1968 by John Marshall in London, who studied 502 women taking daily basal body temperatures. One group was instructed to start coitus at the time of the month when the basal body temperature had been elevated for at least 3 consecutive days and to continue having intercourse daily until the last day of the cycle. The resultant pregnancy rate was a low 6.6 per 100 woman-years (see figure 5-5). When coitus is limited to this period of time, it is referred to as the "strict form" of the temperature method.

A second group in the study allowed intercourse prior to ovulation as well, with the

Figure 5–5. *Limiting coitus to the post-ovulation phase (strict form of the temperature method).*

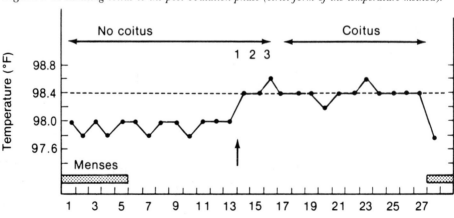

number of coital days determined by subtracting 19 from the number of days in the shortest menstrual cycle that the woman experienced over the previous six cycles. This number gave the day on which abstinence before ovulation should begin. The group experienced a pregnancy rate of 19.3 pregnancies per 100 woman-years.

Most investigators believe that the temperature method produces lower pregnancy rates than the calendar method. Using both methods together should improve the effectiveness of rhythm significantly.

Where can the temperature method go wrong?

Unfortunately one only knows in retrospect when ovulation has taken place. A surprisingly early ovulation is a real threat, even in a woman with previously predictable cycles. Statistically, only 8 percent of women of childbearing age have perfectly regular cycles each month. As previously mentioned, not all women experience the classic temperature dip at the time of ovulation, and, if it does occur, it is not always observable in the early morning when the temperature is taken. The burden of charting temperatures in the early morning when you are only half awake may lead to inaccuracies both in taking and in recording the temperature. One source of confusion may be a temperature elevation in the presence of an unrecognized infection or of tension, or following a sleepless night (see figure 5-3). Smoking a cigarette prior to taking the basal temperature can falsely elevate it, while drinking large amounts of alcohol the night before can falsely lower it.

The temperature change from low to high does not always follow the classic pattern depicted in figures 5-3 and 5-5. As mentioned earlier, the temperature will occasionally rise gradually each day by approximately 0.2°F., or even in steps, such as 0.2° every two or three days. Other deviations from the classic pattern include "zigzag," "double shifted," and "double shifted with a two-day plateau," illustrated in figure 5-6. A woman does not necessarily exhibit the same pattern of variation every month. To use the rhythm method successfully, abstinence is necessary until three consecutive temperatures have been recorded at the highest level.

Figure 5–6. A–E *Variations in the temperature pattern at the time of ovulation.*

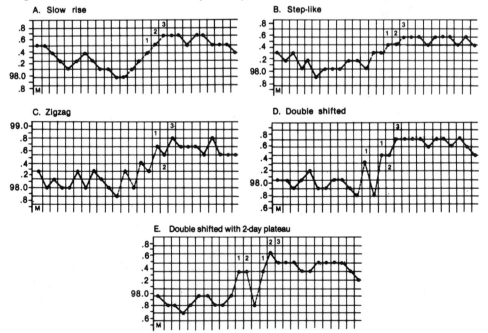

If I am a slow starter in the morning, or in too much of a hurry to take an accurate basal temperature, can I take it at a different time of day?

Most doctors have been taught that the basal (upon awakening) body temperature is the only accurate method to be used in determining ovulation. However, in 1974 Zuspan and Zuspan studied the menstrual cycles of nineteen ovulatory women. These women recorded their basal, 5:00 P.M., and bedtime temperatures. The pattern revealed that the basal was the lowest, the 5:00 P.M. was the highest, and the evening temperature was somewhere in between, but it was easy to interpret the results accurately regardless of when the temperature had been taken. The researchers calculated that if you forget to take your basal temperature, you can take it at 5:00 in the evening instead, and then subtract 0.7°F and record it on the basal body temperature chart for that day. When temperatures are taken at bedtime of the same day, subtract 0.3°F. For many women it is much easier to take either 5:00 P.M. or bedtime temperatures on a regular basis and simply chart them as they are.

How does studying my cervical mucus improve the efficacy of the rhythm method?

The amount and consistency of the mucus secreted by the glands of the cervix is determined by the relative concentrations of circulating estrogen and progesterone during each day of the menstrual cycle. Most women will feel a sensation of dryness if they touch their index finger to their entroitus, or vaginal opening, on the days immediately after the period ends. This dryness is due to the low levels of estrogen in the body at this time (see chapter 1). As the follicle develops in the ovary during each menstrual cycle, it secretes progressively greater amounts of estrogen daily. Most observant women will note a gradual change from dryness to a sensation of moistness over a period of several days. As ovulation approaches, the glands of the cervix, under the influence of greater amounts of estrogen, secrete an abundance of thin, clear, slippery, stretchable mucus. Its appearance is identical to that of raw egg white.

Spinnbarkeit is the term used to describe the stretchability of mucus and its presence is associated with an unmistakable sensation of wetness at the introitus. If you place your index finger at your introitus and withdraw it slowly at this time, and put your thumb and index fingertips together and then slowly separate them, you can usually stretch the mucus to a length of 4 inches. This indicates with certainty that ovulation is occurring, or will occur within twenty-four to seventy-two hours. "Peak symptom" is the term used to describe the last day that this wet and stretchable ovulatory mucus is present, not necessarily the day of maximum stretchability and wetness. The most recent data on this subject have confirmed that ovulation can occur as early as three days before and as late as three days after the peak symptom. On the average, however, ovulation precedes the peak symptom by approximately eight hours.

Following ovulation, the mucus becomes thick, tacky, and opaque, and lacks *spinnbarkeit*. These changes are due to the effect of progesterone produced by the corpus luteum. To avoid conception, abstinence is necessary from the time the thin mucus is first noted until four days after the peak symptom. This method of rhythm, based on analyzing changes in the cervical mucus, is also known as the "ovulation method," "fertility awareness," and the "Billings method," for Evelyn L. Billings and John J. Billings, two of its most ardent proponents who pioneered its use. If you use a speculum (see chapter 1), you can easily learn to recognize your own pattern of cervical mucus secretion, thereby having the knowledge to avoid conception regardless of the length or regularity of each individual cycle. By gently touching the cervical os with a cotton applicator or a long Q-tip and then slowly withdrawing it, you can easily determine how far the mucus stretches between the cervix and the applicator.

The amount of mucus and the amount of *spinnbarkeit* can actually be graded objectively (see the following table). A score of 3 in each category means that ovulation has just occurred or is imminent. It is easy to distinguish between mucus, which has cohesion and elasticity, and other vaginal discharges caused by semen, sexual arousal, or vaginitis, none of which cohere or stretch. Finally, as ovulation approaches some women note a progressive opening of the cervical os.

MEASURING THE AMOUNT AND QUALITY OF CERVICAL MUCUS AND THE OPENING OF THE CERVIX AT THE TIME OF OVULATION

Score	0	1	2	3
Amount of mucus	None	Scant	Dribble	Cascade
		A small amount of mucus can be drawn from the cervical os	A glistening drop of mucus seen in the external os, mucus easily drawn from the cervical canal	Abundant mucus pouring out of the cervical os
Spinnbarkeit	None	Slight	Moderate	Pronounced
		Uninterrupted mucous thread may be drawn approximately one-quarter of the distance between the external os and vulva, or approximately 1 inch (2.5cm).	Uninterrupted mucous thread may be drawn half the distance between the external os and the vulva, at least 2 inches (5cm.)	Uninterrupted mucous thread may be drawn for the whole distance between the external os and the vulva, at least 4 inches (10cm.)
Cervical os	Closed		Partially open	Gaping

SOURCE: *Compiled by the author.*

It has been reported that feeling the cervix daily may be helpful in determining the approximate day of ovulation, by noting changes in its position and consistency. For some women, the cervix is higher in the pelvis on the day prior to ovulation, making it difficult to reach with the examining finger. Following ovulation, it assumes a lower, easier-to-reach position in the vagina, and remains there through menstruation and until a few days before the next ovulation.

The consistency of the cervix at the time of ovulation has been described as feeling like a lip: "rubbery" or "soft" to touch. Within a day or two after ovulation, the consistency of the cervix changes abruptly and becomes firm, like the tip of the nose. Other clues to impending ovulation include breast tenderness, abdominal cramps, and occasionally a spot of blood in the cervical mucus. When all these symptoms are combined with the basal body temperature in determining one's safe and unsafe days, it is appropriately termed the "sympto-thermal" method.

Unfortunately, not all women experience the changes described and, when they do occur, they are often too subtle to predict the day of ovulation with any accuracy.

Are there any recent studies comparing the effectiveness of the Billings cervical mucus method to that of the sympto-thermal method?

Since the sympto-thermal method incorporates the study of the cervical mucus (the Billings method) along with basal body temperatures, the duration of previous menstrual cycles, symptoms of breast tenderness, abdominal discomfort, and the position and consistency of the cervix at ovulation, one would anticipate lower pregnancy rates when it is used correctly. In 1981, doctors at Cedars-Sinai Medical Center in California confirmed that the sympto-thermal method is indeed superior to the Billings cervical mucus method, with pregnancy rates of 13.7 versus 39.7 per 100 woman-years, respectively. Both techniques were associated with poor compliance and high dropout rates among the couples studied, however. In this ambitious study, 1,247 volunteer couples were assigned to practice one of the two methods after an instruction period of three to five months. Before the training period had ended, a disappointing 503 couples had quit, increasing to 726 couples by the end of the first year. In the year following entry into the program, 37 percent of couples using the ovulation method and 26 percent practicing sympto-thermal techniques voluntarily dropped out of the study. Dissatisfaction with the methods, unplanned pregnancies, and problems in identifying mucus changes were listed as the main reasons for leaving the research project. For couples who persisted, pregnancy rates during the year following formal entry into the study improved to 25 per 100 woman-years among the ovulation-method users and 9.4 per 100 woman-years for couples practicing the sympto-thermal method.

Aren't there special test kits to predict when ovulation will occur?

Perfecting the rhythm method has challenged scientists for many years, but until recently no chemical test could accurately predict safe and unsafe days. Over the past five years several companies have manufactured test kits that can measure the sudden surge of luteinizing hormone (LH) which always precedes ovulation by twenty-four to thirty-eight hours (see chapter 1). As previously mentioned, LH is produced by the anterior pituitary gland and is believed to play a vital role in extruding the follicle from the ovary each month. It is known that the length of the LH surge varies from woman to woman, but that each woman has her own predictable and repeatable pattern. Knowing at what point in the cycle your LH surge occurs is helpful, whether you are trying to conceive or trying to prevent pregnancy by perfecting your use of the rhythm method. It should be noted that manufacturers of kits that measure the LH surge are not permitted to advertise their product as a means of enhancing the rhythm method, but you may nonetheless find them helpful for this purpose.

All of the ovulation test kits currently on the market can detect LH levels in the urine ranging in sensitivity between 20 and 40 milli-International Units per milliliter. When the surge of LH appears, they all produce a change in either a test tube or a test strip to an intense blue color. When performed carefully, these tests are between 95 and 100 percent accurate. Examples of the kits are Right-Day, Ovu-Stick, Fortell, First Response, Q Test, and Ovutime. They cost between $35.00 and $45.00 for a packet of six to ten LH readings.

How and when should the LH tests be performed?

The frequency of testing will often depend on a woman's menstrual pattern. If you have regular periods, you should begin testing three to four days before anticipated ovulation and continue every day until you determine the exact day of the LH surge. In the case of the textbook 28-day menstrual cycle, this would mean starting on Day 10. Since ovulation consistently precedes the period by 14 days plus or minus two days, a woman with a regular 35-day cycle would begin testing on Day 17. Though it is more expensive, testing twice daily for three or four days before the expected ovulation is the best way to pick up the sudden rise of LH. It is difficult for a woman with very irregular periods to know when she should begin testing for LH. The best course for her would be to calculate the starting day based on the shortest previous cycle and to keep testing daily until a positive test is obtained. Women with cycle lengths varying by as much as 10 days may require more than one kit to cover all possible days of the LH surge. For these women, relying on test kits can become a very expensive method of birth control.

A blue color change, even if it is not intense, should alert you to abstain or to use barrier contraception and carefully test daily for the LH surge. Since it is known that ovulation will occur within forty-four hours of the LH surge, and that the egg is incapable of being fertilized by forty-eight hours (actually, twenty-four hours at the most) after ovulation, intercourse without contraception should be free of any risk of pregnancy ninety-two hours or more following the most intense color change for LH. This is a conservative estimate, to account for all deviations, a more realistically, it would be safe to resume unprotected intercourse sixty hours after the LH surge.

It is important to note that the greatest accuracy in daily LH testing appears to be between the hours of 11:00 A.M. and 3:00 P.M. Results are least accurate when the test is performed between 7:00 P.M. and 8:00 A.M. In addition, the concurrent use of medications or the presence of protein in the urine due to infection or other causes may invalidate test results.

There have been no scientific studies to show whether the use of ovulation test kits for the presence of LH can improve the success rates of the rhythm method. But if used in conjunction with the sympto-thermal method, one can only assume that the kits will add to the effectiveness of this method. Two notable disadvantages are the time required to run the tests daily, sometimes twice a day as ovulation approaches, and the cost of one or two new kits each month.

What is the CUE Ovulation Predictor and how accurate is it?

The CUE Ovulation Predictor is a device that can predict and confirm ovulation with an accuracy of 93 to 100 percent, according to its manufacturer, Zetek Incorporated of Aurora, Colorado. Unlike other ovulation prediction tests, which detect changes in LH levels, the CUE device electrically measures subtle differences in the salivary and vaginal concentrations of sodium, potassium, and chloride as ovulation approaches. Though the CUE device was originally approved by the FDA in 1985 for couples seeking pregnancy, it is likely to be helpful to women in improving the accuracy of the rhythm method. Though it is not advertised as a method for preventing pregnancy, you can buy or rent the CUE Ovulation Predictor directly from the company for this purpose.

The CUE Ovulation Predictor contains both an oral and a vaginal sensor, or probe, which are attached to a monitor unit by a cable. The monitor, which looks like a calculator, takes information from the sensors and transfers it into a two- or three-digit number which is displayed on the monitor (see figure 5-7). The instrument operates on a standard 9-volt battery.

To take an oral reading, put the round end of the oral sensor on your tongue for about ten seconds; and to obtain a vaginal reading, place the tampon-shaped part of the vaginal probe against the cervix for ten seconds.

Zetek researchers have described different but characteristic measurements for the oral and vaginal probes, as demonstrated in figure 5-8.

The so-called CUE Peak is noted to occur six days before ovulation. This high reading on the monitor is followed by a sharp decline and then a sharp rise two to three days prior to ovulation. The most important aspect of the oral pattern among women tested is that the CUE Peak predicts ovulation by six to seven days. The physiological basis for these changes is unknown, but previous research has demonstrated that estrogen levels in the body alter the chemical components of a woman's

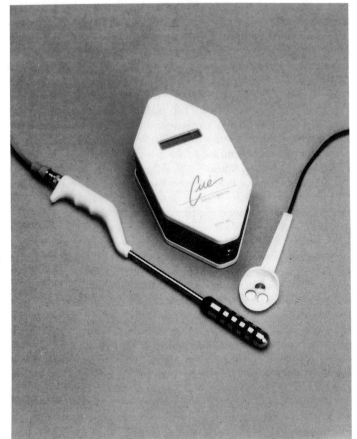

Figure 5–7. *CUE ovulation predictor.*

saliva. The changes in salivary levels of sodium, potassium, and chloride are reflected in this CUE reading (see chapter 11, "The Future").

The vaginal readings have been found to provide a more exact prediction of ovulation than the oral readings. The sharp decline to its nadir, or lowest point, as noted in Figure 5-8, very reliably occurs within a day or two of ovulation, and the subsequent rise is a signal that ovulation is occurring on that day. These changes in the CUE readings are caused by the cervical mucus volume and the concentrations of sodium, chloride, and potassium, which reach their peak at ovulation.

Clinical trials on a limited number of patients to date have demonstrated that the CUE method may prove to be a safe and valuable adjunct to ovulation prediction and natural family planning.

Are there other techniques available to enhance the accuracy of the rhythm method?

If you have access to a speculum and an ordinary low-powered microscope, but preferably a high-powered one, you can easily perform a "fern test" on your cervical mucus on the fourth through sixth days preceding ovulation.

Place a small amount of mucus from the cervical os on an applicator stick and rub it onto a glass slide. When the glass slide is viewed under the microscope at the time of ovulation, a beautiful thick, branching pattern of the mucus, resembling a fern, may

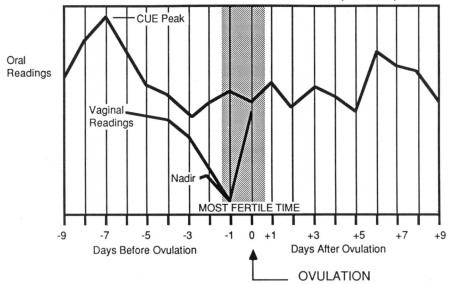

Figure 5–8. *Characteristics of oral and vaginal CUE readings.*

be seen throughout the slide (see figure 5-9). The fern pattern is dependent on the high concentration of salt (sodium chloride) in the cervical mucus at this time.

A scant amount of ferning without branching means ovulation is still not imminent. Following ovulation, under the influence of progesterone, the ferning disappears almost completely within two or three days in practically all women. A fern test may be totally inadequate in the presence of a slight amount of blood in the mucus, which some women experience at the time of ovulation. Inflammation of the cervix, or cervicitis, may also be responsible for an absence of ferning at the time of ovulation.

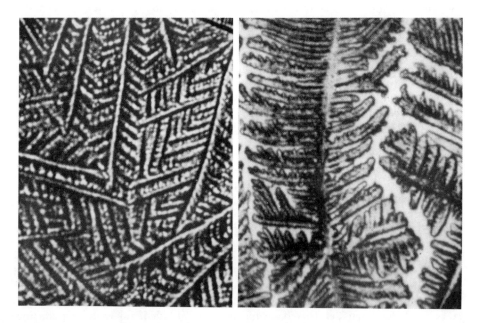

Figure 5–9. *Fern pattern at ovulation.*

Since cervicitis is often an asymptomatic condition, a woman should be evaluated and if necessary treated for it by her gynecologist before relying on the ferning method. Use of lubricants will also hinder this method's success.

The cervical mucus on the glass slide can also be easily tested with the "burn," or "caramel" test, in which the mucus on the slide is allowed to dry and is then heated over a flame for approximately one minute. The slide is then held up to the light, and if it appears transparent, the presence of crystallization and a high chloride concentration associated with ovulation are confirmed. In contrast, light- and dark-brown colors on the slide indicate a lack of crystallization and a mucus that is either pre- or post-ovulatory.

Based on the fact that cervical mucus is rich in sodium chloride at the time of ovulation, researchers have developed a rapid spot test that a woman can perform at home to determine the chloride content of her cervical mucus. In practice, it has proven to be far less reliable than the fern or the burn test.

Some people may consider it absurd to use thermometers, LH determinations, speculums, slides, and a microscope for the purpose of avoiding pregnancy. But among women whose medical condition or religious or moral beliefs dictate against other forms of contraception, such methods may be the only weapon to fight the constant danger of unplanned pregnancy. All available variations of the rhythm method must be explored and offered to women who are willing to use them. The cost of a secondhand microscope seems insignificant in comparison to the cost of an unwanted pregnancy.

What are some of the new methods and devices for improving the rhythm method?

A prerequisite for the endorsement of the rhythm method by a large segment of the population will be the discovery of a rapid, inexpensive, accurate, self-administered method of ovulation prediction. Such a method has not yet been developed.

Over the past few years a variety of inventors have devised exotic instruments, computerized digital thermometers, electrical devices, complicated calendars, and "fertility kits" in attempts to measure more precisely body temperature, the exact day of ovulation, and changes in the consistency and stretchability of a woman's cervical mucus. Some of these devices, which have proven less than satisfactory, are the Ovutimer, Ovulometer, Ovutron, Tachmeter, and Ovu-Guide. Despite the proliferation of such gadgets, none has proven more accurate than the careful observation charted by a woman who has taken the time to familiarize herself with the cyclic hormonal and physical changes that take place in her body each month.

Much of the laboratory research directed at improving the accuracy of the rhythm method is based on the changes in the chemical content of the cervical mucus at different times of the menstrual cycle. In addition to the previously mentioned observation that sodium chloride concentrations increase at ovulation, scientists have observed similar changes in glucose, or sugar, concentrations. Highly touted "fertility test kits" containing Tes-Tape for measuring glucose concentrations can be purchased at most pharmacies. To measure glucose concentrations, simply insert your index finger into the vagina and touch your cervix. A small sample of mucus will usually remain on the fingertip after you have taken your finger out. Greater accuracy will be achieved if you learn to familiarize yourself with visualizing the cervix through a speculum. Touch your fingertip to a one-inch piece of yellow Tes-Tape, and its color will usually turn to dark blue at the time of ovulation. Prior to ovulation, lesser shades of blue and green, representing lower sugar concentrations, will be found. Though this sounds like a simple and safe way to enhance the accuracy of the rhythm method, in actual practice it has proven to be less than ideal. In fact, the majority of investigators now believe that Tes-Tape determinations are of little if any value in predicting "safe" and "unsafe" days.

Protein and enzyme constituents of the cervical mucus also demonstrate specific changes with each menstrual cycle. Despite promising research, however, no test is yet available to aid couples using the rhythm method (see chapter 11, "The Future.")

What are *mittelschmerz* and the "bounce test"?

Mittelschmerz is another name for painful ovulation. The small percentage of women who regularly experience it have the advantage of being alerted to avoid intercourse for twenty-four hours after they experience the pain, when the chances of fertilizing an egg are most likely. These women will also know in retrospect that there is a chance of pregnancy if intercourse occurred less than forty-eight hours before the onset of the pain. The pain can last for as little as a few minutes or as long as twenty-four hours.

The bounce test may help one-third of women who do not experience *mittelschmerz* to determine the day of their ovulation, although it is a bit primitive. Starting six days before the day when ovulation is expected, bounce on a hard surface, such as a wooden chair, by sitting down abruptly three or four times every morning and evening. Occasionally, the pain of *mittelschmerz* will be reproduced when bouncing is performed on the day of ovulation.

If pregnancy occurs while I am using the rhythm method, will there be any danger to the fetus?

There is considerable evidence to suggest that a wide range of pregnancy problems, such as spontaneous abortion and birth defects, may be related to the use of the rhythm method. It has been demonstrated that the optimum chance for normal pregnancy occurs when fertilization of the egg takes place just at the time of ovulation. Users of the rhythm method are more likely to abstain from intercourse at that time and for the few days prior to ovulation. Having intercourse twelve to twenty-four hours after ovulation is more likely to expose an overripe, unhealthy egg to fertilization. Whereas fertilization normally takes place in the portion of the fallopian tube closest to the ovary, late fertilization occurs after the egg has traveled some distance along the tube, or has entered the uterine cavity. This condition of an egg is known as "post-ovulatory," "tubal," or "intrauterine" overripeness. The second type of overripeness is called pre-ovulatory or follicular, and is the result of an egg being retained in the ovary beyond the normal time. As a result, structural defects take place in the egg which may produce an abnormal fetus when ovulation and fertilization finally do occur. Both post-ovulatory and pre-ovulatory overripeness have been held responsible for poor pregnancy outcome.

Statistical data from three different studies conducted in New England have indicated a significantly higher rate of congenital fetal central nervous system defects in the Catholic population than in the Protestant population. In the September 16, 1978, issue of the medical journal *Lancet,* two researchers noted an association between infrequent intercourse and an increased incidence of Down's Syndrome, or mongolism. Down's Syndrome most often occurs when a particular pair of chromosomes do not divide when the egg is being formed. A child born with this condition will have an extra chromosome. The October 21, 1978, issue of *Lancet* published a letter from Marie T. Mulcahy, from the State Health Laboratory Services in Perth, Australia, suggesting that the findings could probably be attributed to the rhythm method of contraception. Ms. Mulcahy cited an epidemiological study of Down's Syndrome patients who were born in western Australia between 1966 and 1975 that showed the incidence among births to Catholic women to be more than double that found in all other religions.

Ms. Mulcahy noted that this high incidence remained more or less constant throughout this ten-year period, that it was apparent in all maternal age groups, and that it was not related to birth rank or to ethnic origin of either parent.

		Down's Syndrome	Incidence Per 1,000
Religion	Live Births	Births	Live Births
Catholic	55,788	108	1.935
Other	150,835	127	0.842

SOURCE: *Mulcahy, Lancet 1987.*

Dr. Richard Juberg of Louisiana State University has recently studied the effects of delayed fertilization among thirty-three parents who have children with chromosomal abnormalities such as Down's Syndrome. Dr. Juberg and his colleagues found twenty-four instances in which there was definite evidence of delayed fertilization. Though other variables may certainly be responsible, it appears likely that the rhythm method may play a significant role in causing some of these chromosomal abnormalities.

CONTRACEPTIVE EFFECT OF NURSING AND RISK OF PREGNANCY FOLLOWING ABORTION AND FULL-TERM DELIVERY

Many women and their doctors are misinformed regarding the time that fertility is restored after full-term pregnancy for both the nursing and non-nursing woman and after abortion. In an excellent statistical review of this information, Dr. Helmuth Vorherr has helped to clarify some of these issues. The data in this section are based on some of his work.

How soon after abortion does fertility return?

Most women regain their fertility within a short time following an abortion. When the terminated pregnancy is between eight and fifteen weeks, the average return of ovulation takes two to three weeks. When the pregnancy is between sixteen and twenty weeks, ovulation usually returns four to six weeks later. The first period following an abortion is usually preceded by ovulation (see figure 5-10).

Figure 5–10. *Return of ovulation and menstruation following abortion.*

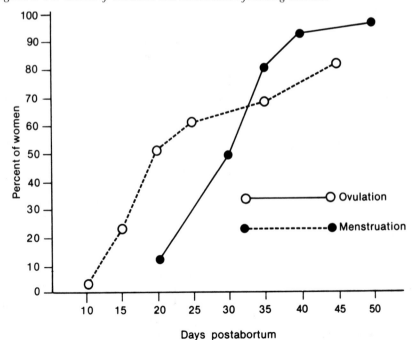

The statistics in the figure make it clear that contraception should be instituted immediately following abortion if repeat pregnancy is to be avoided. There is no such thing as a safe period following pregnancy termination.

What are the chances of conceiving soon after a full-term pregnancy?

Generally, menstruation is not resumed before four to five weeks following childbirth, and the first periods are usually not preceded by ovulation. In both the nursing and non-nursing woman, ovulation rarely takes place before the sixth week following a full-term delivery, though there are documented cases in the medical literature of ovulation occurring as early as twenty-one days postpartum in a non-nursing woman.

Both ovulation and menstruation are more likely to occur earlier with women who do not nurse, as demonstrated in the following table.

COMPARISON OF POSTPARTUM REPRODUCTIVE FUNCTION IN THE NURSING AND NON-NURSING WOMAN

Weeks Until Return of Ovulation	Percentage of Breast-Feeding Women	Percentage of Bottle-Feeding Women
6	5	15
12	25	40
24	65	75
Weeks until Return of Menstruation		
6	15	40
12	45	65
24	85	90

SOURCE: *Vorherr, H. Contraception after abortion and postpartum.* American Journal of Obstetrics and Gynecology *117 (1973): 1002–25.*

The important lesson to be learned from this table is that the likelihood of ovulation, and thus theoretically of pregnancy, may be as high as 25 percent in nursing women twelve weeks following delivery, and 65 percent at twenty-four weeks. These statistics should dispel the myth of reliability on nursing as the sole method of contraception after the sixth postpartum week. Actual conception rates are not nearly as high as indicated by these theoretical risks, however. Among couples using withdrawal, rhythm, and abstinence or infrequent coitus as methods of contraception, the actual percentage of women who conceive will be far below the expected number. Among nursing women, only 1 percent will conceive within three months following childbirth, 5 percent will conceive within six months, and 10 percent within twelve months. Corresponding figures for non-nursing women are 3 percent, 15 percent, and 25 percent.

Despite the fact that nursing is not considered a reliable method of birth control, many American women rely solely on it during the first four to six postpartum months but their numbers may be decreasing. Estimates for 1970 to 1973 are that 34 percent of sexually active nursing women used this method, compared to 24 percent between 1973 and 1976.

Are there ways of improving the efficacy of lactation as a contraceptive?

The length of time before a nursing woman menstruates is quite variable. Often, the determining factor is how frequently and enthusiastically she nurses her baby. It is not unusual for a breast-feeding woman to experience a complete absence of periods for a year or more if she offers the baby no supplemental feedings.

Carefully documented research conducted since 1981 has clearly shown that breast-feeding may work far more effectively as a contraceptive when six or more feedings are given every twenty-four hours, each lasting ten to fifteen minutes, including at least one at night. Nursing practiced in this manner may yield pregnancy rates as low as 1 to 2 per 100 woman-years during the first six to twelve postpartum months. The reason for this protection is that the frequent suckling of the nipple sends impulses to the hypothalamus in the brain, continually blocking the releasing factors responsible for stimulating the LH secretion necessary for ovulation (see chapter 1). Instead, the pituitary gland is consistently stimulated to produce prolactin, and this prevents follicle growth in the ovary as well as preventing ovulation and menstruation. Studies have shown that prolactin levels drop rapidly when a baby is given supplemental feedings.

It is becoming increasingly clear that the continuation of breast-feeding at night may be the major determinant in predicting the return of fertility in lactating women. In one report, doctors found that whenever a woman skipped nursing for a period of ten to twelve hours at night, ovulation was sure to follow within a short period of time. They found that this ten-to-twelve hour hiatus was a more reliable predictor of the return of fertility than were the initiation of supplemental feedings or the return of menses. Another report, published in 1981, found that the first period in a nursing woman who gave no supplemental feedings was never preceded by ovulation.

Though nursing in the manner prescribed may lower a woman's chances of pregnancy, it does take its toll on the time she can devote to other pursuits. For most working women, this schedule will prove unrealistic and impossible to carry out.

Is it possible for a nursing woman to use the Billings or the sympto-thermal method effectively?

Several articles in the past five years have concluded that the Billings and the sympto-thermal methods can be effectively used to predict ovulation in nursing women, even if ovulation occurs sporadically. Using these methods requires careful, daily observations of cervical mucus and other symptoms, however, and attention to such details while caring for a young baby is often difficult. In one recent study only twelve of forty-two nursing women persevered in successfully using these methods.

The vaginal tissues of nursing women are often very thin, resembling those of a postmenopausal woman, because prolactin inhibits the release of estrogen from the relatively inactive ovaries. With prolonged lactation, some women will develop an atrophic vaginitis, characterized by a gray, nonlubricative (lacking mucus), wet discharge. The observant woman will be able to distinguish this condition easily from the cohesive, sticky discharge associated with estrogen release, ovulation, and potential fertility.

DOUCHING: A NONMETHOD

Douching with various solutions is an ancient postcoital contraceptive technique that is totally futile. Current research has demonstrated that sperm can move into the endocervix, beyond the reach of a douche solution, within ninety seconds after ejaculation. This does not mean that the ejaculate is not capable of entering the endocervix as soon as five seconds later, but only that ninety seconds was the fastest the researchers were able to collect and examine the postcoital specimens. In addition, recent studies have located sperm in the fallopian tube ten to forty-five minutes following insemination. Even if a douche is used within ten seconds following ejaculation, it is highly improbable that it could kill all the sperm in the vagina or prevent the ascent through the cervical os of many sperm.

While douching might not decrease a woman's risk of becoming pregnant, there is some evidence that it might increase her chances of an ectopic pregnancy. In an article published in the *American Journal of Obstetrics and Gynecology* in 1986, researchers found that women who douched once or more a week had an average of twice the incidence of ectopic pregnancies as did women who never douched. For unexplainable reasons, those who used a commercial douching preparation were shown to be far more susceptible to ectopic pregnancy than those using water or a noncommercial douching mixture such as water and vinegar.

For the woman in need of postcoital contraception, douching is clearly without value. In the next chapter I will discuss effective methods of postcoital contraception.

6

POSTCOITAL CONTRACEPTION

Estimates of the chances of conception following one act of unprotected intercourse at the time of ovulation vary from a low of 2 to 4 percent, to a high of 20 percent. You may have forgotten to take adequate contraceptive precautions, or the method itself may have failed. The possibility of slippage or tears of a condom and the expulsion of an IUD from the uterus or of a TODAY sponge from the vagina emphasizes the need for effective "morning-after" contraception. Pregnancy prevention following rape represents one of the most acute and pressing needs for this form of postcoital therapy.

Effective postcoital contraception is now available in the form of hormonal preparations, the "morning-after IUD," and menstrual extraction. These practical and popular methods have given women the opportunity to terminate safely both the suspected and the diagnosed pregnancy following unprotected coitus. Unfortunately, little if any information about this invaluable form of emergency contraception has been disseminated to the general public. The FDA and the American College of Obstetricians and Gynecologists have not alerted the public to the fact that this option is available.

MORNING-AFTER HORMONAL PREPARATIONS

What is the "morning-after pill"?

Though several hormonal preparations have been used effectively as postcoital contraceptives, most gynecologists associate the "morning-after pill" with the infamous drug diethylstilbestrol, or DES. Unlike other estrogens, DES is classified as a nonsteroidal synthetic estrogen. This is a fancy way of saying that it is made in the laboratory and not in the body, and is of a chemical structure totally different from the steroidal shape of natural estrogens and those contained in birth control pills.

In addition to DES, many other hormonal preparations have proven to be highly effective in preventing the survival of the fertilized egg when administered within seventy-two hours following unprotected intercourse at the time of ovulation (see table). Currently the most popular of these products is Ovral, a commonly prescribed birth-control pill. This pill contains the synthetic estrogen ethinyl estradiol and the progestin norgestrel (see chapter 2). Ethinyl estradiol is the estrogen component of many other oral contraceptives. It has been used alone, without the progestin, as a highly successful morning-after pill. Similarly, the progestins norgestrel and quingestanol acetate have been used alone as postcoital contraceptives.

POSTCOITAL HORMONES

Drug	Trade Name	Dosage
Diethylstilbestrol (DES)	——	25 milligrams twice a day for five days
Ethinyl estradiol	Estinyl	2.5 milligrams twice a day for five days *or* Ten 0.5-milligram tablets a day for five days
Conjugated estrogens	Premarin	10 milligrams two or three times a day *or* Intravenous 50 milligrams a day for two days
Esterified estrogens	Evex, Menest	10 milligrams twice a day for five days
Estrone	Ogen	5 milligrams twice a day for five days
Ethinyl estradiol (0.05 milligrams) and norgestrel (0.5 milligrams)	Ovral	Two tablets immediately and repeat in twelve hours
Norgestrel	——	One dose of 1.0 to 3.35 milligrams
Quingestanol acetate	——	One dose of 1.5 milligrams

SOURCE: *Compiled by the author.*

How do morning-after medications prevent continuation of a pregnancy?

Morning-after hormones act as interceptors, meaning that they prevent implantation of the egg after fertilization has taken place. It is theorized that they may act as pregnancy interceptors at several locations. One of their main effects appears to be on the corpus luteum, causing it to malfunction and produce inadequate amounts of progesterone which is essential for support of an early pregnancy. The decline of progesterone is occasionally reflected by a premature drop in the basal body temperature during the second half of the menstrual cycle (see chapter 5). The premature breakdown of the corpus luteum is referred to as the *luteolytic* effect of these hormones.

A second, very likely site of morning-after medication activity is in the endometrium, where it causes a deficiency of an enzyme called *carbonic anhydrase*. Without this enzyme, the fertilized egg can't dispose of its carbon dioxide waste products and therefore dies. Studies of the endometrium have also noted microscopic retardation of growth following morning-after medications, in addition to the lack of another enzyme, *alkaline phosphatase*.

In the past it was theorized that these hormones, especially DES, were responsible for both slowing down and speeding up the passage of the fertilized egg down the fallopian tube. A "tube-locking" effect was believed to be responsible for a higher incidence of ectopic (tubal) pregnancy in women who conceived despite the morning-after treatment. However, it is now generally believed that these hormones prevent intrauterine pregnancy, not tubal pregnancy. Therefore, when pregnancy does take place, it has more of a chance of being in the tube, though the actual number of tubal pregnancies among such women is no higher.

What are some of the side effects associated with postcoital contraceptives and how can they be averted or alleviated?

The extremely high dose of estrogen contained in most postcoital medications is reported to cause nausea in approximately 70 percent of users and vomiting in over 33 percent. Postcoital doses of Ovral have been associated with a 19 percent incidence of vomiting and the same 70 percent likelihood of nausea. Ovral also has the advantage of reducing the duration of therapy from five days to a mere twelve hours, and the number of pills consumed to only four, compared with as many as fifty with other medications.

Dr. Hans Lehfeldt, in his 1976 review in *OB/GYN Digest,* noted a lower incidence of side effects such as headache, nausea, and vomiting with ethinyl estradiol. His technique is to give 5 milligrams a day of ethinyl estradiol for five days. To reach the 5-milligram dose, however, a woman must take a total of ten 0.5-milligram tablets throughout the entire day. As a result, only 10 percent of Lehfeldt's patients were nauseated and only 2 percent vomited.

If pills, rather than intravenous estrogens, are taken, it is a good idea for your doctor to prescribe a few more tablets than the required dosage. Vomiting within four hours after the pill is swallowed necessitates taking another pill, since there is a chance that not all of the medication will have been absorbed into the body prior to this time. It is also advisable for your doctor to prescribe medication to prevent nausea and vomiting, to be taken one hour before each tablet. If vomiting secondary to oral estrogen can't be controlled, pregnancy will become a real threat unless your doctor prescribes intravenous Premarin, 50 milligrams daily for two days. When Premarin is taken orally in a dose of 10 milligrams three times daily for five days, nausea will occur 50 percent of the time and breast tenderness will affect 37 percent of the women using this medication.

Other side effects reported with morning-after hormones include headaches, dizziness, and menstrual irregularities. As many as 20 percent of women will experience some type of menstrual irregularity, suggestive of pregnancy, during the cycle that the postcoital hormones are taken. Often the flow is delayed or lighter than normal, which should reassure women who fear that the DES they took did not successfully intercept a pregnancy. To be on the safe side, however, a sensitive pregnancy test should be performed on all women with light or delayed menses following a course of postcoital hormones.

If you are medically unable to take the estrogen in birth-control pills—due to hypertension, migraines, epilepsy, liver disease, phlebitis, or breast cancer—you will certainly not be able to take the enormous dose of estrogen in postcoital contraceptives. Sudden onset of symptoms such as blurring of vision, severe headache, chest pain, severe leg cramps, cough, or shortness of breath while using these medications necessitates stopping them immediately and seeking medical evaluation.

Women who are unable to take estrogens can use postcoital progestins such as norgestrel and quingestranol acetate, with the drawback that slightly higher pregnancy rates and abnormal bleeding have been associated with these preparations.

How effective are postcoital contraceptives?

DES, the infamous synthetic estrogen used in the 1950s and 1960s to prevent miscarriage (see page 159), has proven to be an effective postcoital contraceptive. In a review combining the results from several DES studies totalling 5,593 women, twenty-six pregnancies were reported. The authors estimated that without DES 1,100 women, or 20 percent of those exposed, would have conceived. More recent reports have sampled more than 1,000 women using DES without a single pregnancy.

While DES is an excellent postcoital contraceptive, other estrogen preparations have fared equally well. Yussman treated 200 rape victims with 50 milligrams of intravenous conjugated estrogens (Premarin) for two days without a pregnancy, while others have administered Premarin orally, 10 milligrams three times a day for five days, to 359 women with only one pregnancy reported. The incidence of nausea appears to be less frequent with Premarin than with DES, especially when it is given intravenously.

In a 1980 study, doctors at the Centers for Disease Control compared the effectiveness of ethinyl estradiol and conjugated estrogens as postcoital contraceptives. Almost 1,000 women took one of the two estrogens following unprotected coitus at midcycle, with a pregnancy rate of only 0.7 percent noted for those treated with ethinyl estradiol compared with 1.6 percent for women who took conjugated estrogens. Nausea and vomiting, however, were significantly more frequent among those who took ethinyl estradiol. Though prescribed within seventy-two hours of unprotected intercourse, postcoital contraception in this study and several others was found to be almost twice as likely to succeed when it was started within twenty-four hours after unprotected intercourse. The most recent addition to postcoital contraception is the use of the birth-control pill Ovral. Researchers at the University of Western Ontario reported a pregnancy rate of only 0.16 percent when two Ovral tablets were taken soon after unprotected intercourse followed by a repeat dose twelve hours later.

What effects will morning-after hormones have on the developing fetus if they fail to intercept the pregnancy?

The effects on a fetus that is only a few hours old are unknown, but since organ development does not take place for several weeks, it is highly unlikely that these hormones will be responsible for causing anomalies. When inadvertently taken after pregnancy is already a few weeks along, the risk of fetal anomalies will increase significantly. Deformities associated with the use of ethinyl estradiol and norgestrel contained in Ovral are discussed in chapter 2. In the highly publicized experience with DES, both male and female fetuses have been reported to suffer a wide range of genital abnormalities when the drug is taken after the seventh week from the last menstrual period. An advantage of using ethinyl estradiol, conjugated estrogens, estrone, and esterified estrogens is that they are all steroidal in structure. As a result, they are not likely to initiate the changes characteristic of nonsteroidal estrogens such as DES.

How does DES taken by a mother affect the risk of vaginal cancer in her daughter?

Practically all medication given to a mother crosses the placenta and reaches the fetus. Between 1940 and 1971, DES was widely used to prevent miscarriage, especially for women with poor obstetrical history, diabetics, and others who experienced vaginal bleeding early in pregnancy. It has been estimated that approximately two million pregnant women took DES or two other equally harmful nonsteroidal estrogens, dienestrol and hexestrol. In most instances, treatment with these substances began in the seventh week of pregnancy. Coincidentally, that is the time when vaginal and cervical development and demarcation becomes most active in the female fetus.

In 1972, three Boston physicians noted a sudden increase among young women in the number of previously rare cancers of the vagina and cervix, called clear-cell adenocarcinomas. Upon further investigation they discovered that the majority of the mothers of these young women had taken nonsteroidal estrogens during their pregnancies. In addition, benign though highly abnormal changes were observed in the cervix and vagina of many of the daughters exposed to DES, dienestrol, and hexestrol. The Registry of Clear-Cell Adenocarcinoma of the Genital Tract of Young Females was formed in 1972 with the purpose of reporting all such tumors in women born in the United States and abroad after 1940. In 1977, the name of the Registry was changed to the National Cooperative Diethylstilbestrol Adenosis Project, or DESAD.

To date at least 250 vaginal and 100 cervical adenocarcinomas have been reported. Of these, use of nonsteroidal estrogens by the mothers has been confirmed in approximately 65 percent. More than fifty of these women have died of adenocarcinoma, while others have undergone radical and mutilating operations to prevent the spread of the disease. Fortunately, our worst fears of an epidemic of genital cancer have not been realized. The risk of development of clear-cell cancer is estimated to be no more than 1.4 per 1,000 and possibly as few as 1.4 per 10,000 exposed daughters. The peak incidence appears to occur at the age of nineteen, with a precipitous decline noted after the age of twenty-four. The occurrence of adenocarcinoma after the age of twenty-seven is extremely rare.

What are the benign cervical and vaginal changes caused by DES?

Using sophisticated diagnostic techniques, including colposcopy, skilled gynecologists have noted adenosis in anywhere from 80 to 97 percent of daughters exposed in utero to DES. *Adenosis* refers to the presence of strawberry red, mucus-secreting glandular tissue on the outer part of the cervix and vagina. These glands are normally located inside the cervix and are usually not readily seen with a speculum.

In addition to adenosis, the cervix in approximately 40 to 50 percent of these women often appears characteristically deformed, so that the diagnosis of maternal DES ingestion can be made simply by viewing its unusual shape during a routine examination. One of these distorted shapes, called a vaginal hood or collar, is seen as a circular fold in the upper vagina into which the cervix containing adenosis appears to merge. Another is the classic cock's comb, a small triangular protuberance seen at the upper pole of the cervix. In addition to abnormalities of the cervix and vagina, uterine abnormalities were first described by doctors at Baylor College of Medicine in 1977, including underdevelopment of the uterus combined with a peculiar T-shaped configuration of the uterine cavity, and constricting bands in the uterine cavity along the horizontal arm of the T. These abnormalities are easily found by a technique in which dye is injected through the cervix and outlines the uterine cavity and fallopian tubes. This procedure is called a *hysterosalpingogram*. More recent investigation has determined that the presence of irregular or "shaggy" margins of the endometrial cavity outline that show up on X rays is often associated with prenatal exposure to DES. About two-thirds of DES-exposed women have uterine anomalies on hysterosalpingogram even though the external configuration of the uterus may appear normal when viewed through the laparoscope (see laparoscopy). In one study of DES-exposed women, 86 percent of those with characteristic cervical anomalies were noted on X ray to have a uterine defect. In contrast, women spared cervical and vaginal abnormalities will not, in almost 100 percent of all cases, have a uterine deformity such as a T-shaped or constricted uterus.

Do these abnormalities of the cervix and uterus in DES daughters adversely affect their chances of a successful pregnancy?

There is no doubt that women who are exposed in utero to DES are more likely to experience several types of reproductive difficulties. But it has not been conclusively shown that the anatomic abnormalities caused by DES are responsible for infertility. In a 1980 study, doctors compared the fertility of 618 women who had had prenatal exposure to DES with 618 control subjects; they noted no significant differences in their ability to conceive. In contrast, doctors at the University of Chicago, comparing 226 DES-exposed and 203 controls, observed that twice as many in the DES group reported infertility. Researchers at the University of North Carolina reported infertility among 31 of 106 DES-exposed women and also noted that they were more likely to experience irregular menstrual cycles and longer and heavier periods.

Much of the ongoing research related to the fertility and reproductive outcome of the pregnancies of DES-daughters has been conducted by Raymond H. Kaufman, M.D., and his associates at the Baylor College of Medicine in Houston, Texas. In their 1986 study, published in the *American Journal of Obstetrics and Gynecology*, they found a strong relationship between DES exposure in utero and subsequent infertility: 36 percent of their patients with hysterosalpingogram evidence of DES abnormalities had difficulty conceiving. If constrictions of the uterine cavity combined with a T-shaped uterus, a woman's inability to conceive was, on average, twice as great. A surprising and unexplainable discovery in this report was that 37 percent of DES-exposed women with normal uterine X rays also experienced infertility. Why infertility rates were equal between women with normal and abnormally shaped uteri in this study is not understood. Perhaps there is some other, unknown factor common to all DES-exposed women.

In the April 1986 issue of *The Journal of Reproductive Medicine*, researchers at Beth Israel Hospital in Boston compared fifty DES-exposed and fifty control women who had been experiencing infertility for one to two years. Only two of the fifty DES women as opposed to twenty-two of the fifty control women conceived. While the question of infertility remains controversial, experts agree that the pregnancy of a DES-exposed woman must be classified as high-risk. In July 1978, Dr. Donald Goldstein of Harvard Medical School reported on the pregnancies of five women exposed to DES in utero. All had typical abnormalities of the cervix and all experienced symptoms characteristic of an "incompetent cervix," meaning one that is weakened and unable to carry the weight of a growing pregnancy. It usually results in a spontaneous and premature dilatation, or opening, of the cervix followed by miscarriage during the second or third trimester (see chapter 7, "Abortion"). Dr. Goldstein attributed this to underdevelopment of the cervixes *(hypoplasia)* of these young women and suggested that the chances of successful pregnancy could be enhanced by suturing the cervix just after the twelfth week of pregnancy, before it began to dilate. In a 1980 study, Dr. Goldstein and Dr. Merle J. Berger reported a dismal 31 percent spontaneous abortion rate among DES-exposed women, a 5 percent incidence of ectopic pregnancy (see ectopic pregnancy) during the first trimester, and an additional 18 percent miscarriage rate during the second trimester. Sadly, only 34 percent of all the DES-exposed women in two recent studies eventually achieved a successful full-term pregnancy.

In a 1984 project, combining the research of doctors from Baylor college of Medicine and the Mayo Clinic, 676 DES-exposed women underwent hysterosalpingogram. The pregnancy outcome for almost half of these women was related to the severity of their uterine defects noted on X ray. The presence of a T-shaped uterus, uterine constrictions, or a "shaggy" appearance of the endometrium were all associated with a higher incidence of premature birth, ectopic pregnancy, and an overall unfavorable pregnancy outcome when compared to women with normal uterine X rays. Even with a normal uterine configuration, a DES-exposed individual was slightly more likely than other women to have an unfavorable pregnancy outcome.

On the brighter side, up to 80 percent of all the DES-exposed women in two recent studies eventually achieved a successful pregnancy. This encouraging fact should be conveyed to all the unfortunate women who were exposed to DES in utero. Even if you fail to carry one or two pregnancies successfully, the odds are still in your favor that your persistent attempts will be rewarded. Another cause for optimism is a 1980 study from Boston's Beth Israel Hospital in which doctors found that some of the vaginal and cervical abnormalities attributed to DES may decrease spontaneously and even disappear in time.

How does a doctor diagnose areas of adenosis that are too small to be seen with the naked eye?

The simplest method of diagnosing adenosis is by applying a special iodine solution over the cervix and vagina, and biopsing (taking a piece of tissue from) those suspicious areas that do not absorb the iodine stain. Another method of detecting adenosis or cancer is with an instrument called a colposcope (see figure 6-1). When used skillfully, the colposcopic magnification of abnormal areas allows painless evaluation of adenosis in either a clinic or a doctor's office. Many doctors believe that they achieve maximum accuracy by combining use of the colposcope and iodine techniques.

Does the week of pregnancy in which a woman first takes DES determine the likelihood of developing adenosis?

The table that follows demonstrates the likelihood of adenosis based on when in the pregnancy DES is first taken.

PERCENTAGE OF WOMEN WITH ADENOSIS
BASED ON WEEK IN PREGNANCY
(FROM LAST MENSTRUAL PERIOD)
THAT DES WAS STARTED

Week of Pregnancy in Which DES Was Started	Percentage of Women with Adenosis
7–8	100
9–10	89
11–12	70
13–14	20
15–16	Less than 15

SOURCE: *Compiled by the author.*

It appears unlikely that a fetus can develop adenosis when the first dose is taken after the eighteenth week of pregnancy. Surprisingly, the amount of DES ingested is of less importance than when in the pregnancy it was begun. For example, adenosis has been known to develop after women used very small amounts of DES for only a few days during the critical seventh week of pregnancy.

Should adenosis be treated?

This question is a source of great controversy among gynecologists. The aggressive therapeutic approaches that some doctors support are based on the assumption that benign adenosis has the potential to become clear-cell adenocarcinoma. Though it is true that adenosis has been found in almost all women with clear-cell carcinoma, a direct transition from adenosis to cancer has never been observed under a microscope. For this reason, other physicians believe that adenosis is not precancerous but is present coincidentally along with cancer in only a few unfortunate women. These doctors argue that if adenosis were precancerous, there would be many more DES-exposed daughters afflicted with cancer than the very low 1 per 1,000. Extensive studies, such as that from the University of Southern California, have included hundreds of women with adenosis with not one instance of clear-cell adenocarcinoma being diagnosed. Since the oldest patients exposed to DES are now only in their forties, it is too soon to give a prognosis for the chances of adenosis becoming malignant.

Figure 6–1. *Colposcope.*

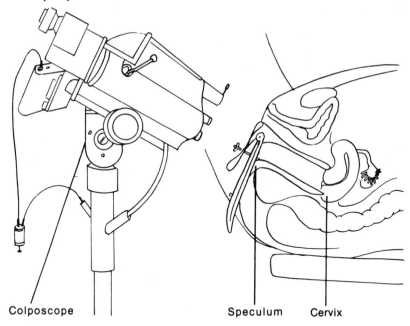

Colposcope   Speculum   Cervix

Dr. Arthur Herbst, one of the physicians who originally reported the relationship between DES and cancer, warns that iatrogenic damage from overtreatment might well be worse than the adenosis itself. He advises careful and frequent examination rather than aggressive forms of therapy for women with adenosis. Dr. Duane Townsend, another authority, speaks of the prevailing opinion in dealing with adenosis as one of "cautious optimism and careful observation."

How often should an adenosis patient see her doctor?

It is suggested that a woman with adenosis have a pelvic exam and Pap smear at least every six months. The frequency of the colposcopic exam will vary according to the amount and severity of the adenosis, but should be no less often than once per year. The iodine staining technique may be performed at the same time as the colposcopy, though it is certainly not advised that the iodine technique be the sole method of examination. If your gynecologist does not have a colposcope or is inexperienced with it, seek out a skilled colposcopist who performs several such examinations a week. The fee for colposcopic examination may vary from $50.00 to $200.00, and most insurance policies pay for the procedure as long as the following information is noted on the insurance form: "Mother took DES during pregnancy. Possible precancerous cervical and vaginal changes noted requiring colposcopy and further follow-up." Insurance policies will usually also pay for a biopsy that is taken at the time of the colposcopy, since this is a surgical procedure. Many large teaching hospitals have special colposcopy clinics, where the fee is often lower than that of a private practitioner. If biopsies are required, the pathologist who studies them will usually charge an additional $50.00 to $100.00, also usually covered by most insurance plans.

The minority of doctors who believe in aggressive management of adenosis have claimed success with various methods including cauterization (burning), cryosurgery (freezing), carbon dioxide laser, and progesterone suppositories. More radical techniques have included excision (cutting out) of the adenosis, or even partial vaginectomy, or removal of part of the vaginal wall.

At what age should a girl exposed to DES undergo her first pelvic examination and colposcopy?

Of the first 170 patients with adenocarcinoma reported to the Registry (see page 159), only 16, or 9 percent, were girls aged twelve years or younger. Most authorities suggest that the examination be delayed until the onset of menses, or at the age of fourteen if menstruation has not yet begun. It is highly unlikely that DES was prescribed to prevent miscarriage by any sane obstetrician after 1972, therefore this problem should no longer be encountered in girls of fifteen years of age or less. Immediate examination is indicated if any abnormal bleeding or discharge is noted in a DES daughter at any time. The examination in a virginal woman sometimes requires anesthesia in a hospital operating room in order for a doctor to visualize carefully and accurately the entire vagina and cervix.

The good news is that the overall cure rate following treatment for DES-related adenocarcinoma is approximately 80 percent. Early detection increases survival to better than 90 percent. A tumor that has a more benign or curable appearance is seen most often in women over nineteen years of age, rather than in those who are younger.

Though the youngest patient reported with adenocarcinoma has been seven years old, and the oldest thirty-four, the peak incidence appears to be at nineteen years of age. As previously stated, it is encouraging to note that the incidence of adenocarcinoma drops significantly after the age of nineteen, and is most unusual after the age of twenty-four.

Are DES-exposed daughters more likely to develop abnormal Pap smears, dysplasia, or carcinoma-in-situ of the cervix and vagina?

As mentioned in chapter 2, over 90 percent of cervical cancers originate in the outer "squamous" cells of the cervix at the junction where they meet the inner glandular cells. Before life-threatening invasive squamous-cell carcinoma occurs, the squamous cells pass through a series of microscopic changes known as dysplasia and carcinoma-in-situ. These preinvasive changes often progress over a period of several years.

Epidemiologists initially predicted that the incidence of abnormal Pap smears and squamous-cell abnormalities of the cervix and upper vagina might develop in as many as 20 percent of DES-exposed daughters. They based this estimate on the observation that these young women have large areas of glandular cells on the outer cervix and upper vagina rather than at the more usual location near the inner part of the cervix. They reasoned that the greater surface area between the glandular and squamous elements would result in an increased risk of squamous-cell abnormalities. While subsequent studies have not demonstrated a risk as high as 20 percent, in one report from Boston, dysplasia was found in almost 8 percent of DES daughters. In three other studies published between 1976 and 1981, doctors reported that the risk of dysplasia and carcinoma-in-situ of the cervix and vagina was five to ten times greater for DES-exposed daughters than for those whose mothers were not exposed to DES. In the largest study to date, researchers from the National Collaborative Diethylstilbestrol Adenosis Project studied the incidence of cervical and vaginal dysplasia in almost 4,000 DES-exposed young women from several medical centers in the United States. Their report, published in the *Journal of the American Medical Association* in 1984, found that biopsy-proven dysplasia occurred with a frequency of 15.7 per 1,000 woman-years for DES daughters versus 7.9 per 1,000 woman-years for nonexposed daughters. This two-times-greater risk emphasizes the importance of careful follow-up and periodic examinations and Pap smears for all DES daughters. A knowledgeable gynecologist who is familiar with the history of DES will diagnose more cases of dysplasia and carcinoma-in-situ if he or she takes the Pap smear from the periphery of the cervix rather than its center. The former location is more likely to yield cells from the critical junction between the glandular and squamous cells.

How can I find out if I was given DES during my pregnancy?

Contact the obstetrician who treated you during the pregnancy. Many obstetricians have sent notices to patients who were given diethylstilbestrol in order to alert them. If the doctor is deceased or retired, another doctor often has access to the original doctor's records. Women who were hospitalized during the pregnancy in question may be able to obtain transcripts of their old records, which are occasionally kept on microfilm in hospital record rooms. Despite these avenues, most women will be unable to know for sure whether they received DES. If there is a reasonable suspicion that they did receive it, examination is essential.

As a result of the well-established relationship between DES use in pregnancy and malignancy and reproductive problems in subsequent female offspring, many individual and class-action lawsuits have been brought against the six drug companies responsible for distributing nonsteroidal estrogens in the 1950s and 1960s. Since women who took DES and other such drugs are often unable to recall the name of the specific manufacturer, several states have based product liability settlements on how much of a share of the market each manufacturer had at that time. In situations where the statute of limitations against suing has run out, several states have passed new laws extending the original time limits for pursuing a DES claim. As the population of DES daughters has moved into the childbearing years, so-called "third-generation" DES lawsuits have been filed on behalf of children born prematurely or with permanent disability resulting from the abnormalities of their mothers' reproductive organs.

Can a daughter who was exposed to DES in utero use birth-control pills?

Whether or not abnormal changes in the vagina and cervix may be precipitated by the hormones in birth-control pills is still not known. Some doctors believe that alternative contraception should be prescribed for DES offspring. Other authorities, such as the well-known Dr. Adolf Stafl, see no indication for denying birth-control pills to these women.

If a woman uses DES as a morning-after pill, is it possible that she may increase her chances of malignancy at a later date?

It does not appear that a woman taking DES over a short period of time will experience any harmful effects at a later date. Though no extensive studies have been conducted on women who took DES throughout several months of pregnancy, their incidence of vaginal and uterine cancer has not been significantly higher than that of other women. At the University of Chicago a study published in 1978 compared the incidence of breast malignancy among 693 women who used DES during their pregnancies in the 1950s with a group of 668 women who never used the drug. Dr. Arthur L. Herbst, the author of this study, noted no statistical difference in breast cancer rates between the two groups. Review of the incidence of ovarian and cervical cancer among DES mothers also proved negative.

Smaller studies of DES mothers have reached conflicting conclusions. One report from Dartmouth Medical School found that DES-treated and untreated mothers showed about the same incidence of breast cancer for the first twenty-two months after the drug was administered. After that time, however, the treated women showed almost twice their previous rate, and this rate increased over a period of twenty years or more. Women over sixty who previously took DES in pregnancy were found to have a continually increasing breast cancer risk. This trend is usually not observed in the general population.

The Department of Health and Human Services 1985 DES Task Force reviewed the recent literature on this subject and cautioned that there is now "greater cause for concern" about a breast cancer risk among women who received DES during pregnancy. The same report states that a causal relationship between DES use and cancer has not been established. Though it's difficult to interpret the Task Force's conclusions, one can't argue with their suggestion that women who took DES during pregnancy should examine their breasts monthly, have a yearly breast examination, and undergo periodic mammography.

If I take DES early in pregnancy and then give birth to a son, what problems may I anticipate?

Research conducted at the University of Chicago in 1981 on 308 DES-exposed men has revealed abnormalities of the genital tract in 31 percent. Of these, approximately half had cysts of the epididymis, the tube that carries sperm from the testes. Other genital defects noted were abnormally small testes, undersized penises, and thickening of the capsule of the testicle. Moreover, 18 percent showed severe pathologic changes in sperm shape, concentration, and motility, compared with only 8 percent in a control group. Similar findings have been noted in a smaller study by doctors at New York's Beth Israel Medical Center. It is still too early to determine whether lesions comparable to vaginal and cervical adenocarcinoma will develop in these males, though it appears unlikely. However, 65 percent of the DES-exposed men with abnormally small testes had a history of undescended testes, and it has long been known that such men may be at increased risk of developing cancer of the testes at a later date. In a report published in the *Journal of the American Medical Association* in 1983, doctors from Tufts–New England Medical Center in Boston described the case of a twenty-eight-year-old DES son who was found to have a malignant testicular tumor called a *seminoma*. Though this one case does not constitute epidemiological evidence of a relationship between DES and testicular cancer, the peak incidence of this tumor occurs when men are in their thirties. Since DES use was most prevalent in the late 1950s and 1960s, it is possible that the group at greatest risk would be expected to contract cancer in the late 1980s and early 1990s.

By far the most encouraging report concerning exposure of males to DES in utero was published by doctors from the Mayo Clinic in 1984. They compared 828 exposed men and 676 controls for genito-urinary anomalies, infertility, and testicular cancer, and found no differences between the two groups. In trying to explain why their findings were in such contrast to those of other groups, the Mayo Clinic doctors theorized that the study designs of previous programs were faulty in several ways. In addition, the men in their study might have been exposed to lower doses of DES than men in other studies who were found to have low sperm counts and genital anomalies.

The suggestion of doctors at the University of Chicago and the Beth Israel Hospital is that all DES-exposed men undergo a complete urological examination. Though data is scarce, researchers have found no evidence of effects on a third generation of males following DES exposure.

A psychosexual study, conducted at Stanford University on boys exposed to DES in utero, concluded that they were significantly "less masculine" than a comparative group not exposed to this drug. Psychiatrists rated six-year-olds and twenty-year-olds according to masculinity factors, such as athletic coordination, behavioral movements, heterosexual experience, masculine interests, and aggression-assertion attitudes. While the potential inaccuracies and biases of such a study are readily apparent, it does suggest that hormones may be capable of influencing some aspects of postnatal psychosexual development in boys.

In 1983, the *British Journal of Obstetrics and Gynecology* published the findings of doctors at Radcliffe Infirmary who had studied 264 sons and 266 daughters of women who had taken DES during their pregnancies. They found that DES offspring had a higher incidence than unexposed individuals of a wide range of psychiatric illness including depression, anxiety, and anorexia. Larger studies are needed to confirm or refute these findings.

POSTCOITAL IUD

What is the "morning-after IUD"?

For women who are unwilling or medically unable to tolerate DES, insertion of an IUD after unprotected intercourse will effectively prevent pregnancy. Since fertilization takes place in the tube followed by a three-day journey of the egg to the endometrium, the IUD usually sets up an inflammatory reaction in the endometrium capable of destroying the egg as it reaches its destination. Used in this way, the IUD probably causes early abortion.

In one study, ninety-seven women had a Cu-7 inserted following unprotected intercourse. Seventeen women had it inserted within 24 hours; thirty within 48 hours; seventeen within 72 hours; seventeen within 96 hours; fourteen within 120 hours; and two within 144 hours. There were no pregnancies. The advantage of an IUD over DES and the morning-after pill is that it causes no nausea, vomiting, or potentially dangerous side effects. In addition, it may be left in the uterus for contraception during future cycles. Unfortunately, all IUDs with the exception of the Progestasert (see chapter 3) have been removed from the U.S. marketplace. Theoretically, the Progestasert should work well as a postcoital device, but there are no studies to confirm its success.

MENSTRUAL EXTRACTION

What is menstrual extraction?

Menstrual extraction is a highly successful method of fertility control in which tissue is removed from the endometrial cavity through a small, flexible, plastic "cannula" attached to a source of suction. The suction source may be either a machine (see chapter 7) or a specially designed syringe. Menstrual extraction is usually performed on a woman whose period is late, and who fears pregnancy but prefers not to know whether or not she is pregnant.

It should be noted that the criterion for calling a procedure a "menstrual extraction" rather than an "abortion" is not whether a pregnancy test is positive or negative. If your uterus is of normal size or only slightly enlarged, and if you are three weeks or less beyond a missed period, the criteria for a menstrual extraction are satisfied regardless of pregnancy test results. In some areas of the country, however, a positive pregnancy test is required before a doctor will perform a menstrual extraction. Outside those states, if your psychological and religious well-being is best served by menstrual extraction without a pregnancy test, then your doctor is obligated to abide by your wishes.

Menstrual extraction is also known as menstrual induction, menstrual planning, menstrual regulation, instant period, miniabortion, and minisuction.

Where and how is menstrual extraction performed?

Menstrual extraction may be safely performed in a doctor's office or in a clinic that also performs abortions. The doctor inserts a speculum and then washes the cervix with an antiseptic solution. The cervix is then held in position by means of an instrument called a *tenaculum* (see figure 6-2). Application of the tenaculum may cause a slight pinching sensation.

Novocain, or a Novocain-like medication, is then injected into the area around the cervix. This paracervical ("around the cervix") block is painless when administered

Figure 6–2. *Tenaculum attached to cervix.*

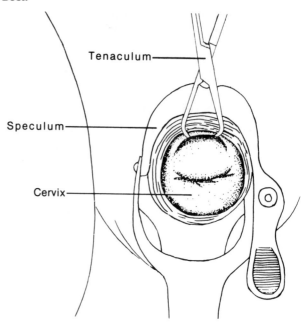

correctly, and it significantly reduces the discomfort that accompanies the procedure. Chloroprocaine hydrochloride (trade name Nesacaine) is a relatively new local anesthetic that is used for most menstrual extractions and abortions, since it is safer and quicker acting than other local anesthetics (see chapter 7, "Abortion").

After allowing the anesthetic to take effect for one to two minutes, the doctor inserts a 4-, 5-, or 6-millimeter plastic cannula, well lubricated with K-Y Jelly, through the cervix and into the uterine cavity. Dilatation of the cervix is usually not necessary for menstrual extraction, but when it is, it can best be performed with Pratt dilators. The largest Pratt dilator that should ever be used for menstrual extraction is numbered 17–19, equivalent to a diameter of approximately 6 millimeters.

The cannula is then attached to suction, and is moved around the endometrial cavity with an in-and-out motion until the tissue is removed. The cannula moves against the walls of the endometrium, creating a characteristic grating sound, and the professional who is performing the extraction will encounter a feeling of resistance on the part of the patient. That phase of the menstrual extraction may be totally painless, but more often than not a woman will experience menstruallike cramps. For some women, especially those who have never borne children, the pain may be quite intense, even following an adequate paracervical block.

The total operating time is usually no longer than ten minutes, and you can leave the office unaided within thirty minutes. If you need contraception, birth-control pills may be started on the same day. Insertion of an IUD at the time of menstrual extraction is not advised, however, because in the case of postoperative bleeding or fever, your doctor will not be able to determine whether the symptoms are attributable to the IUD or to retained tissue fragments from the menstrual extraction. In any case, it is best to avoid intercourse for at least a week, or until there is no evidence of bleeding.

What determines the size of the cannula that a doctor will use?

Because of its larger diameter, the 6-millimeter cannula is more likely than the 4-millimeter cannula to cause pain when introduced through the cervix. When there is abundant tissue, or when the uterus is slightly enlarged, however, the larger cannula will more rapidly and more efficiently empty the uterine cavity. Incomplete evacuation of the uterus is the most common complication of menstrual extraction, occurring in 2 to 12 percent of cases. Retention of pieces of pregnancy tissue often causes secondary infection and bleeding, necessitating antibiotics, repeat extraction, D and C, or sometimes even hospitalization. This complication is far more likely to occur with a 4-millimeter cannula than with a 6-millimeter one. In one large study of menstrual extraction performed on women with a positive pregnancy test, the pregnancy remained completely intact and uninterrupted in 5 percent of those on whom the 4-millimeter cannula was used. With a 6-millimeter cannula, the continuing pregnancy rate was a very low 0.7 percent. Regardless of the cannula size used, both a pregnancy test and a reexamination should be performed two weeks following all menstrual extractions in order to be certain that the pregnancy has been successfully terminated.

Will the fetus that survives a menstrual extraction be injured?

Fetuses surviving a failed menstrual extraction have an intact gestational, or pregnancy, sac, and there is no need to fear a deformity or an injury. However, the insertion of instruments into the uterine cavity at the time of the attempted procedure can occasionally cause a severe infection of the pregnancy tissues. Symptoms of this complication are almost always exhibited within one week and include a temperature over 38°C (100.4°F), a foul-smelling vaginal discharge which may be blood-tinged, and lower abdominal cramps. If not treated rapidly, the infection may spread to the lower pelvis, tubes, and ovaries, causing permanent damage, adhesions, and impaired future fertility. Bacteria may also enter the bloodstream and attack other organs and even cause death. These potentially dangerous complications can be avoided with immediate hospitalization, high doses of intravenous antibiotics, and termination of the pregnancy with a D and C. Attempts at salvaging a pregnancy in the presence of a uterine infection are foolhardy and doomed to failure.

All Rh-negative women should receive an intramuscular injection of immune globulin (RhoGAM) within seventy-two hours after a menstrual extraction, in order to prevent formation of antibodies against Rh-positive fetuses during future planned pregnancies. (The one exception to this rule is when the father is known to be Rh-negative, in which case the medication need not be given.) If you are Rh-negative and a menstrual extraction has not terminated your pregnancy, rest assured that an injection of RhoGAM will not cause harm. In fact, it will probably help in preventing you from forming antibodies against your Rh-positive fetus.

Should I take any other precautions following menstrual extraction?

Taking your temperature twice a day for one week will allow early detection of a fever over 100.4°F. Approximately 3 percent of all women undergoing menstrual extraction note such an elevation, which often indicates retained tissue fragments or an inflammation of the endometrium, called *endometritis*. A foul-smelling vaginal discharge accompanied by lower abdominal cramps may also signify inflammation. All of these symptoms necessitate immediate reexamination and treatment by a physician.

Medications containing aspirin should not be taken either before or after menstrual extraction and abortion. Aspirin significantly prolongs the bleeding time and decreases platelet activity, thereby increasing blood loss. Aspirin also lowers body temperature and as a result will mask a fever that might be caused by retained tissue and endometritis. Aspirin is also an antagonist of prostaglandins, the substances used to induce second-trimester abortions (see chapter 7).

The flow following a menstrual extraction should be no heavier than a normal menstrual period. Heavy bleeding, defined as having to replace a sanitary pad or a tampon more than once an hour, is abnormal and must be evaluated by a doctor.

Is it true that many women undergo menstrual extraction unnecessarily, since they are not pregnant?

It has been determined that when menstrual extraction is performed prior to the seventh day after the missed period, only 50 percent of these women are actually pregnant. Between the seventh and fourteenth day about 85 percent of them are pregnant, while after that time the number increases to 95 percent. In one study of 500 menstrual extractions, 177 women were shown not to have been pregnant when the removed tissue was studied under a microscope. Though the accuracy of home pregnancy tests leaves something to be desired, newer blood and urine tests performed in doctors' offices have an accuracy of 100 percent when performed eight days following conception. This means that a woman can know if she is pregnant before her period is even missed. To avoid unnecessary menstrual extractions, an early pregnancy test is desirable for women who would prefer to know whether they are actually pregnant.

Can I perform menstrual extraction on myself or on a friend if I have the proper equipment?

A small minority of radical feminists have advocated monthly menstrual extraction both as a form of contraception and as a method of shortening the number of days of the menstrual flow. This notion has been soundly discredited by most other feminists and by all health professionals. The risks of endometritis, hemorrhage, and even perforation of the uterus are far too great for this procedure to be performed on a monthly basis, especially by a novice. Even occasional self-administered menstrual extraction must never be attempted.

What is the cost of menstrual extraction?

The fee for a menstrual extraction should be less than that for an abortion, and may range from a low of $50.00 to a high of $200.00. For the 15 percent of women who are Rh-negative, the expensive RhoGAM injection will increase the total cost by $40.00 to $50.00. The cost of this procedure in terms of your future reproductive capacity is still in question. Weakening of the cervix during subsequent pregnancies (see chapter 7) appears unlikely, since the cervix is not significantly dilated during a menstrual extraction. In those rare cases when endometritis appears, infertility can be prevented if the infection is treated immediately and vigorously with antibiotics.

When pregnancy is terminated beyond the mini-abortion, or menstrual extraction, stage, it is classified as an early abortion. Chapter 7 deals with the methods and complications of early and late pregnancy termination.

7

ABORTION

The historic 1973 *Roe v. Wade* Supreme Court decision that legalized abortion did not stop this subject from being one of the most volatile and divisive issues confronting Americans today. Unplanned pregnancies constitute a major epidemic in the United States. Of the estimated 3 million unplanned pregnancies each year, approximately one-half end in elective abortion.

The newest members of the Supreme Court have been chosen by presidents Nixon and Reagan in part specifically because of their opposition to abortion. In addition, legislators and religious leaders have worked fervently at the local, state, and national levels to restrict and ultimately eliminate a woman's right to abortion. For example, Pennsylvania and twenty-eight other states have passed laws requiring physicians to inform women seeking abortion of the "detrimental physical and emotional" effects of the procedure, to describe fetal development in detail, and to let women know of agencies willing to provide financial help should they decide against abortion. Some states have placed additional obstacles before women and their physicians. Fortunately, in a 1986 ruling the Supreme Court struck down the Pennsylvania restrictions, thereby setting an important precedent for the other twenty-eight states as well. In the majority opinion, Justice Harry Blackmun said that "states are not free, under the guise of protecting maternal health, to intimidate women into continuing pregnancies." He added: "Few decisions are more personal and intimate, more properly private, or more basic to individual dignity and autonomy than a woman's decision . . . whether to end her pregnancy. A woman's right to make that choice freely is fundamental."

The tactics of some anti-abortionists have included picketing abortion clinics and harassing and threatening women who enter these facilities. In some cities, doctors who perform abortions have been boycotted and intimidated, while a small number of fanatics have repeatedly resorted to bombings and other violent forms of vandalism at abortion clinics.

Sadly and predictably, the individuals who suffer most from anti-abortion legislation have been poor women. The passage of the Hyde Amendment by Congress in 1976 denied federal funds for abortion to Medicaid recipients unless the life of the mother was at risk. Some individual states have assumed this financial burden, but the majority of states have not. Anti-abortionists have claimed that cutting off public funds for abortion would be a great cost-saving measure. Though this reasoning has influenced many a lawmaker, just the opposite is true. Researchers at the Alan Guttmacher Institute have clearly demonstrated that every dollar the state spends providing abortions for Medicaid-eligible women saves about four dollars in medical and welfare expenditures. This can be translated into hundreds of millions of dollars saved annually by public funding of abortions. It is ironic that those who speak most vociferously against "all those welfare mothers" are often the same individuals who oppose public funding of abortions.

How widespread is the problem of unplanned pregnancy among teenagers in the United States?

The United States has the shameful distinction of having the highest teenage pregnancy rate among all developed countries. In 1981, there were approximately 160 pregnancies for every 1,000 teenagers between the ages of fifteen and nineteen, with 90 of 1,000 girls in this age group giving birth and 70 of 1,000 having elective abortions. Fourteen percent of births in the United States are to teenage mothers. These statistics are not surprising in view of the fact that 50 percent of all teenagers do not use contraception during first intercourse, and female teens wait an average of six months to one year after the initiation of sexual activity before seeking medical advice.

Fear of parental discovery and fear of betrayal by a health care provider are the two main reasons why teenagers delay in seeking contraception. The absence of frank and accurate sexual education programs in the pre–high school setting only compounds teenagers' ignorance about birth control. Finally, the cost of seeking private medical care and contraception is often too great for a teenager who needs it. Though many clinics such as Planned Parenthood will accommodate young women or couples with financial hardships, these facilities are not readily available to all women. A 1984 survey by the Alan Guttmacher Institute clearly demonstrated this problem. They found that 78 percent of the counties in the United States, with 28 percent of the American women between the ages of fifteen and forty-four, offered no abortion services. Furthermore, only one-third of abortion providers in the United States were willing to perform abortions after the twelfth week of pregnancy.

Though it may be difficult to believe, a handful of young women continue to die each year as a result of illegal abortions. Lack of accessibility to an abortion facility and inability to afford a legal abortion were cited as the two main reasons why these tragedies still occur in the United States.

Can a doctor perform an abortion on a minor without parental consent?

In a 1979 decision, the Supreme Court declared unconstitutional a statute that required unmarried minors to ask their parents for consent prior to an abortion. The Court maintained that it *was* constitutional for a state to require a physician to notify the parents of a dependent and immature minor who is living at home. Several states have used this ambiguous ruling to enact legislation requiring unmarried minors to obtain the consent of both parents or the confidential authorization of a judge before being granted an abortion. In most states where this law has been in effect, judges have granted abortions to nearly every girl under eighteen years of age who has requested it. In one survey from Massachusetts, of 156 girls under eighteen who elected to go to court rather than ask their parents' consent for an abortion, the court granted their petitions in all but two cases. It is unfortunate that any woman seeking an abortion should ever have to beg for it or to be forced to tell her story to a court-appointed lawyer, thereby destroying the confidentiality and privacy demanded of such a difficult and personal decision. So far, several challenges to this legislation in federal courts have been upheld, and the Supreme Court is scheduled to clarify its previous rulings on this subject.

Even in states with no restrictive legislation, some doctors have the notion that it is their moral obligation to inform parents that their daughter is pregnant if she is below the age of eighteen. Without the girl's consent, such communication is a betrayal and runs contrary to the principles of the Hippocratic oath. A physician should certainly encourage a young woman to have her parents share in the decision on abortion, but if she is unwilling to do so, a doctor is stepping beyond his or her bounds to act otherwise.

In my view, a report published in 1974 of the Committee on Education in Family Life of the American College of Obstetricians and Gynecologists, entitled "The Management of Sexual Crises in the Minor Female," is right on target:

> However, when she [a minor] is unwilling to tell her parents that she is sexually involved, or that she is pregnant, the physician may not be free to do what he believes is in the best interest of the patient, because the law is either restrictive or unclear. In such situations, the physician has three choices: he may refuse to help the girl unless she agrees to inform her parents; he may himself inform them, thus betraying her confidence; or he may agree to give her advice and help without the parents' knowledge. The third choice probably represents a less serious violation of the physician's duty than either of the other two.

In situations where the physician judges that the minor who refuses to tell her parents is incapable of making a rational decision, the committee recommends that he or she not act on personal judgment but carefully select as a consultant a medical colleague or a member of another helping profession, such as a clergyman or a psychologist, and share the decision and responsibility with that colleague and the young girl.

Can my husband legally prevent me from having an abortion?

The 1973 Supreme Court decision liberated women in early pregnancy from any form of state control. Since the state has no direct authority to prevent a woman from having an early abortion, neither does it have indirect authority to prevent abortion because a husband disapproves of his wife's decision. Since husbands have no enforceable right to deny abortion, their consent is not legally required prior to abortion during the first trimester.

When a second-trimester abortion is performed in a hospital, the situation may be different, because each hospital sets its own guidelines for abortion consent. A hospital is within its legal right to request a husband's consent prior to performing abortion—or any other surgical procedure. In addition, the state may also exert influence over the hospital since it has the authority to regulate second-trimester abortions.

What procedures should be carried out prior to a first-trimester abortion?

Some women make the mistake of neglecting to have a pregnancy test performed before an early abortion, because they feel certain that they are pregnant. I have personally examined several nonpregnant women referred to my office for an abortion solely on the basis of missed or late periods. I have also examined women who had had false-positive results from a home pregnancy test. The newer urinary and blood pregnancy tests performed in laboratories, abortion clinics, and doctors' offices are far more accurate than their over-the-counter versions and can detect pregnancy even before a period is missed.

First-trimester abortion, or abortion performed during the first three months of pregnancy, may be carried out in clinics, doctors' offices, or hospitals. Choosing the right facility and the most qualified doctor to perform the abortion requires some investigation. Sometimes clinics such as Planned Parenthood can provide confidential abortion and contraceptive counseling as well as refer you to the nearest sympathetic doctor, clinic, or hospital. An equally good way to find a competent clinic or a qualified, licensed physician is to call the National Abortion Federation at their toll-free hotline: (800) 772-9100. Despite the accessibility of these services, 6 percent of all women who have abortions do so outside their home state because of the unavailability of abortion services in many areas of the United States.

Regardless of where the abortion is performed, the procedure should be thoroughly explained to you beforehand, all possible complications discussed, and all questions answered to your satisfaction. Counseling should include a discussion of the possible options, such as continuing with the pregnancy and either keeping the child or giving the child up for adoption. Significantly, 5 to 6 percent of women who apply for abortion actually reconsider their decision and elect to continue with the pregnancy. It is for this reason that some authorities suggest that the counseling session not take place on the day that the abortion is scheduled. For the majority of women who do go through with the procedure, two or three days of reflection may prove invaluable in convincing them that the decision they made is the correct one. If the final decision is to proceed with the abortion, most facilities require a letter of informed consent to be signed, indicating that the method of abortion and its potential complications have been fully explained. Most abortion clinics discuss contraceptive techniques before, as well as after, the procedure is completed.

It is imperative that all women relate a complete medical history and receive a physical examination before an abortion. Essential laboratory tests include a hemoglobin and hematocrit test to check for anemia, urinalysis, a test of the blood type and Rh factor, and a Pap smear for cancer detection. Some clinics also perform a routine chest X ray and cervical cultures for detecting gonorrhea and chlamydia.

Regardless of the type of anesthesia used (see anesthesia), make sure you don't eat or drink for at least eight hours prior to the abortion. If an emergency dictates the use of general anesthesia, an empty stomach ensures that the potentially dangerous risk of food regurgitation into the windpipe, or trachea, will be avoided. If general anesthesia is requested, a preoperative dose of atropine is sometimes given to help dry up excessive secretions in the mouth which may cause breathing difficulties. If local anesthesia is used, some facilities give a preoperative intramuscular or intravenous injection of a tranquilizer. Many abortion clinics and most doctors' offices do not use general anesthesia, so you should check beforehand if that is the method you prefer. Women who are opposed to the use of both local and general anesthesia should inquire about the newer "dissociative anesthetics." These agents are capable of producing a trancelike state without inducing sleep. Women selecting this method usually report total amnesia of the abortion procedure. A number of clinics insert laminaria (see laminaria) or other hygroscopic (water-absorbing) cervical dilators from four to twenty-four hours prior to the abortion, which allow the cervix to open gradually without painful or forceful dilatation at the time of the procedure. Patients who have laminaria inserted should report to their doctors any temperature elevation, severe cramps, or bleeding.

Finally, a woman should be sure to determine the policy of fee collection at the facility she chooses. Practically all abortion clinics and doctors' offices require most, if not all, of the payment before they perform the abortion. Some clinics include in the fee the Rh immune globulin (RhoGAM) injection for Rh-negative women, but most do not. The smaller, 50-microgram dose is more than adequate to protect a woman against Rh sensitization. For a second-trimester abortion, the larger, 300-microgram injection is recommended since more fetal blood cells could enter the maternal circulation and induce antibody formation. All laboratory tests are usually included in the fee. There is usually an additional bill for general or dissociative anesthesia. The total cost of an abortion may vary significantly from one clinic to another, and it is a good idea to do some comparison shopping before making a selection. Some clinics base their fee on the number of weeks of pregnancy, as determined by the size of the uterus, and the larger the size, the more expensive the procedure. I know of no abortion clinic that accepts personal checks.

How is abortion performed during the first trimester of pregnancy?

Of the approximately 1.5 million elective abortions that were performed in the United States in 1985, more than 90 percent were terminated during the first trimester.

In the first eight weeks of pregnancy, measured from the first day of the last menstrual period, an abortion may be easily accomplished with a 6-millimeter plastic cannula in a manner identical to that described for menstrual extraction (see chapter 6). Because a greater amount of suction is needed for an abortion than for menstrual extraction, the cannula should be attached to a suction machine rather than to a syringe (see figure 7-1).

If the pregnancy has advanced further than eight weeks, dilatation with Pratt dilators is almost always necessary in order to allow insertion of larger suction cannulas or curettes, called vacurettes. These instruments may be curved or straight; the largest size necessary for first-trimester abortions is 12 millimeters. Metal suction cannulas are also used, but they lack the flexibility of the softer, disposable plastic types. Theoretically, the metallic cannula would appear to increase the risk of uterine perforation. But one study that compared these two cannulas found no difference in the incidence of complications.

The uterine cavity is completely evacuated within five minutes when the curette is gently moved in, out, and around the uterine cavity (figure 7-2). The same grating sound and the tightening of the uterine muscle after menstrual extraction is also observed following abortion. Rapid tightening or contraction of those muscles is essential in preventing excessive bleeding. The process may be improved by intramuscular or intravenous injections of oxytocin, or intramuscular injections of ergotrate, two uterine-muscle-contracting drugs.

The contraction of the uterine muscles may cause moderate to severe cramps during the first two minutes following the abortion. They usually subside within twenty minutes, and pain medication given intramuscularly or orally should relieve the discomfort. Medications such as Darvon Compound, Percodan, Fiorinal, and Darvocet-N 100 are best avoided since they all contain aspirin, which may interfere with the coagulating ability of the blood. Most abortion facilities have a well-equipped recovery room staffed by nurses, where postabortal patients are observed for a period of two hours or more. Most women are able to get dressed and to leave within a half hour if local anesthesia is used. Following dissociative anesthesia, general anesthesia, or in situations where a substantial dose of preoperative tranquilizer was adminis-

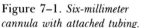

Figure 7–1. *Six-millimeter cannula with attached tubing.*

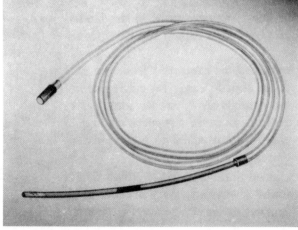

tered, a woman who is sensitive to the effects of medications may feel drowsy for longer than two hours.

Most abortion facilities dispense a total of six ergotrate tablets, with instructions to take one every four hours for the first twenty-four hours to keep the uterus contracted and to diminish the amount of bleeding. Uterine cramping is to be expected after taking each tablet. Ergotrate tends to elevate the blood pressure and should thus not be prescribed to hypertensive women.

Antibiotics are widely prescribed following an abortion. In one survey it was found that they are given prophylactically to prevent infection in 70 percent of all abortion clinics in the United States. Though many physicians believe it is unscientific to treat everyone for the possibility of a small number of infections, several recent studies, including a 1985 report from the Centers for Disease Control, have demonstrated that the risk of postabortal infection can be reduced by as much as one-third when prophylactic antibiotics are used.

Most women will experience a menstruallike flow following an abortion. The bleeding should be no heavier than your heaviest menstruation. It is sometimes dark in color and may be accompanied by passage of an occasional clot. It is not uncommon for the bleeding to stop completely and then return a few days later. The need for four or five sanitary napkins per day for the first ten postabortal days is considered

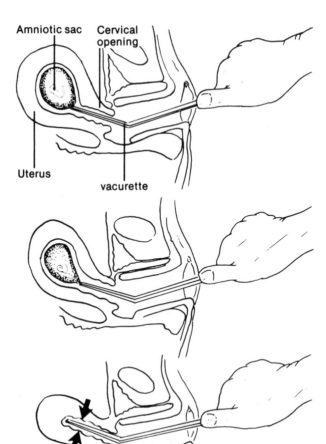

Figure 7–2. *Evacuation of early pregnancy with 8-millimeter curette.*

normal. The passage of several clots over a short period of time, or the soaking of two napkins with bright red blood in less than an hour, however, is cause for concern and must be reported to a doctor.

Rest is advisable on the day of the abortion, but most women are able to resume normal activities, including work, on the following day. Douching and intercourse should be avoided for two weeks, and sanitary napkins are preferable to tampons during the first postabortal week. Showers and baths are both permissible. Contrary to popular belief, you can't introduce infection into the vagina by taking a bath, but for aesthetic purposes some women may want to avoid baths during the first few days, when the bleeding is heaviest.

In addition to reporting heavier-than-normal bleeding, other symptoms requiring medical attention are severe cramps which begin later than a day after the abortion; an oral temperature exceeding 100.4°F; a greenish, foul-smelling vaginal discharge; and burning on and frequency of urination.

Fertility rapidly returns following a first-trimester abortion, with 60 percent of women ovulating within the first twenty-five postabortal days. Normal menses return between four and eight weeks, and 80 percent of women menstruate prior to the fifth postabortal week. These statistics demonstrate the urgency of starting adequate contraception immediately. If the Pill is the contraceptive of choice, it may be started on the day of the abortion. Some clinics will insert IUDs at the time of the abortion, but most do not (see chapter 3). A pelvic examination should be performed two weeks after the abortion, and a woman who wants an IUD can have one inserted at that time. Postabortal exams are usually included in the abortion fee, though insertion of an IUD or the fitting of a diaphragm during the visit usually involves an additional fee.

After Week 8 of pregnancy, it is customary for physicians performing abortions to use a vacurette with an outside diameter equal to, or two millimeters less than, the number of weeks of the pregnancy, counting from the first day of the last period. Many skilled physicians can use the smaller 6-millimeter cannula for terminating pregnancies even as advanced as ten weeks (see figure 7-1). The curette size should never be greater in diameter than the number of weeks of pregnancy. A ten-week gestation requires a 10-millimeter cannula, which is the equivalent of a number 31 Pratt cervical dilator, or smaller. It is not unreasonable to ask your doctor the cannula size that he or she intends to use. If the reply is a 9-millimeter cannula and you have been pregnant for six weeks, seek abortion at another facility.

What are some of the more common complications of first-trimester abortion?

Hemorrhage is the most common immediate complication, and it occurs in 2 to 10 of every 1,000 undergoing abortion. A very small percentage of these women may bleed to the point of needing a blood transfusion.

Hemorrhage usually occurs when the endometrial cavity is not completely emptied of its pregnancy tissue or when, for some unknown reason, the uterine muscle becomes flaccid and fails to contract immediately following the abortion. The latter condition, called *uterine atony,* is more likely to occur in a uterus of twelve weeks' size than in one of six or eight weeks' size. It usually responds to intravenous oxytocin. Statistically, the average blood loss resulting from an abortion at five weeks is about 3 tablespoons, while at twelve weeks it is equal to 16 tablespoons.

Perforation of the uterus may occur when the end of a sound, a dilator, or a vacurette accidentally passes through the uterine wall and into the ligaments on either side of the uterus or even in the abdominal cavity. Estimated to occur in approximately 1 in 1,000 abortions, it is an extremely dangerous complication. The amount of hemorrhage caused by perforation may be severe, and the presence of a suction curette in the abdominal cavity can easily cause damage to the intestine.

Perforation rates are inversely related to the skill and care taken by the doctor, and directly related to the size of the uterine cavity. As a pregnancy advances, the enlarging uterine muscle becomes softer and thinner, making it much more susceptible to perforation. The 10- or 12-millimeter vacurette is a much more dangerous instrument to use in it than the small, flexible 6-millimeter Karman cannula.

When perforation is suspected, the doctor should stop the procedure immediately and transfer the woman to a hospital. Blood should be made available for transfusion, and exploratory surgery may be in order if the bleeding appears to be heavy or if intra-abdominal hemorrhage is suspected. At the time of surgery the site of perforation can usually be located and easily sutured. Occasionally surgery may be more complex, involving *ligation*—tying of the larger blood vessels near the area of the bleeding. On rare occasions, hysterectomy may be the only method of controlling the hemorrhage.

When the blood loss following perforation is not excessive, the suction curettage may be completed safely and successfully in the hospital by one doctor, while another views the perforated uterus through a laparoscope (see chapter 9). Laparoscopic visualization helps to determine whether the perforation site is actively bleeding and whether the vacurette is in danger of again perforating or injuring a piece of intestine. Such use of the laparoscope may obviate the need for major exploratory surgery.

A doctor who does not dilate the uterus in a slow, gradual manner may cause laceration and hemorrhage from the cervix. This is more likely to occur in a young woman with a small, rigid cervix who has never had a previous abortion or pregnancy. Cervical laceration may occur in as many as 1 percent of cases and usually requires suturing to stop the bleeding. In a 1983 study of over 15,000 women undergoing first-trimester abortions, doctors found that cervical injury was 27 times less likely to occur when laminaria are inserted prior to abortion (see laminaria); when the procedure is performed by an attending physician instead of a resident physician; and when local rather than general anesthesia is used.

Bleeding that begins several days following an abortion is often the result of retained fragments of pregnancy tissue, a complication that has been noted to occur between 3 and 11 times for every 1,000 abortions performed. It usually requires a repeat suction curettage or a D and C to remove the fragments. As with menstrual extraction, a fever that accompanies the bleeding means that the retained tissue has become infected, and antibiotics must be prescribed.

When a D and C is performed for removal of infected abortal tissue, it is vital that the curettage, or scraping, of the endometrium be done very gently. Otherwise permanent scarring of the endometrium may be a late complication. This condition, called Asherman's syndrome, though rare, can lead to permanent sterility.

Infection is one of the most common and potentially one of the most serious complications faced by women who undergo first-trimester abortion. Various studies demonstrate that the risk of fever may range between 0.6 and 6.0 per 100 first-trimester abortions. Fever, lower abdominal pain, and a yellowish vaginal discharge in the absence of bleeding may signify endometritis (inflammation of the endometrium). Endometritis complicates the first-trimester abortions of as few as 8 and as many as 35 women out of 1,000, but can usually be cured by antibiotics without curettage. Endometritis is also more common as the size of the uterus increases. As previously mentioned, to reduce the incidence of postabortal infections some doctors prescribe antibiotics to all their patients. Others consider this "shotgun" method to be unscientific. To date, seven different reports, including a 1985 study of over 26,000 women by the Centers for Disease Control, have demonstrated that the use of prophylactic antibiotics can decrease the incidence of postabortal fever by as much as one-third.

The total complication rate of first-trimester abortion—including hemorrhage, perforation, retained pregnancy tissue, and endometritis—has been estimated to affect an average of 22 per 100,000 women. It is clear that the number and severity of complications greatly increase with each week of pregnancy, as demonstrated in figure 7-3.

What is the chance of death following first-trimester abortion?

Deaths following early abortion are extremely rare, but they are not rare enough. In one study combining statistics from California and New York, 759,647 abortions resulted in twenty deaths, for a fatality rate of 2.6 per 100,000 women. Other studies have shown the rate to be 1.7 per 100,000 women. The most recent statistics from the Centers for Disease Control demonstrate that complications of anesthesia are now the leading cause of death from first-trimester abortion. A close second and third are infection and hemorrhage.

What is the safest type of anesthesia for first-trimester abortion?

Without doubt, paracervical block, occasionally supplemented by small amounts of intravenous or intramuscular tranquilizer, is the safest form of anesthesia. In a 1981 study of national abortion statistics, Dr. Herbert B. Peterson and his associates at the Centers for Disease Control in Atlanta, Georgia, determined that deaths attributed strictly to general anesthesia (after eliminating all other factors) were 0.37 per 100,000 abortions. In contrast, the rate for local anesthesia was 0.15 per 100,000. Dr. Peterson concluded that general anesthesia was associated with a twofold and possibly as much as a fourfold increase in death risk when compared to local anesthesia.

Some abortion clinics, and almost all ambulatory abortion facilities in hospitals,

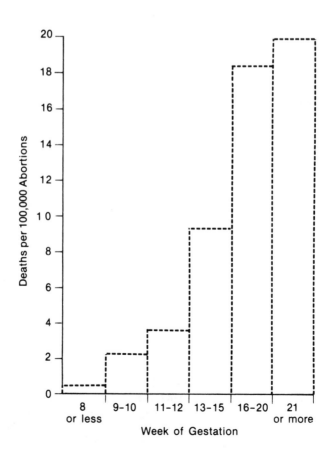

Figure 7–3. *Deaths per 100,000 abortions based on week of gestation.*

offer a choice of paracervical block, dissociative anesthesia, or general anesthesia. The sensible choice in nearly all cases should be paracervical block.

It is important to realize, however, that no anesthetic is 100 percent safe, and even the local anesthetics used for paracervical block have the potential for danger. There are women who have died from paracervical block used for first-trimester abortions. Some of these deaths were caused by improper injection of the anesthetic into the bloodstream, while others may have been caused by rare allergic reactions. The use of chloroprocaine hydrochloride (trade name: Nesacaine), the most rapidly metabolized local anesthetic, has reduced the risk associated with longer-lasting drugs such as lidocaine (trade name: Xylocaine) and procaine hydrochloride (trade name: Novocain). Because of the threat of toxic levels in the blood, the smallest effective volume and the lowest concentration of local anesthetic should be used.

Ringing in the ears, numbness in the mouth area, and the sense of impending disaster are often the first signs of an overdose of local anesthesia. If you are undergoing an abortion under local anesthesia and begin to experience any of these sensations, immediately tell the doctor to stop injecting the anesthetic into your cervix. Rapid accumulation of an anesthetic in the bloodstream can cause hyperactive behavior, tremors, and respiratory difficulty which in turn may be followed by a convulsion. The result could be central nervous system depression, a life-threatening slowing of the heart rate, and circulatory and respiratory collapse.

Because of the constant risk of local anesthesia toxicity, doctors should administer paracervical anesthesia only when resuscitative drugs and equipment and skilled personnel are on hand.

With general anesthesia, a short-acting barbiturate is injected intravenously, which puts you to sleep. A mask is placed over your face, and a light anesthetic gas, such as nitrous oxide, is administered. Upon completion of the abortion, recovery is usually quite rapid. General anesthesia is preferable only if you are sensitive or allergic to local anesthetics or if your extreme apprehension may make even a routine examination difficult, if not impossible, for the doctor to perform.

Risk of death is increased 2 to 4 times with the use of general anesthesia in first-trimester abortion. Cardiac arrest under general anesthesia may occur, for totally unexplained reasons, as often as 1 in 2,500 operations performed on hospitalized patients. This statistic includes people of all ages and health conditions, but cardiac arrest does not occur as frequently among younger and healthier women who undergo early abortion. It still remains a threat to this group, though, as statistics confirm. At the 1986 meeting of the National Abortion Federation, doctors reviewed maternal deaths in New York City between 1980 and 1984 that were related to elective abortion. Of the ten reported deaths, seven were caused by cardiac arrest associated with the use of methohexital sodium (trade name: Brevital sodium), a short-acting barbiturate. In response to this investigation, the Centers for Disease Control reviewed its data on the 193 abortion-related deaths in the United States from 1972 to 1985. They concluded that 27 of these deaths involved complications of general anesthesia. Of these 27 deaths, 21 were associated with the use or misuse of short-acting barbiturates such as Brevital and Pentothal (pentothal sodium). These statistics underline the importance of careful administration of these drugs by trained anesthesia personnel.

If general anesthesia is used, it is essential not to eat or drink anything for at least eight hours prior to the procedure. This assures adequate emptying of food from the stomach and prevents the potentially fatal risk of food regurgitation into the windpipe while you are under anesthesia.

Ketamine hydrochloride is a relatively new nonbarbiturate anesthetic, classified as a neuroleptic, which can be administered intravenously or intramuscularly. This drug has been gaining great popularity because, unlike barbiturates and general anesthesia, it does not impair reflexes in the pharynx and larynx or cause choking or respiratory depression. Instead, ketamine produces an almost trancelike state in which a person appears to be awake but experiences no pain, an effect called "dissociative anesthesia" because it selectively interrupts pain pathways to the brain without altering other nervous reflexes. For most patients, the anesthetic effect is rapid, lasts but a few minutes, and produces total amnesia of the abortion procedure. No anesthetic is perfect, though, and ketamine is certainly not an exception. It can elevate the blood pressure, and women with heart disease and hypertension must be carefully monitored. One of the most serious and common problems associated with ketamine use is bizarre psychological behavior, a reaction reported to occur in as many as 12 percent of women who are anesthetized with this drug. Reactions may range from a pleasant dreamlike state to hallucinations and delirium. Though no permanent psychological effects have been reported, the bizarre behavior pattern may last for a few hours and in rare cases for as long as twenty-four hours. To reduce the risk of hyperactive behavior, many anesthesiologists prefer to add a tranquilizer such as Valium when administering ketamine.

Should first-trimester abortions be performed in a hospital rather than in a clinic or a doctor's office?

Several studies have demonstrated complication rates to be *lower* when abortions are performed in clinics rather than in hospitals. The explanation for the excellent results may be that many clinics and offices use only paracervical anesthesia. In addition, doctors who work in abortion clinics perform a large number of abortions daily, and naturally become proficient at them.

Certain potentially dangerous bacteria live in a hospital environment and are resistant to many antibiotics. The chance of infection from these resistant bacteria is much lower in a setting outside the hospital.

It should be noted that when a complication does occur in a clinic or office, the patient is transferred to the hospital. If she dies there, the hospital and not the clinic is recorded as having been responsible for the complication. For this reason, clinics may have deflated complication rates. Doctors from the Centers for Disease Control have found that when death rates are adjusted for the presence of preexisting medical conditions and other factors, the death rate for first-trimester abortion is 0.7 per 100,000, whether the procedure is performed in a hospital or a clinic.

Are there any medical conditions that might make a hospital setting preferable for a first-trimester abortion?

It is my opinion that a hospital abortion is not called for when the uterus measures twelve weeks' size or less, counting from the onset of the last menstrual period. However, there are gynecological and medical conditions that occasionally dictate that certain first-trimester abortions be carried out in a hospital. For example, the uterus may be filled with fibroids (see chapter 10, "Hysterectomy"), making it difficult to determine accurately the length of the pregnancy. Often it is necessary to perform ultrasound to ascertain the exact pregnancy length as well as the position of the pregnancy sac within the uterus. Fibroids may also distort the endometrial cavity, making it difficult for the doctor to insert the dilators or curettes. Abortion under such conditions is sometimes best performed in a hospital. Some women are born with congenital abnormalities in the shape of the uterus and may actually have a septum, or wall, between the two halves of the uterus, or even have two separate uteri with separate endometrial cavities. If the doctor is lucky enough to detect such a condition prior to surgery, he or she would most likely choose to perform the abortion in the hospital.

It is best for women with serious medical problems to be hospitalized for an abortion also. Problems might include diseases such as hypertension greater than 160/100 (see birth control pills and hypertension); diabetes requiring insulin; heart disease or significant heart murmur as a result of previous heart disease; a history of deep vein phlebitis or pulmonary embolus (see chapter 2); blood coagulation disorders; chronic debilitating diseases; and anemia. A normal hemoglobin level for women ranges between 11 and 15 percent grams per 100 milliliters of blood, and any measure below 11 signifies anemia. If the hemoglobin is less than 10 percent grams per 100 milliliters, abortion in the hospital is preferred and should be preceded by laboratory tests to determine the cause of the anemia. A significant number of women with severe psychiatric problems are also best managed in a hospital environment.

Isn't a woman's risk of infertility and ectopic pregnancy in the fallopian tube greater following an abortion?

Theoretically, if an abortion is complicated by a severe postoperative pelvic infection involving the fallopian tubes, it could lead to tubal occlusion and higher rates of infertility and tubal pregnancies. Immediate reporting of a postabortal fever, abdominal pain, or foul-smelling discharge, followed by appropriate treatment by your doctor, should prevent this complication.

Fortunately, in actual practice these complications do not occur. Seven separate studies, the most recent one in *Obstetrics and Gynecology* in 1984, have failed to demonstrate any relationship between abortion and subsequent infertility. Similarly, a Columbia University College of Physicians and Surgeons report in 1986 noted no association between abortion and future ectopic pregnancy. Despite these facts, there appears to be a prevailing myth among doctors and patients that elective abortion poses great risks in this regard. In fact, I know of several instances in which women have decided to continue with an unplanned and unwanted pregnancy simply because they feared that an abortion would lead to infertility or a hazardous outcome of a future planned pregnancy.

What complications might be encountered during a pregnancy that follows a first-trimester abortion?

To avoid most complications, the ideal time to perform a first-trimester abortion is probably between the sixth and ninth weeks of pregnancy, as measured from the last menstrual period. After the tenth week, complications such as hemorrhage, retained placental fragments, and infection increase significantly.

A great controversy currently exists among gynecologists over the important question of whether dilatation of the cervix at the time of an abortion is responsible for an incompetent, or weakened, cervix during subsequent pregnancies. A woman with an incompetent cervix will suffer from repeated second-trimester spontaneous abortions and premature births because her cervix will be unable to support the weight of her growing uterus. Though the cause of cervical incompetence is usually unknown, trauma in the form of forceful dilatation may be the problem in some women, and several researchers believe that women who undergo repeated abortions are more likely to have an incompetent cervix.

In a fascinating experimental study reported in the *British Journal of Obstetrics and Gynaecology,* dilators were passed through the cervixes of surgically removed uteri in an attempt to detect the stage of dilatation at which microscopic tissue rupture could first be detected. In almost 50 percent of the specimens tested, evidence of tissue damage was apparent at a dilatation of 9 to 11 millimeters. The investigators concluded that use of a dilator of 8 millimeters or less caused a harmless dilatation of the cervix, while dilators larger than that critical size were more likely to cause damage.

Though it is possible to question the applicability of this experimental data, the lesson to be learned is obvious: the smallest possible dilators should be used for a suction curettage if the potential problem of an incompetent cervix is to be avoided. The effects of midtrimester (second-trimester) abortion on future cervical incompetence are of greater concern than those of first-trimester abortion (see midtrimester abortion), since greater dilatation of the cervix is required in the former.

Clinical studies investigating the relationship between first-trimester abortion and subsequent spontaneous abortion and premature labor are somewhat contradictory. In an impressive study from the University of Washington in 1977, researchers compared the obstetrical records of more than 500 women who had previously had an induced abortion and a similar control group who had not experienced the procedure. They concluded that there were no significant differences between the two groups. Furthermore, the incidence of spontaneous abortion and premature birth was not affected by the number of previous abortions or by the week of pregnancy in which the previous abortion was performed. A 1980 report from Hawaii, involving over 2,000 women, reached similar conclusions, but noted that the risk of miscarriage was far greater when pregnancy occurred within one year after either an induced abortion or a full-term birth. Similarly, Michael B. Brachen, M.D., of Yale University School of Medicine, found that babies tended to be of lower birth weight when the time interval between the abortion and the next conception was less than one year. Aside from this, Dr. Brachen, in his 1986 report published in *The American Journal of Epidemiology,* noted no relationship between birth weight in later pregnancies and the abortion technique that was used, the complications that were encountered, or the week of pregnancy in which the abortion was performed.

In contrast to these studies, doctors at Boston's Brigham and Women's Hospital concluded that women who had had two or more induced abortions were two to three times as likely to miscarry during subsequent pregnancies. Interestingly, the technique used during the abortions did not appear to be an important contributing factor, in direct conflict with several other studies that stressed the importance of the abortion method in determining the success or failure of future pregnancies. Data from the World Health Organization, encompassing the statistics of seven European nations, showed that the use of a sharp curette, rather than the more gentle and modern suction apparatus, increased the likelihood of a future midtrimester spontaneous abortion. Of further interest is that the World Health Organization data suggest that dilatation with an instrument larger than 9 millimeters increases the incidence of incompetent cervix, babies with low birth weight, and premature labor. In 1981, Dr. Susan Harlop and her associates noted that if a woman's cervix was dilated to 12 millimeters or more at the time of an induced abortion, she was more likely later to give birth to a premature infant, compared to a woman whose cervical dilatation was 11 millimeters or less. Based on her findings, Dr. Harlop cautioned women to have induced abortions performed as early as possible in order to minimize cervical dilatation and subsequent weakening of the cervical tissues.

Placenta previa is a condition in which the placenta or afterbirth covers the cervix rather than assuming its normal position high in the uterus. Placenta previa may be responsible for severe hemorrhage late in pregnancy. While two small studies have suggested that induced abortion may be a risk factor for a later occurrence of placenta previa, doctors from Grady Memorial Hospital in Atlanta, Georgia, found no such association in their extensive 1984 report that studied more than 29,000 abortions.

In a 1979 article published in the *British Medical Journal,* doctors at the Welsh School of Medicine found a higher than normal incidence of spina bifida, a neural tube defect, among children of women with a history of two or more previous abortions. Specifically, the rate was 8.4 per 1,000 births among those studied, versus 2.3 per 1,000 for those who had never undergone abortion.

Is there any way to decrease the risk of trauma to the cervix during elective abortions?

Laminaria digitata is dried seaweed that has been used, both legally and illegally, as a cervical dilator for more than 100 years. Due to its hygroscopic, or water-absorbing, ability, a stem of laminaria, when inserted into the cervix, absorbs its secretions and

Figure 7–4. *Insertion of laminaria into the cervix.*

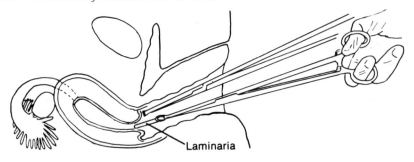

increases its diameter by three to five times over a period of six to twelve hours. The effect is to dilate the cervix slowly and painlessly prior to first- or second-trimester abortion (see figure 7-4).

The insertion of laminaria into the cervical canal causes only minimal discomfort and does not require a local anesthetic. It allows for suction curettage with minimal if any dilatation several hours later. Three or four laminaria inserted into the cervix will greatly facilitate a second-trimester D and E (dilatation and evacuation). For a late second-trimester abortion, it is often best to insert a second or a third set of laminarias within twenty-four hours after the first set is inserted, to allow maximum cervical dilatation with minimal trauma. When several laminaria are inserted fourteen to nineteen hours prior to prostaglandin or saline abortion, the interval between injection of these solutions and abortion has been noted to be shortened by an average of six hours compared to no laminara.

Though the incidence of cervical injury may be greatly reduced with laminaria, the incidence of cervical and uterine infection may be slightly higher because opening the cervix prior to abortion could introduce potentially harmful bacteria. This is especially true when the laminaria is inserted more than twenty-four hours prior to abortion.

Lamicel is the trade name for a new synthetic polyvinyl sponge saturated with alcohol containing 450 milligrams of magnesium sulfate. Its manufacturer, Cabot Medical Corporation, claims that Lamicel has several advantages over laminaria, including a more rapid, gentle, and predictable dilatation of the cervix. There are no large studies that have compared these two products, but one disadvantage of Lamicel is that its minimum diameter is 3 millimeters, compared with only 1 millimeter for laminaria. Lamicel's larger diameter limits its usefulness as a cervical dilator in very early pregnancies, since it is more painful on insertion. In addition, some doctors have noted that Lamicel is not capable of achieving the greater cervical dilatation needed for performing late midtrimester D and E. Insertion of several laminaria more easily accomplishes this goal.

Another synthetic dilator named *Dilapan* consists of a hydrogel polymer rod. Though reports of large clinical trials have not been published, the manufacturers of this device claim that it dilates the cervix more rapidly than laminaria. In some clinical tests, this product was found to fragment upon removal and to shorten as it expanded, leaving the inner cervix undilated. In addition, this soft, slippery rod may occasionally pass into the uterus rather than remain in the cervix and then have to be removed with the suction device at the time of the abortion. The laminaria does not have this problem, because it has a plastic shield over its end that prevents it from entering the uterus.

Prostaglandins in the form of vaginal suppositories and intra-amniotic and intramuscular injections have been employed successfully for midtrimester abortions. They induce uterine contractions followed by expulsion of the fetus and placenta (see midtrimester abortion). Unfortunately, prostaglandins often cause unpleasant side effects such as nausea, vomiting, diarrhea, and fever. Newer analogs, or chemical derivatives, of prostaglandins in the form of vaginal and intracervical gels and tablets have been tested in clinical trials and appear to soften and dilate the cervix effectively without causing painful uterine contractions or severe adverse side effects. The most popular prostaglandins for this purpose are derivatives of prostaglandin E2 or PGE2 and 15-methyl PGF2$^\alpha$. Both appear to be promising alternatives to laminaria as a painless and safe method of dilating the cervix prior to a first- or second-trimester abortion.

In a 1984 study published in *The Journal of Reproductive Medicine,* doctors at Mount Sinai School of Medicine in New York City administered either a PGE2 or PGF2$^\alpha$ analog in the form of a suppository to 46 women prior to first-trimester abortion. Within one or two hours of insertion, both analogs were found equally effective in dilating the cervix an average of 3 millimeters in all the women. The results of this preliminary study are encouraging because they demonstrate that preabortion cervical priming with either of these prostaglandin analogs can help prevent the cervical injuries associated with forceful mechanical dilatation of the cervix.

Isn't it true that acupuncture has been used to dilate the cervix prior to abortion?

In a report published in *The Journal of Reproductive Medicine* in July 1985, Yu Kang Ying, M.D., and his associates at Nassau County Medical Center in New York used acupuncture on twenty women immediately prior to first-trimester abortion. By placing one needle on loci of each hand and one on each leg, they were able to bring about significant cervical dilatation in eighteen of the twenty women. While the mechanism by which acupuncture accomplishes cervical dilatation is not understood at the present time, it would appear to be a method worthy of further investigation.

How do I choose the right clinic and doctor to perform my abortion?

You should choose a doctor's office or an abortion clinic that is within ten minutes' drive of a hospital in which the doctor has operating privileges. Don't be timid. Ask to inspect the treatment and recovery area, the availability of intravenous equipment, a tray of emergency drugs, oxygen and mask for resuscitation, cleanliness, and adequate staffing with registered nurses supervising.

The following list has been prepared by Planned Parenthood to delineate the physical facilities an abortion clinic must have if it is to be considered acceptable:

1. Adequate, private space specifically designated for interviewing, counseling, and pregnancy evaluation.
2. Conventional gynecologic examining or operating accessories, drapes, and linen.
3. Approved and electrically safe vacuum aspiration equipment, and conventional instruments for cervical dilatation and uterine curettage.
4. Adequate lighting and ventilation for surgical procedures.
5. Facilities for sterilization of instruments and linen, and for surgical scrub for all personnel.
6. Laboratory equipment and personnel (or immediate access to laboratory facilities) for preoperative and emergency determinations and for tissue diagnosis of uterine contents.
7. Postoperative recovery room, properly supervised, staffed, and equipped.
8. Adequate supplies of drugs, intravenous solutions, syringes, and needles, including four to six units of plasma volume-expander liquids for emergency use (until blood is available).
9. Dressing rooms for staff and patients, and appropriate lavatory facilities.

10. Ancillary equipment and supplies, including stethoscopes, sphygmomanometers (for taking blood pressure), anesthesia equipment—including oxygen and equipment for artificial ventilation and administration of anesthetic gases—and resuscitation equipment and drugs.
11. Ability to transfer a patient without delay to a conventional operating theater and a written letter of agreement from a full-service hospital regarding transfer of emergency patients.
12. Special arrangements for patient emergency contact (on a twenty-four-hour basis) for evaluation and treatment of complications, or postoperative follow-up and examination, and for family planning services.

Some doctors still perform first-trimester abortions with a sharp curette (see chapter 2) rather than with a suction apparatus. The curette causes greater blood loss, almost triples the incidence of retained pregnancy tissue, and causes intolerable and prolonged pain even when local anesthetic is used. If there is no suction apparatus in the office, find another doctor. If there is a suction apparatus, then ask the doctor what size dilator and curette he or she intends to use (see page 177).

Though many doctors perform abortions, not all are Board-certified obstetricians and gynecologists. Though certification by that specialty board is not an absolute guarantee of a doctor's competence or manual dexterity, it does show that he or she has completed an approved residency program and has demonstrated the ambition and knowledge to pass extensive qualifying examinations. I would be more inclined to recommend that a Board-certified obstetrician-gynecologist treat a potential complication of an abortion, rather than a family practitioner or general surgeon.

A telephone call to a local family planning clinic, such as Planned Parenthood, may be helpful in locating a competent physician. These centers receive follow-up evaluations from women who are referred for abortions. If treatment has been below par, it is unlikely that the doctor or clinic will remain on the referral list for long. Several Planned Parenthood affiliates perform first-trimester abortions. All personnel at these facilities must meet very high standards of care and undergo a thorough inspection before they are approved. Furthermore, those Planned Parenthood affiliates that do not perform abortions themselves will not usually refer you to a physician's office or abortion clinic unless they have sent a representative to personally inspect it beforehand.

A call to an operating room nurse or an obstetrical resident at a local hospital will often be the most helpful in securing a qualified physician. A senior resident in an approved obstetrics and gynecology program is often the best judge of the relative talents of the attending staff physicians.

What is the cost of a suction curettage?

When an early abortion is performed in a clinic or a doctor's office, the fee should not exceed $300.00, though a more reasonable fee would be $150.00 to $200.00. Very few clinics include RhoGAM (see page 174) in the fee. If you know you are Rh-negative, find out beforehand whether the cost of an injection of RhoGAM is included. If not, it will usually cost between $35.00 and $50.00, with an additional fee for general anesthesia. Most abortion clinics request payment in full prior to the abortion, and some can be very blunt about collecting every last dollar. The fee should include a reexamination two weeks later, as well as contraceptive counseling both at the time of the abortion and at the two-week visit. Insertion of an IUD and fitting of a diaphragm will entail an extra fee.

The ambulatory facilities at most hospitals are more than adequate, but are usually twice as expensive as those of a clinic or doctor's office. However, many insurance companies provide full or at least partial payment for abortions performed in a hospital, as well as for those in a clinic or office.

For the indigent woman who cannot pay for an abortion, local family planning centers usually make special financial arrangements with a clinic or a private doctor. Because most hospitals in the United States do not meet their obligations in caring for such women, the majority of their abortions are now being performed in private clinics and offices.

How can a pregnancy that has advanced beyond twelve weeks be terminated?

Approximately 9 percent of all abortions are performed after the pregnancy has reached its twelfth week. A second-trimester, or midtrimester, abortion is one that takes place between the thirteenth and the twenty-fourth week. For some women, this decision is reached following detection of an inherited disease or a genetic defect diagnosed by amniocentesis performed during the sixteenth week of pregnancy. For others, however, the delay in seeking abortion is the result of a host of deep-seated psychological conflicts, immaturity, and in many cases even denial that a pregnancy exists.

More often than not, when a pregnancy has progressed beyond twenty weeks, a woman will be unable to specify the date of her last menstrual period or the date of conception. To be sure that the pregnancy has not progressed beyond the critical legal limit of twenty-four weeks, she must undergo an ultrasound examination to verify the exact length of the pregnancy. Late second-trimester abortion has become one of the most troubling problems of the abortion issue. Technological advances in pediatrics continue to lower the threshold of viability for newborns, so that there is often a fine line between a late second-trimester abortion and the premature birth of a potentially viable fetus. Modern neonatology and prenatal care have improved to the point that a fetus may soon be considered capable of surviving outside the uterus when it has been twenty-four to twenty-six weeks since the mother's last menstrual period. The ethical conflict between the interest of the pregnant woman and that of the fetus escalates as the pregnancy progresses and as the fetus develops a capacity for independent life.

There is now convincing data to show that dilatation and evacuation, or D and E, when performed by an experienced and skilled physician, is the safest way to terminate a midtrimester pregnancy. Currently, D and E accounts for almost 70 percent of all midtrimester abortions. This method involves use of suction curettage with vacuum cannulas as large as 16 millimeters combined with special forceps and other instruments to remove fetal and placental tissue. Within twenty-four hours prior to a D and E, most doctors prefer to insert several laminaria or other cervical dilators into the cervix on one or more occasions to dilate it slowly and safely and facilitate the procedure (see laminaria, page 183). Though there are no large studies demonstrating that this precaution decreases the incidence of cervical incompetence in a future pregnancy, it is a widely held belief that it does. While some believe that it is safest to perform D and E under general anesthesia, one recent study has found that complication rates are lower when local anesthesia is used.

A skilled doctor can perform a D and E in an outpatient clinic with equal and possibly even greater safety than when it is performed in a hospital. Unfortunately, not many doctors in the United States have the skill to perform a D and E to terminate a midtrimester pregnancy. Therefore, in a large number of medical centers, pregnancies beyond the twelfth week are aborted by injecting solutions such as hypertonic saline or a combination of prostaglandins and urea into the amniotic sac surrounding the fetus. These substances work effectively to cause uterine contractions, labor, and expulsion of fetus and placenta. Intra-amniotic procedures may require one to five days of hospitalization at considerably more cost than a D and E, but since D and E's performed late in the second trimester require substantially more professional experience and expertise than those done between the thirteenth and fifteenth weeks, the relative number of intra-amniotic saline and prostaglandin installations increases after the sixteenth week.

As discussed earlier, prostaglandins in the form of vaginal suppositories, gels, and intracervical tablets have also been used to induce abortion (see prostaglandins). Vaginal PGE2 suppositories (trade name: Prostin E2) have a distinct advantage over intra-amniotic injections because they can be inserted during the critical twelfth to sixteenth weeks when there is not yet enough amniotic fluid to allow intra-amniotic injection. In fact, extensive research with PGE2 suppositories has shown that they are capable of effectively inducing uterine contractions and abortion from early in the first trimester until late in the second. And, unlike intra-amniotic injection, insertion of prostaglandin suppositories every three to five hours requires no special medical skill.

Regardless of the method chosen to terminate a pregnancy during the second trimester, we must not lose sight of the fact that abortion at this time is a far more dangerous procedure than it is when performed during the first trimester. Statistically, while midtrimester abortions account for only 9 percent of all abortions performed in the United States, they are responsible for 50 percent of all abortion-related deaths. An analysis of abortion mortality in the United States from 1972 to 1981 showed that there were 4.9 deaths per 100,000 abortions for midtrimester D and E, and 9.6 per 100,000 for intra-amniotic installation procedures such as hypertonic saline or prostaglandins and urea. Major complications such as hemorrhage, infection, pulmonary embolus (see chapter 2), amniotic fluid embolus, and surgery to remove retained placental fragments are all more likely to occur in midtrimester abortions. In one study from the Centers for Disease Control in Atlanta, Georgia, doctors reported an overall serious complication rate for D and E of 1 in 400 procedures; in contrast, the incidence for hypertonic saline was 1 in 40 and that for intra-amniotic prostaglandins was 1 in 80. For comparison, fewer than 1 in 1,000 women undergoing a suction curettage procedure suffered serious complications.

What is hypertonic saline?

Hypertonic saline is a highly concentrated 20 percent salt solution which, when injected into the amniotic cavity, causes fetal death, labor, and the expulsion of the fetus and placenta. Until ten years ago, it was the most popular method of terminating second-trimester pregnancies in the United States. With the perfection of D and E and a variety of prostaglandin techniques, however, hypertonic saline is now used for only 3 percent of all midtrimester abortions. It was first introduced in Japan, but it is no longer used there because it was found to be associated with some very serious complications. These complications have been observed in this country as well. Though many doctors have performed hundreds of saline abortions and have claimed only minimal side effects, the procedure is not without its dangers. In fact, the total complication rate for women undergoing saline abortion in various studies has been estimated at 20 to 26 per 100 women. The death rate has varied between 12 and 18 per 100,000 abortions, which means it is many times more likely than suction curettage to cause death.

To induce a hypertonic saline abortion, the solution must be injected into the amniotic fluid surrounding the fetus. This fluid is contained in the amniotic sac, or bag of waters, and increases in quantity as pregnancy advances. An adequate quantity of amniotic fluid must be present before saline can be safely injected, usually not before the sixteenth week of pregnancy, when the uterus is enlarged to a height slightly more than half the distance between the pubic symphisis bone (see chapter 1) and the umbilicus. For the woman who is slightly more than twelve weeks pregnant and must wait four weeks to terminate her pregnancy with hypertonic saline, this method is psychologically devastating.

How is a hypertonic saline abortion performed?

The first step involves urinating immediately before receiving the injection, to ensure that the needle will not perforate a distended urinary bladder lying in front of the uterus (see chapter 1). The skin overlaying the enlarged uterus is then cleansed with antiseptic solution, and a local anesthetic such as chloroprocaine hydrochloride (trade name: Nesacaine) is injected into the skin.

A long needle is then inserted through the anesthetized skin and the uterine muscle, into the amniotic sac. A moderate amount of pain will be felt below the skin, but it can be greatly relieved if the needle is inserted rapidly. Correct placement of the needle is confirmed by a free flow of clear amniotic fluid through the tip of the needle.

At this point, some doctors prefer to thread a plastic catheter through the needle and into the amniotic sac, and then remove the needle, leaving the catheter in place. Withdrawal of amniotic fluid and injection of hypertonic saline is accomplished by attaching a syringe to the catheter. Other doctors prefer to inject the solution from the syringe attached to the needle.

The advantage of a plastic catheter is that it can be left in place, taped to the abdomen, so that if the initial injection is unsuccessful in producing abortion within twenty-four to forty-eight hours, reinjection will be simplified. The disadvantage is that a plastic catheter may increase the risk of infection both on the skin and along the path of the catheter. If a plastic catheter is not used and reinjection is necessary, the longer, painful needle must be used again.

Within a variable interval of several hours following the injection, contractions usually begin, followed by labor and eventual expulsion of the fetus and placenta. Some gynecologists incorrectly refer to this stage as a "minilabor," slightly more painful than severe menstrual cramps. Nothing could be further from the truth. Despite the small size of the fetus, the labor is often prolonged and very painful, usually requiring liberal amounts of pain medication.

What are the most common complications of saline abortion?

The first potentially serious complication experienced with hypertonic saline may occur while it is being injected. If the doctor accidentally injects the solution into a uterine blood vessel, rather than into the amniotic fluid, the *hypernatremia,* or increased levels of salt solutions in the blood, can cause instant death. This complication has been estimated to occur in less than 0.4 percent of all women undergoing saline abortions, and may be avoided by very slow injection of the saline with frequent withdrawal of the syringe handle to ensure that clear fluid, and not blood, returns into the catheter. If there is even a trace of blood in the catheter or syringe, no more saline should be injected until the fluid becomes perfectly clear again. It takes approximately 200 cubic centimeters of saline to produce abortion, roughly equivalent to the volume of a drinking glass. With such a large amount, there is a chance of accidental intravenous injection, so while the solution is being injected the doctor must constantly watch for early signs of hypernatremia: headache, restlessness, numbness of the fingers, a sensation of increased body warmth, and excessive thirst. The procedure must be stopped immediately when any of those warning signs are noted. A woman must be fully awake and alert, never sedated, before and during the saline injection.

If the needle is accidentally placed in the muscle of the uterus and saline is then injected, necrosis, or death of the muscle, may occur. That complication, though very rare, may require hysterectomy, but it should not happen if the doctor strictly adheres to the precautions just outlined. Rarer still is the placement of the needle into the abdominal cavity rather than into the amniotic sac. Injection of saline into the abdominal cavity usually causes immediate and severe pain. No harm will result if the injection is stopped immediately.

Following accurate placement of the saline into the amniotic sac, some of it is absorbed into the bloodstream over a period of several hours. For a woman with medical problems such as heart disease, the increased salt load and expansion of the blood volume may be quite dangerous.

A temperature greater than 100.4°F may occur in as many as 16 percent and as few as 2 percent of women undergoing saline abortion. The temperature elevation is usually due to either necrosis or death of tissue, but may also be a result of infection. When infection is the cause of the fever, it can become a potentially lethal complication and, as previously noted, it is the leading cause of saline abortion death.

The incidence of hemorrhage has been calculated at 2.6 percent, and 1 to 2 percent will hemorrhage to the point of requiring a blood transfusion. An unexplained but very serious complication of saline abortion is a decrease of several blood coagulation (clotting) factors. Without these factors, uncontrolled hemorrhage may occur in 1 of every 1,200 women receiving saline.

Finally, 10 to 16 percent of women who abort the fetus retain the placenta and do not, as should be expected, pass it within one to two hours. This complication necessitates the removal of the placenta either by hand or with a sharp curette and other instruments under anesthesia. All these complications, while rarely mentioned to patients by their doctors, are potentially very serious and serve to emphasize the dangers that may occur with hypertonic saline abortions.

Is there any way to reduce the incidence of complications with hypertonic saline?

If difficulty is encountered while the doctor is trying to insert the needle into the amniotic sac, it may be overcome by direct visualization with an ultrasound machine.

Shortening the time between injection of the saline and passage of the aborted fetus may reduce the incidence of some complications. In their extensive review of the literature, Drs. Lonnie S. Burnett, Ian Colston Wentz, and Theodore M. King noted that when oxytocin was given in an intravenous solution following saline injection, 48 percent of women aborted within twenty-four hours, compared with only 22 percent when saline was used alone. After forty-eight hours, 93 percent of the saline-plus-oxytocin group had aborted, compared with 85 percent in the saline-only group. In addition, the incidence of fever and infection was reduced by one-third, while there was a significant drop in the number of women with retained placentas, from 16 to 2 percent. On the negative side, the incidence of hemorrhage actually tripled, and the risk of hemorrhage from diminished coagulation factors was increased to 1 in 300 women, from 1 in 1,200 women.

What are prostaglandins, and how are they used to induce abortion?

Prostaglandins are lipids, or fatlike chemicals, found in their natural state in the bodies of all men and women. It is their presence in the endometrium that is thought to be responsible for causing painful uterine contractions during menstruation. Many different types of prostaglandin derivatives, or analogs, have been synthesized in the laboratory, classified according to chemical structure. Two such prostaglandins, $PGF2^{\alpha}$ and PGE2, have been used successfully to induce abortion since both are capable of stimulating intense uterine labor contractions which usually result in the expulsion of the fetus and placenta. $PGF2^{\alpha}$ has been approved by the FDA for intra-amniotic injection and has been used successfully in this manner for many years. A small minority of doctors have claimed success by injecting $PGF2^{\alpha}$ or PGE2 gel extra-amniotically (outside the amniotic sac). After insertion of a catheter between the amniotic sac and the uterine wall and injection of these substances, contractions will ensue within twelve hours. PGE2 has had even greater success as a vaginal suppository because it can be used as an alternative to a D and E abortion between the critical thirteenth and sixteenth weeks of pregnancy, during which time not enough amniotic fluid is present to inject the $PGF2^\alpha$ solution safely. While the insertion of a 20-milligram PGE2 suppository every three to five hours will produce strong uterine contractions and expulsion of the fetus, reducing the dose to only 3 milligrams will cause softening, or "ripening," of the cervix without uterine contractions.

Intracervical tablets and vaginal PGE2 gels have been used to dilate and thin the cervix gently and painlessly prior to first- and second-trimester suction curettage.

Since the insertion of a vaginal suppository requires no medical skill, it has been suggested that a woman could use prostaglandins in her own home to bring on a late period, termed a "menstrual extraction" (see previous chapter), or for a self-adminis-tered termination of an early pregnancy (see above and chapter 11, "The Future"). Though results of several studies are encouraging, more work is needed before this method can be endorsed. In one report from Oxford University, PGE2 suppositories were given to 300 women whose menses were delayed from three to thirty-five days. Of 275 confirmed pregnancies, 229 were successfully aborted, and of those only 6 percent required D and C for prolonged bleeding or retained tissue fragments. In another study of 60 women who had been pregnant for 56 days or less, successful abortion was accomplished in 55 cases with use of a vaginal suppository containing a prostaglandin analog named 15 methyl prostaglandin F2 methyl ester. Four women required hospitalization and D and C for retained tissue fragments. California physi-cians using the same analog reported successful pregnancy termination in 16 of 20 women who were less than 50 days pregnant. Their 1983 report was followed by another in which this compound was used in 60 patients whose pregnancies were advanced to between 6 and 15 weeks. Abortion did not ensue, but 42 percent of the women had perceptible cervical dilatation sufficient to allow suction curettage abor-tion without further mechanical dilatation of the cervix.

Neils H. Laursen, M.D., and Zoe R. Graves, Ph.D., of Mount Sinai Hospital in New York City, administered suppositories of either the analog 9-dexo-16, 16-dimethyl-9 methylene PGE2, or the analog 15 (s)-methyl $PGF2^\alpha$ to 46 women prior to first-trimester abortion. In their 1984 publication, they reported that these agents had been equally effective in painlessly increasing the dilatation of the cervix by an average of 3 millimeters within one to two hours. In the doses used, all of the women demon-strated some degree of cervical dilatation with minimal prostaglandin-associated side effects. The authors concluded that both of these analogs showed great promise for avoiding the 1 percent incidence of cervical injury reported with first-trimester abor-tions.

In 1987, doctors at the University of North Carolina tested a PGE1 analog, named ONO-802, on 121 women undergoing first-trimester abortion. Sophisticated equip-ment was used to measure cervical resistance and softening before and three hours after insertion of a suppository containing ONO-802. While a slight effect was noted among women who had previously given birth, no such changes could be seen in the firmer cervixes of those who had never had a child.

Intravenous and intramuscular $PGF2^\alpha$ has also been used to induce abortion. In one study of 815 women with pregnancies ranging between six and twenty-four weeks, doctors administered an analog of $PGF2^\alpha$ every one and one-half to three hours. Abortion occurred in over 96 percent of the women treated, but over 20 percent required D and C in order to remove retained pregnancy tissue.

Though prostaglandins can cause contractions of the uterus, bring on a late period, and induce abortion during the first few days of a pregnancy up until the end of the second trimester, the main drawback to their extensive use remains their unpleasant side effects (see page 193). The ideal analog, devoid of these problems, has yet to be developed.

How successful are prostaglandin suppositories in inducing abortions between the twelfth and sixteenth weeks of pregnancy?

In December 1977, the FDA approved the use of PGE2 as a vaginal suppository for the termination of pregnancy from the twelfth gestational week through the second trimester. The drug is marketed by Upjohn under the name Prostin E2. A 20-milligram suppository is inserted in the vagina at three- to five-hour intervals until fetal expulsion occurs. In one study of 102 patients, complete evacuation of the uterus occurred in 100 patients in a mean time of nine hours, with an average total dose of just under three suppositories. Only two patients retained placental fragments requiring a D and C. The most frequent side effects were vomiting, in two-thirds of the women; temperature elevation of more than 2°F, in one-half; diarrhea, in one-third; and nausea, in one-tenth. One-tenth of the patients also experienced a transient though significant drop in blood pressure.

A skilled physician can terminate a pregnancy between the thirteenth and sixteenth weeks more safely and with less pain and uncomfortable side effects with a D and E than with PGE2 suppositories. Unfortunately, not all doctors have the expertise to perform D and E's. PGE2 suppositories are a safe alternative which require no special skill on the part of the person inducing the abortion.

Specifically, why is D and E better than other methods of midtrimester abortion?

Joel Robins, M.D., and Edward J. Surrago, M.D., of the Nassau County Medical Center, compared the results of 400 consecutive abortions by dilatation and evacuation at thirteen through fifteen weeks of gestation with results previously obtained in 112 women at the same period of pregnancy who had been aborted with PGE2 vaginal suppositories. Their study, reported in *The Journal of Reproductive Medicine* in July 1982, clearly demonstrated the advantages of D and E over prostaglandin suppository abortion. While D and E patients spent an average of sixteen painless minutes under general anesthesia, it took an average of fourteen hours from the insertion of the first prostaglandin suppository to the expulsion of the fetus. During this time the women often suffered in painful labor compounded by distressing prostaglandin reactions such as vomiting (37 percent), diarrhea (31 percent), and temperature elevation (24 percent). Though one D and E patient required a D and C two weeks later for retained fetal tissue, this complication occurred three times more often with prostaglandins. The total hospital stay for the D and E group was shorter by slightly more than one day.

In 1984, doctors at the Centers for Disease Control in Atlanta, Georgia, compared the safety of over 9,500 D and E abortions at thirteen to twenty-four weeks with 4,700 saline abortions and 2,800 abortions performed by installation of urea and prostaglandin $F2^{\alpha}$ into the amniotic sac. Though the overall risk of serious complications associated with urea and prostaglandins was almost two times greater than with D and E, most of these differences occurred at sixteen weeks or less. But between sixteen and twenty-four weeks, the rates of serious complications were almost comparable. These statistics, however, do not take into account the vital fact that those undergoing prostaglandin abortion had to endure long and painful labors complicated by the previously noted side effects. In a 1982 report, the same doctors analyzed almost 4,000 midtrimester abortions performed by D and E, installation of intra-amniotic $F2^{\alpha}$ without urea, and intra-amniotic hypertonic saline procedures. D and E was shown to be five times less likely than prostaglandins and ten times less likely than saline to be associated with a serious complication such as hemorrhage, retained products of conception, or infection. In this study, even when D and E was performed at seventeen weeks' gestation or later, it was associated with a lower rate of serious complications than either prostaglandins or saline. The risk of injury to the cervix was slightly higher with D and E than with prostaglandins or saline, though.

How does PGF2$^\alpha$ compare to hypertonic saline when used for intra-amniotic midtrimester abortion?

Several studies have confirmed five definite advantages of PGF2$^\alpha$ over hypertonic saline:

1. Only 8 cubic centimeters (40 milligrams) has to be injected into the amniotic fluid to induce abortion. When compared with the 200 cubic centimeters of saline that is needed, there is much less chance of PGF2$^\alpha$ entering the bloodstream.

2. Prostaglandins have a much more rapid injection-to-abortion interval. In the 1984 Centers for Disease Control study previously discussed, the outcome of almost 5,000 saline abortions was compared to that of 2,800 women given intra-amniotic urea and prostaglandins. The urea-prostaglandin abortions required an average of fourteen hours to complete, whereas the saline abortions took nearly twenty-six hours. The use of laminaria significantly shortened the completion time of the urea-prostaglandin procedures, but made no difference in the saline abortion time. Practically speaking, less time is spent in the hospital, and therefore less expense is incurred, when prostaglandins are used. (The injection-to-abortion interval could be lengthened if pain medication containing aspirin is taken to relieve the discomfort of contractions, because aspirin is a prostaglandin antagonist. Never take commonly used pain medications such as Darvon Compound or Percodan when undergoing prostaglandin abortion.)

3. Prostaglandins do not cause significant changes in the blood volume or salt load, and can therefore be given with greater safety to women who have cardiac or other coexisting medical problems.

4. Prostaglandins do not alter blood coagulation factors. In the 1984 Centers for Disease Control study, hemorrhage occurred in 0.32 per 100 procedures for prostaglandins, versus 1.7 per 100 for saline.

5. If prostaglandins are given incorrectly, there is no risk of death from hypernatremia or necrosis of the uterine muscle. In the Centers for Disease Control study, saline was associated with a 2.3 times greater risk of serious complications than was the combination of prostaglandins and urea.

Are there any adverse reactions when prostaglandins are used for an abortion?

The most frequent side effect is vomiting, which has been reported to occur in at least 50 percent and at most 75 percent of all women, and there is a 25 percent incidence of extreme nausea without vomiting. A transient temperature elevation, without apparent fever, has been noted 6 percent of the time. These symptoms do not usually appear until several hours after the initial injection. A rectal suppository sometimes proves helpful in alleviating these symptoms before they occur, but diarrhea has been a problem for 16 percent of the women who have tried this measure.

The most frightening side effect for both patient and doctor occurs as often as 1 to 3 percent of the time: the immediate onset of an asthmalike shortness of breath, nausea, vomiting, restlessness, drop in blood pressure, slowing of the pulse, irregularities of the heartbeat, and even seizures. These symptoms are believed to be caused by inadvertent passage of the prostaglandins directly into the circulatory system. Fortunately, the prostaglandins are metabolized rapidly by the body and all symptoms disappear within twenty minutes. Because of the danger of this side effect, it is recommended that prostaglandins not be used in aborting asthmatic women.

The uterine muscle contractions caused by prostaglandins are often so strong that they can cause lacerations, or tears, of the lower cervix in approximately 0.5 percent of all patients. The cervix must be carefully inspected following prostaglandin abortion, and all lacerations sutured immediately. This complication is more likely to occur in young women who have never experienced childbirth. Currently available prostaglandins cannot be considered for inducing full-term pregnancies, as an infant subjected to such potent contractions would have a strong likelihood of being severely damaged.

In a study of 600 prostaglandin abortions, it was noted that 30 percent of the women did not go into labor within twenty-four hours but required reinjection with one-half of the initial 40-milligram dose. In addition, 140 women retained placental fragments following passage of the fetus. Ten of these placentas were successfully removed in bed; 117 required removal in a nearby treatment room; and 13, or 2.2 percent, required removal in an operating room. A total of 25 of the patients in this study were later readmitted because of retained placental fragments and bleeding, while 5.3 percent of the 600 women experienced bleeding equal to or greater than one unit of blood (500 cubic centimeters).

A report published by the Centers for Disease Control compared 1,200 prostaglandin abortions with 10,000 saline abortions. The authors of this study concluded that prostaglandins had the advantage of a more rapid injection-to-abortion interval, but the disadvantage of a higher rate of fever, uterine infection, retained placental fragments, and rehospitalization for complications following the procedure.

Finally, it should be noted that the injection of intra-amniotic saline causes fetal death almost instantly. In contrast, when prostaglandins are used without urea a fetus may occasionally be born alive and survive for minutes or even hours. This understandably presents great emotional and moral concern for the woman, her physician, and the medical staff. To induce fetal death, many doctors inject hyperosmolar urea into the amniotic sac when the prostaglandins are administered. Urea has the added advantage of reducing the necessary amount of prostaglandin, thereby reducing the incidence of its unpleasant side effects.

Are prostaglandins harmful to women with sickle-cell trait?

Though an earlier study suggested that prostaglandins were more likely to increase the rate of sickling in blacks with sickle-cell trait, two subsequent reports by other researchers have refuted this claim. In one of these studies, the blood from eighty patients with sickle-cell trait was mixed with a prostaglandin substance; in another, prostaglandins were administered directly to eight patients with sickle-cell trait. In neither instance was sickling increased. Though the use of prostaglandins in terminating the pregnancy of a woman with sickle-cell trait or sickle-cell disease is probably safe, D and E or injection of hypertonic saline may be considered logical alternatives.

What are the risks of an incompetent cervix and premature birth following a midtrimester abortion?

Little is known about the effects of second-trimester abortion on future pregnancies. The limited available information on obstetric outcomes after installation of intra-amniotic solutions, such as saline and prostaglandins, suggests no significant increase in the risk of low birth weight or prematurity. But the fact that cervical lacerations and fistulas (abnormal openings) have been linked to prostaglandin abortions is reason for concern that cervical incompetence may occur in a small percentage of women.

Concern has been expressed in the medical literature that the large 16-millimeter cannulas used for D and E may cause permanent damage to the cervical tissues. It has been theorized that this could lead to cervical incompetence, spontaneous abortion, and premature delivery in subsequent pregnancies. In one study, investigators compared the incidence of low birth weight among children of women who had had cervical dilatation of 16 millimeters for midtrimester abortion with that among babies whose mothers had had previous cervical dilatation of 14 millimeters. They found that the former group were at a 2.5 times greater risk of delivering a low birth weight infant than were women in the latter group. For this reason, the use of laminaria and other products that slowly and atraumatically dilate the cervix prior to D and E are now used extensively in the United States. And new prostaglandin analogs in the form of vaginal suppositories and gels to dilate and soften the cervix painlessly prior to abortion show great promise as a way of avoiding cervical injury caused by mechanical methods of dilatation (see page 183).

What is hysterotomy?

Hysterotomy means termination of a pregnancy through a cesarean-section-like incision in the uterus. The mortality rate from hysterotomy has been estimated to be at least twelve times greater than it is for D and E, and six times greater than it is for installation of prostaglandins or hypertonic saline into the amniotic sac. In some studies the death rate associated with hysterotomy has ranged from a low of 30 to an astronomical high of 200 per 100,000 women. Total complication rates vary between 25 and 50 per 100 women aborted. In addition, future full-term pregnancies usually necessitate cesarean section because of the weakening of the uterine muscle caused by the hysterotomy. While the trend in modern obstetrics is to allow women with previous cesarean sections to attempt vaginal delivery during subsequent pregnancies, this is not the case with hysterotomy because the incision is made in the upper part of the uterus rather than in the lower part as occurs with cesarean section. Incisions of this type are much more likely to rupture if subjected to the stress of labor during a subsequent full-term pregnancy. Hysterotomy should rarely, if ever, be used today as a means of terminating a pregnancy.

How expensive is a second-trimester abortion?

Because midtrimester abortions are often associated with many serious complications, a doctor's fee will almost always be significantly higher than for suction curettage. The minimum fee is usually $300.00 to $400.00 but it may run as high as $700.00 to $800.00. Second-trimester D and E, especially if performed between the thirteenth and sixteenth weeks of pregnancy, has been proven safe when carried out in either a hospital or an outpatient clinic. Hypertonic saline or prostaglandins that are used intra-amniotically usually require hospitalization, often for a period of three or four days which will cost several hundred dollars. If a D and C is necessary to remove the placenta, anesthesia and operating room fees must be added to the already-high total. Some insurance policies cover part or all of the hospitalization costs. There are smaller hospitals that specialize in performing midtrimester abortions, and actually offer a fixed fee for the entire hospitalization. At some hospitals the set fee for midtrimester abortions at less than twenty weeks may be less than $800.00.

In the past, attempts have been made to reduce the cost of intra-amniotic hypertonic saline and prostaglandin abortions by performing them in outpatient clinics. Other attempts have been made to reduce the total hospital stay by injecting prostaglandins or saline in a clinic or office and then admitting these women to the hospital only when labor is well established. These have proven to be very dangerous and unacceptable practices. In a report from the Medical Society of New York, doctors demonstrated that the risk of death was three times as great for women undergoing second-trimester abortion without remaining continuously in the hospital from the time of induction of the abortion until its completion. Some 43 percent of statewide maternal deaths were due to hemorrhage, many of which could have been prevented if the women had been in a hospital with an adequate blood bank and transfusion facilities.

Are women who undergo abortion likely to experience emotional problems and guilt feelings later on?

One study at Johns Hopkins University Hospital evaluated a total of 373 women for psychological aftereffects from abortion. One group had been aborted with suction curettage, another had been aborted with saline, and a third group had carried their pregnancies to term. In comparing the three groups, no significant variation was found in "sense of alienation from society" or "self-esteem." Furthermore, subsequent sexual enjoyment and marital happiness appeared unchanged in all three groups. A second psychological study of 380 women who underwent abortion in New York revealed that almost 79 percent were happy with the decision, while only 7 percent experienced some self-anger, and 1.5 percent were very angry with themselves and negative about their decision. Among Catholics, it was noted that guilt and difficulty with the decision to abort occurred somewhat more frequently than among non-Catholics, but even here negative feelings were minimal. In a study published in the *British Medical Journal,* doctors found only one case of postabortion psychosis among almost 4,000 women who had undergone the procedure, and that individual had had a previous history of depression following two previous full-term pregnancies. The authors concluded that postpartum psychosis is six times more likely to occur than postabortion psychosis.

Several studies have shown that religion did not seem to play an important part in the general population's use of abortion facilities. In fact, Catholics tend to be slightly overrepresented in abortion patient groups relative to their population percentage in the states of Maryland, Colorado, New York, Connecticut, and Hawaii. Catholic women are less likely to try to prevent pregnancy or to define it as unwanted when it occurs, but when the pregnancy is defined as unwanted, they seek abortion as readily as non-Catholic women.

In conclusion, there is a small percentage of women who do experience mild, transient depression following first- and second-trimester abortion. There are no data to support the claim that serious psychological problems will develop in a normal woman who has an abortion.

Does easy access to abortion make a woman less likely to use adequate contraception?

On the contrary, several studies have shown that more women are using effective contraception than ever before. Unfortunately, teenagers continue to lag behind older women in this regard.

The statistics from a New York City study conducted from 1970 to 1974 demonstrate beyond a doubt that most women who undergo abortion will, in the future, use adequate contraceptive techniques. A study of white, Puerto Rican, and black women aborted in 1970 revealed that members of all three groups used adequate contraceptive techniques when they were reevaluated in 1974. Though black women were noted to have a slightly higher repeat pregnancy rate, it was not nearly as high as it would have been if adequate contraception had not been used. The conclusion reached was that a "very consistent level of use of the most effective contraceptive measures" was practiced among all three groups. In analyzing U.S. abortion statistics in the 1980s, epidemiologists have demonstrated that women at risk of a repeat abortion use similar or slightly better methods of contraception than do women at risk of a first abortion. Following one abortion, women are more likely to depend on the Pill or on sterilization, the two most effective methods. This should dispel the prevailing myth that many women irresponsibly use abortion as a primary method of birth control.

In a 1984 report from Montreal, almost 600 women undergoing first or repeat abortions were compared, based on the results of extensive two-hour psychological interviews. The conclusion reached was that the two groups were similar in personality and in conscientious use of contraception. Age and frequency of intercourse were the only important distinguishing traits between the two groups. The women undergoing a repeat abortion had a mean age of twenty-seven, compared to a mean age of twenty-four among those having a first abortion. The repeaters had had intercourse an average of eleven times in the month during which they conceived; those having their first abortion averaged eight acts of coitus during this time.

By far the safest method of preventing unwanted pregnancy is permanent sterilization. In the next two chapters we will address the subject of male and female sterilization.

8

VASECTOMY

In the last five years, permanent sterilization techniques for men and women have assumed a role of increasing importance in the United States as well as in other countries throughout the world. It is estimated that the total number of sterilized adults in this country is more than 16 million, with approximately 1 million operations currently performed each year. Surveys have indicated that sterilization has replaced birth-control pills as the most commonly selected method of fertility control for married couples more than thirty years of age.

The total number of surgical sterilizations and the proportion of vasectomies to tubal ligations have fluctuated over the years, with the key determinant often being the dissemination of inaccurate information about the supposed dangers of vasectomies. Following a great deal of adverse publicity, the number of vasectomies performed in the United States dropped from 510,000 in 1980 to approximately 400,000 in 1981. A further decline to an all-time low of 299,000 took place in 1982, the first time in twelve years that the total number of male and female sterilizations dropped below 1 million: 69 percent of them were tubal ligations, compared with only 31 percent vasectomies. This disproportion was the result of the negative publicity about vasectomy and the increasing popularity of the laparoscope for tubal sterilization. This two-year downward trend reversed itself dramatically in 1983 with a 52 percent increase, from 299,000 to 455,000, a rise that can be directly attributed to the many new studies confirming the safety of vasectomy. But there is room for pessimism: In 1984, the last year for which statistics are available, the number declined to 418,500. The majority of sterilization procedures continue to be performed on women. In 1984, 64 percent of the 1,149,599 operations were tubal ligations and only 36 percent were vasectomies. In view of the fact that vasectomy is acknowledged to be a safer, simpler, and less expensive procedure than tubal ligation, these statistics are somewhat disturbing.

Despite the overwhelming evidence proving the safety of vasectomy, a large segment of our population views this operation with fear, skepticism, and ignorance. Many men still mistakenly believe that vasectomy causes ill effects such as the inability to ejaculate, the loss of virility, the inability to achieve orgasm, hair loss, premature aging, and a change in voice pitch. Vasectomy has even been accused of causing skin disease; kidney, lung, heart, and liver diseases; narcolepsy (inability to stay awake); and multiple sclerosis. Sadly, such misinformation has been responsible for the choice of many men to avoid this simple and relatively harmless procedure.

198

What evidence is there that vasectomy is safer than female sterilization?

In spite of what you may have heard to the contrary, vasectomy is without doubt a safer operation than any method of female sterilization. The most recent statistics, published in the *American Journal of Public Health* in 1985, clearly prove this point. In this report by prominent researchers in the United States, the safety of vasectomy was compared with that of tubal ligation performed either through the laparoscope or with an abdominal surgical incision. They found that deaths occurred at a rate of 4.72 per 100,000 procedures by laparoscopy, and 2.29 per 100,000 through abdominal surgery. In contrast, there were no deaths associated with vasectomy. The investigators defined major complications as the need for intravenous antibiotics, the presence of hemorrhage requiring transfusion, or operative difficulties or trauma leading to hospitalization. For every 100,000 abdominal tubal ligations, 6,170 resulted in major complications, compared with 2,100 for laparoscopies, and 43 for vasectomy. Failure rates, defined as operations followed by either pregnancy or the persistence of motile sperm in the ejaculate, occurred at a rate of 326 per 100,000, 276 per 100,000, and 160 per 100,000, respectively.

What is vasectomy?

Vasectomy means cutting of the *vas deferens*, the two tubes that carry sperm from each testicle (see figure 8-1). It is a minor surgical procedure, sometimes referred to as "clipping the cords," and is the simplest, surest, and safest surgical or medical method known for preventing unwanted pregnancy.

The first vasectomy was performed more than 300 years ago, but it did not begin to be used routinely as a means of sterilization until 1925. It can be performed with equal ease in hospitals, clinics, and doctors' offices. The preference of some doctors for hospital vasectomy is influenced by the very small chance of encountering bleeding if the veins near the vas deferens, called the *pampiniform plexus* (see figure 8-1), are accidentally cut. Hospitals have better facilities for treating such bleeding problems.

Most vasectomies in the United States are performed by urologists, though general surgeons and family practitioners also do a considerable number of them. When rare complications do occur, a Board-certified specialist in urology will usually be better able to deal with them.

What steps should my doctor take prior to performing vasectomy?

It is vital that your doctor take a complete history and perform a thorough physical examination prior to surgery. The history should include inquiries about all previous illnesses and surgical procedures. If prolonged bleeding or clotting problems have

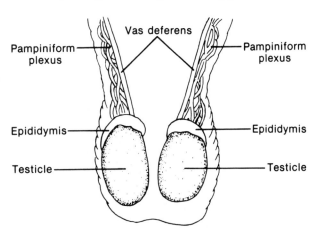

Figure 8–1. *Male genitalia, showing epididymis and vas deferens.*

Vas deferens

Pampiniform plexus

Pampiniform plexus

Epididymis

Epididymis

Testicle

Testicle

accompanied other operations or dental work, it could indicate a possible abnormality in blood clotting factors or platelets. This would require further testing before surgery. Some medications can cause prolonged bleeding; aspirin, or any medication containing aspirin, must not be taken for at least five days prior to surgery. A family or personal history of sensitivity or allergy to general or local anesthesia should be noted and investigated, and appropriate precautions taken before and during surgery. A history of heart disease, hypertension or high blood pressure, diabetes, sexually transmitted disease, phlebitis (see chapter 2), anemia, or liver disease may indicate a need to cancel surgery or at least to perform it in the safe confines of a hospital rather than in an outpatient clinic or doctor's office.

In addition to a general physical examination, your doctor should examine your genitals for signs of a local infection, penile discharge, inguinal hernia, scarring from previous surgery, an undescended testicle, a fluid-filled sac (called a *hydrocele*), or abnormally dilated veins (called a *varicocele*). A preoperative blood count, urinalysis, and clotting profile are often helpful tests.

Your doctor is obligated to inform you thoroughly of the details of the surgical procedure as well as all possible operative and postoperative complications that may occur. Though some men may consider such a discussion too graphic, it is in your best interests to have no misunderstanding prior to vasectomy. The feasibility of all alternative methods of contraception should be part of every informed consent discussion between you and your doctor. Despite modern microsurgical methods of reversing or re-anastomosing a previously cut vas deferens, you should consider the operation irreversible. If you wish to maintain the option of having children in the future, you should never undergo vasectomy.

How is vasectomy performed?

Vasectomy is easily accomplished using local anesthesia. A tranquilizer or sedative may be taken one hour before surgery, and then the area where the incision will be made is shaved. Some doctors prefer one midline scrotal incision; others use two

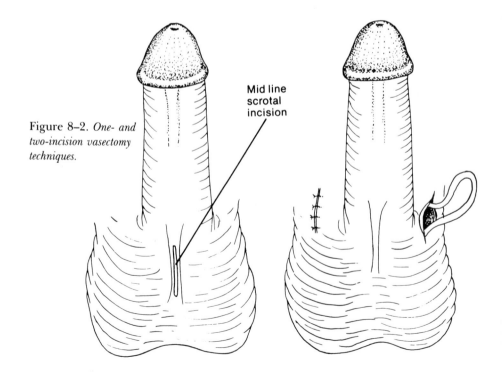

Figure 8–2. *One- and two-incision vasectomy techniques.*

Mid line scrotal incision

Figure 8–3. *Tantalum clips applied to cut ends of vas deferens.*

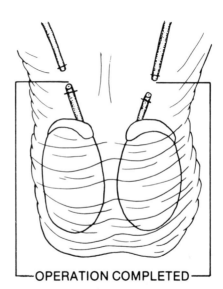

Vas divided
& Tantalum
Clips applied

incisions, one over each vas deferens (see figure 8-2). The scrotal incision usually measures less than one inch in length and is made after adequate amounts of local anesthestic, such as lidocaine (trade name: Xylocaine) and chloroprocaine hydrochloride (trade name: Nesacaine), are injected into the skin. The two vas deferens are then located, pulled out through the incision, and cut. The two loose ends of each vas may then be closed with a suture, cauterization (burning), or special metallic tantalum clips (see Figure 8-3).

Most doctors remove a small portion of each vas deferens, to keep the loose ends apart. The skin is then closed with absorbable sutures which dissolve in seven to ten days. Upon completion of a successful operation, the sperm produced by the testes will be blocked from passing beyond the point of surgery (see figure 8-4).

What instructions should I be given following vasectomy?

Most men experience a moderate amount of pain on the day of surgery and the following day. It is best to spend the day of surgery in bed. If possible, keep an ice pack on the scrotum intermittently for at least six to eight hours after surgery, to

Figure 8–4. *Appearance of completed vasectomy.*

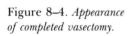

OPERATION COMPLETED

reduce the chances of swelling, bleeding, and discomfort. Returning to work is not advisable until three days after surgery, if you have a sedentary job; seven days, if you perform manual labor. Heavy lifting and strenuous athletic activities should be avoided for seven days. It is also a good idea to wear an athletic supporter for about a week. It will provide scrotal support and help prevent swelling and pain over the operative area. Many doctors prefer that you not shower or bathe for the first forty-eight hours following a vasectomy. Warm baths after this time for approximately twenty minutes, two to four times daily, will often assist in the healing process. Pain medications that do not contain aspirin may be taken periodically during the first week following surgery.

It is best to keep a small gauze bandage over the stitches for a few days in order to avoid irritating the skin. The dressing should be changed every two days and kept clean. Some swelling and oozing of a clear liquid from the incision is not unusual, but if the amount of swelling is greater than the diameter of a quarter it may mean that there is an infection or a *hematoma,* a collection of blood in the area just under the skin. Slight discoloration of the skin, resembling an abrasion, is not unusual.

How soon after vasectomy can a man resume coitus?

Coitus with use of contraception may be resumed after seventy-two hours. If you experience discomfort, wait a full seven days. Before a couple can rely on vasectomy for permanent contraception, spermatozoa must first be emptied from the upper part of the vas deferens and from the seminal vesicles (see chapter 1 and figures in this chapter). This may take as many as fifteen ejaculates, though the usual number is six to eight. Following the surgery, your doctor must examine sperm specimens until two ejaculates in succession contain no active sperm. At that point, additional contraception will no longer be needed.

Following vasectomy, sperm production in the testes continues, but at a slower rate than before the operation. Fewer mature sperm will be produced, and those that reach maturity will disintegrate in the testes and the epididymis.

Many men fear vasectomy because they believe it will significantly diminish the volume of ejaculate. Actually, more than 90 percent of the fluid in the ejaculate comes from accessory glands, such as the seminal vesicles and the prostate. These glands are unaffected by vasectomy, so the 10 percent diminution in total semen volume is never even noticed.

What are some of the complications of vasectomy?

The complication rates for vasectomy are very low in comparison to other surgical procedures, and most of the complications are minor. They include swelling, discoloration, and discomfort lasting a few days. Several studies—including one of 1,500 men and another of 2,700 men undergoing vasectomy—have demonstrated a death rate of zero. Complication rates have been consistently 5 percent or lower. In one study from Baylor College of Medicine, major complications were reported in 4.1 percent, and minor complications in 1.7 percent, of all men undergoing this procedure. *Epididymitis,* or inflammation of the epididymis, was responsible for 1 percent of all major complications. This condition can usually be cured within a week with heat, scrotal support, and occasionally antibiotics. Adhesion of the vas deferens to the scrotal skin complicated surgery in another 1 percent. Abscess or infection caused by the stitches around the tied vas deferens occurred in slightly less than 1 percent of the men, but was absent when metallic clips were used instead of sutures.

The remaining 1.2 percent of complications included *hematoma,* or blood clot formation, at the surgical site; *orchitis,* or inflammation of the entire testicle; and *recanalization,* or reopening and recommunication of the two cut ends of the vas. This last condition occurred in 10 of the 2,700 patients, for a failure rate of 0.37 percent. Even when surgery is performed by an expert, between 0.1 and 0.4 percent of the time the two cut ends will amazingly find each other and reestablish communication, resulting in an unwanted pregnancy.

In 0.3 percent of all cases a painful nodule or lump may be found at the site of surgery. This is called a *sperm granuloma* and appears to be caused when some of the products of the dead sperm actually leak through the wall of the ligated vas deferens and epididymis. The granuloma produced is actually a localized immune or allergic reaction, and it may take weeks or even months to subside. When the granuloma does not subside, it can be treated with ice packs and anti-inflammatory drugs. Granulomas that are painful or increase in size must be surgically removed.

Can other allergic reactions to sperm occur following vasectomy?

It was first noted in 1964 that some men develop antibodies against their own sperm following vasectomy. This is believed to happen when some of the products of the dead sperm, unable to pass through the closed vas, become absorbed into the bloodstream. The circulating sperm products then stimulate the body to produce antibodies against them. More recent investigations have demonstrated that as many as 50 to 65 percent of men will have elevated antibody levels in the first year following vasectomy. After that, the antibody concentration will decrease to very low levels. In some cases, this immunological response lasts ten years or longer. Although there has been widespread publicity and fear about the presence of sperm antibodies in vasectomized men, there is no scientific evidence to show that it causes disease or medical complications. It should be noted that some fertile men, who have never undergone vasectomy, for some reason also have antibodies to their own sperm.

Can vasectomy be responsible for diminishing the sexual drive and potency in some men?

On the contrary, most men report that their sexual potency is the same as or greater than before the operation. In a study of 189 men undergoing vasectomy at the Margaret Sanger Research Bureau, two-thirds reported an increase in sexual desire, attributed mainly to removing the anxiety of a possible pregnancy. One sixty-year-old man reported diminished sexual desire. Some 98 percent of the patients stated that they would recommend the operation to others.

There is no physiological basis for any adverse psychological response to vasectomy. The available evidence suggests that a normal, sexually well-adjusted man experiences no significant psychological changes after sterilization if he has been given an opportunity to express his fears and have his questions answered in advance by the physician performing the surgery.

Testosterone, a hormone produced by the testes, is believed to be responsible for a man's normal sexual drive as well as for maintaining his male characteristics. Blockage of the vas deferens does not alter testosterone release, which takes place directly into the bloodstream from the testes. Several studies have measured blood testosterone levels before and after vasectomy without noting any change. Some studies of vasectomized men have been undertaken for periods of up to ten years following surgery. In addition to noting normal testosterone levels, researchers have confirmed that there were no changes in the pituitary hormones LH or FSH (see chapter 1) or in other steroid hormones produced by the testes and adrenal gland.

As previously mentioned, some men incorrectly look upon vasectomy as the termination of their masculinity. It has been demonstrated that most men who experience sexual problems following vasectomy have had underlying psychological problems prior to the surgery. For this reason, it is the responsibility of doctors to carefully evaluate each patient preoperatively. If doubt exists about an individual's mental status, psychiatric consultation should be obtained prior to surgery.

What is the relationship between vasectomy and a man's later risk of heart disease?

As discussed in chapter 2, atherosclerosis is the formation of fatty plaques deposited in the walls of arteries. Complete occlusion of a coronary artery by atherosclerosis often results in myocardial infarction—heart attack. Two studies performed on a small number of vasectomized monkeys in 1975 and 1978 indicated that they developed atherosclerotic plaques in their coronary arteries at a greater rate than did nonvasectomized monkeys. The authors of these research papers were unable to explain this phenomenon, but they theorized that it was triggered by the formation of antisperm antibodies which are frequently noted following vasectomy (see vasectomy complications). They hypothesized that the leakage of antigens from the spermatozoa into the bloodstream following vasectomy led to this immune response in the coronary arteries.

These articles received extensive coverage in both scientific journals and the lay press, and they discouraged thousands of men from undergoing vasectomy. Many doctors declined to perform the procedure on any of their patients, while others excluded those with a personal or family history of heart disease or any immune disease. The reason for this fearful response is that the monkey, unlike other laboratory animals, is closely related physiologically to man and has similar responses to disease.

Unfortunately, little if any publicity has been given to an article published in *The Journal of Reproductive Medicine* in 1983 that totally refuted this research. When Niels H. Lauersen, M.D., and his associates at the Mount Sinai School of Medicine in New York City placed five vasectomized monkeys and five control monkeys on identical high-cholesterol diets, they found that both groups developed equally high cholesterol levels. At autopsy ten months later there was no difference in the occurrence of atherosclerotic plaques between the vasectomized and control group, despite the presence of sperm antibodies in the bloodstreams of the vasectomized monkeys.

Monkeys aside, several epidemiological studies from the United States and several European countries have been unable to demonstrate a relationship between vasectomy and atherosclerosis. In fact, while the number of vasectomies has increased over the past fifteen years, there has been a definite decline in the number of cardiovascular deaths in the United States.

In 1983, *The New England Journal of Medicine* published two epidemiologic studies from England. The first report matched 1,500 men younger than fifty-five years of age who had been hospitalized with a diagnosis of myocardial infarction, stroke, or hypertension with 3,000 controls hospitalized for other conditions. Overall, 2.4 percent of the controls and 2.7 percent of the study group were found to have undergone vasectomy, an insignificant difference. In the second study, 1,700 men who had had vasectomy were compared with men who had undergone a variety of other surgical procedures. During an average follow-up of six and one-half years, there was no evidence of an elevated risk of cardiovascular disease among the vasectomized men when compared with the control group. In a report from the Kaiser-Permanente Medical Group in Oakland, California, doctors followed 1,600 men for ten or more years after vasectomy and found no difference in their incidence of heart disease when compared with a group of nonvasectomized men. Researchers in Seattle followed almost 1,400 vasectomized men for an average of fifteen years and also found no increase in coronary heart disease.

The largest and most comprehensive study to dispel the fears of possible harm following vasectomy was conducted in 1983 by researchers at the National Institute of Child Health and Human Development. In this report, the incidence of more than fifty diseases was compared among more than 10,000 vasectomized men and an equal number of nonvasectomized men. The majority of individuals had had their operations eight to ten years earlier, and 2,000 had been vasectomized ten or more years prior to the study. After analysis of the statistics, the emphatic conclusion was that vasectomy was not associated with any serious medical condition. Surprisingly, the number of men with diabetes and heart attack was significantly lower in the vasectomy group. In addition, only one-half as many vasectomized men died annually from cancer, and less than two-thirds as many died of heart and blood vessel disease. Based on these statistics, the authors of this report correctly concluded that their findings were "highly reassuring."

All of these positive studies have had the effect of reversing the recent decline in the use of vasectomy as a method of birth control. As news of study data has circulated among doctors and the public, the number of vasectomies in the United States has increased dramatically. The Association for Voluntary Sterilization reports an increase from approximately 299,000 in 1982 to 418,500 in 1984.

What type of man is most likely to request vasectomy?

It has been demonstrated that men with higher incomes and more schooling than that of the general population are most likely to want vasectomy. Minority groups, especially blacks, have been consistently underrepresented in choosing vasectomy as a form of contraception. Reasons cited have included the fear of loss of masculinity, fear of genocide, fear of surgery, and the predominant feeling among less-educated black men that the ability to father children is intimately related to their masculine role.

There also appear to be significant regional differences among men who choose vasectomy and those who do not. In one study conducted in 1970, the lowest rate of vasectomies was noted in the mid-Atlantic states, and the highest in the Pacific states. Among indigent couples, the West again demonstrated the highest rates, while the South had the lowest incidence of vasectomy.

How successful are surgical efforts to reverse vasectomy?

Approximately one out of 2,000 vasectomy patients will decide at a later date to undergo surgery in order to have more children. This usually happens when a man remarries following either divorce or the death of his wife. The unforeseen death of a child may also precipitate this decision. The operation for reuniting the cut ends of the vas deferens is called *vasovasotomy*. To perform this operation, an incision is made over the previous vasectomy site. The ends of the vas are located, opened, and sewn together with very fine suture material under an operative microscope (see figure 8-5).

The operation to reverse vasectomy under the microscope requires special training, sophisticated equipment, and suture material that is so fine as to be difficult to see with the naked eye. The destruction to the *lumen,* or the opening of the vas deferens, may be quite extensive, and the caliber of one end may be different from that of the other, making repair difficult. Following surgery, reappearance of the sperm in the ejaculate may be noted in as few as 35 percent and as many as 84 percent of men. However, sperm in the ejaculate does not always guarantee success in achieving pregnancy. In some studies as few as 33 percent of men with viable sperm following vasectomy were capable of impregnating their partners. One of the most successful surgeons in this field is Sherman J. Silber, M.D., of St. Luke's Hospital in St. Louis. Using the most up-to-date microsurgical techniques on 200 vasovasotomy patients, he reported normal sperm counts and sperm with good motility (movement) and morphology (shape) in 90 percent of his patients. In addition, Dr. Silber achieved pregnancy rates of 70 percent. In another microsurgical review from Australia, 100 percent of the men undergoing vasovasotomy had viable sperm present, and 70 percent were able to impregnate their partners within two years.

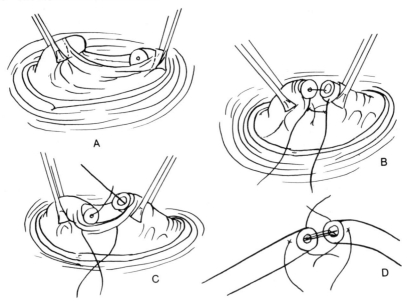

Figure 8–5. *Vasovasotomy technique.*

What is the cost of vasectomy?

When performed in a doctor's office, the fee may range from $150.00 to as much as $800.00. Hospital costs are usually much higher and include use of the operating room, anesthesia, and the fee for the pathologist if a portion of the vas deferens is removed and sent for analysis. Insurance policies usually cover all or most of this expense.

Vasovasotomy with the use of microsurgery is a far more expensive procedure, with fees ranging from a low of $1,200 to a high of as much as $2,500.

Aren't there special banks where men can store their semen prior to vasectomy?

For men who want "fertility insurance" prior to vasectomy, there are special sperm banks where ejaculates are frozen in liquid nitrogen at a temperature of −196°F for months or even years. If a man decides at a later date to have children, those specimens may be thawed and artificially inseminated into his partner's vagina. The number of ejaculates stored in this "cryobanks" is usually five to eight for each man, and the fertilizing capacity of the frozen specimen is two-thirds of that expected when fresh semen is used. The initial cost of sperm storage varies from one bank to another but averages between $35.00 and $50.00 per specimen, with an annual storage fee of $35.00 to $60.00 dollars per year.

Freezing does not appear to cause harm to the sperm cell. The incidence of miscarriage and abnormal births is actually lower when frozen semen is thawed and used. Some investigators believe that this is because freezing helps eliminate the unhealthy and fragile sperm. To date, published reports have documented hundreds of normal infants resulting from clinical use of frozen semen. The greatest success has been achieved with specimens stored for less than six months, though pregnancy has been reported following storage of sperm for as long as ten years. Though it had initially been predicted that semen banks would become a great success in the United States, the response of American men to the idea of fertility insurance has been disappointing. Several commercial sperm banks have closed for lack of financial success.

Though human sperm banks have been in existence for almost twenty years, a man should not delude himself into believing that he can deposit his semen into one of these facilities and return a few years later with the guarantee of fathering children with these stored specimens. To quote the National Medical Committee of Planned Parenthood-World Population: "The promise of fertility insurance to be achieved by storing semen may be misleading. Moreover, it may lead to the persuasion of immature or poorly motivated individuals to undergo vasectomy."

9

TUBAL LIGATION

The increase in voluntary sterilization among women during the 1970s and early 1980s has been attributed to the development of newer, more sophisticated instruments and techniques, as well as to the removal of most legal barriers preventing permanent contraception. The negative publicity surrounding postoperative complications of vasectomy (see chapter 8) has also added to the number of couples selecting tubal ligation. As laboratory and clinical studies published in the early 1980s convincingly demonstrated the safety of vasectomy, more men began to request this procedure. The year 1983 was a landmark—the first time since 1969 that the number of female sterilizations actually decreased, even though it was by a mere 4 percent. The trend was quickly reversed in 1984 (the last year for which statistics are available), when the number of female sterilizations soared to 731,000, compared with 418,500 vasectomies. Perfection of surgical techniques and the introduction of laparoscopic and "minilap" procedures have greatly simplified tubal sterilization and probably account for its popularity. Another reason why female sterilization remains the method selected by the overwhelming number of American couples is that fewer operations are being performed as hospital procedures. This is reflected in the statistics for 1984 showing a 14 percent decline from 1983 in the number of tubal sterilizations done in hospitals as opposed to outpatient facilities.

Despite these advances, the inescapable fact is that, even under the best of circumstances, 2 women will die for every 100,000 operations performed. In contrast, even the largest surveys on vasectomy have failed to demonstrate a single surgically related death.

What is tubal ligation?

By definition, *tubal ligation* means ligating, or tying, the fallopian tubes (see figure 9-1). The more general term of tubal sterilization refers to any procedure that prevents fertilization of the egg by the sperm within the tube. Traditional methods have often involved ligation combined with excision, or cutting out a piece of the tube. Newer techniques have utilized coagulation, or burning, as well as the placement of elastic bands and clips around a segment of the tube. Tubal sterilization immediately following childbirth is called *postpartum* or *puerperal sterilization,* while *interval sterilization* refers to the procedure when it is not associated with pregnancy. Tubal sterilization may also be performed in combination with an abortion.

What is the difference between abdominal and vaginal tubal ligation?

Abdominal tubal ligation, performed by means of an abdominal incision, is still the most commonly used method of tubal sterilization in this country. It is by far the most popular method employed in the immediate postpartum period. Methods of vaginal

208

Ligation of Fallopian tube

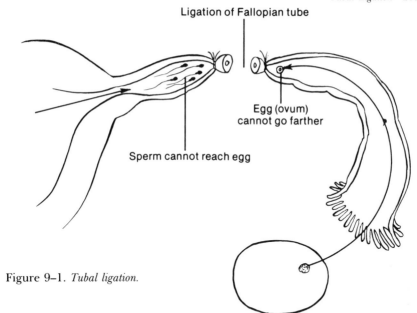

Egg (ovum)
cannot go farther

Sperm cannot reach egg

Figure 9–1. *Tubal ligation.*

tubal ligation (see page 229, on colpotomy and culdoscopy), in which the surgery is performed via the vagina, are also used, though never as postpartum procedures. The doctor's fee for abdominal or vaginal tubal ligation can range from $500 to $1,500.

What procedures are followed before tubal ligation is performed?

Prior to surgery the area over the proposed operative site is shaved and scrubbed with an antiseptic solution. If the incision is to be made just above the pubic hairline, most or all of the pubic hair is removed.

All solid foods and liquids are restricted for eight hours prior to surgery, to ensure that the stomach is empty in the event of inadvertent retching under general anesthesia. (If the stomach is full, food particles and liquids may be aspirated into the trachea, or windpipe, producing a potentially dangerous situation.) Intramuscular medication is given one hour before surgery and usually consists of a tranquilizer. Some centers combine the tranquilizer with *atropine,* a drug that helps dry up excessive secretions in the mouth and throat which could cause breathing difficulties under general anesthesia.

Though abdominal tubal ligation is most commonly performed under general anesthesia induced with intravenous pentothal, patient preference and medical indications occasionally make other methods more attractive. Local anesthesia may be easily injected into the incision, though there is usually some discomfort when the tubes are grasped. Spinal and epidural anesthesia have also been used successfully; they both involve injection of an anesthetic into the lower back, resulting in complete absence of pain at the operative site. Of the two, epidural is usually preferred because it allows movement of the legs as opposed to the complete paralysis produced by the spinal. In addition, epidural anesthesia doesn't cause the sometimes excruciating postoperative headache that may follow a spinal anesthetic. The only disadvantage of the epidural is that it is more difficult to administer, and not all anesthesiologists have the experience and the delicate touch needed to achieve consistent success with it. In the last few years, "dissociative anesthesia" has also gained in popularity (see chapter 7).

Many doctors prefer their patients' lower bowels to be empty prior to surgery, and routinely order a preoperative enema. Although this is rarely if ever necessary, old customs die slowly. Catheterization of the urinary bladder immediately before surgery allows better visualization of the uterus, which lies behind it. However, the introduction of a catheter increases the risk of a postoperative urinary tract infection. Catheterization can usually be avoided if a woman completely empties her bladder immediately before entering the operating room.

ABDOMINAL TUBAL LIGATION

How is an abdominal tubal ligation performed?

When abdominal tubal ligation is performed within two days following childbirth, a one-inch skin incision is usually made just below or through the lower border of the umbilicus, or navel. This is the level at which the top of the enlarged uterus is located. The resulting scar will be hardly noticeable.

For interval abdominal tubal ligation (not performed soon after childbirth), the skin incision is usually longer and is located in a lower position on the abdomen, just below the upper part of the pubic hairline. The incision may be vertical or horizontal.

After the abdominal cavity is entered, as many as a hundred different methods may be used to tie the tubes. Most methods of tubal ligation are named after the physicians who devised them. The easiest and most popular is the Pomeroy technique, in which a loop of tube the size of a knuckle is elevated and a catgut suture is tied below the loop (figure 9-2).

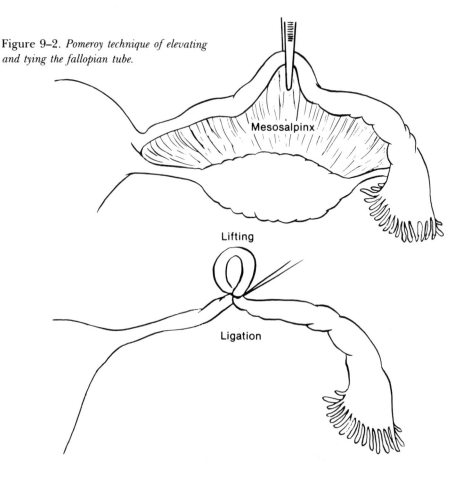

Figure 9–2. *Pomeroy technique of elevating and tying the fallopian tube.*

Mesosalpinx

Lifting

Ligation

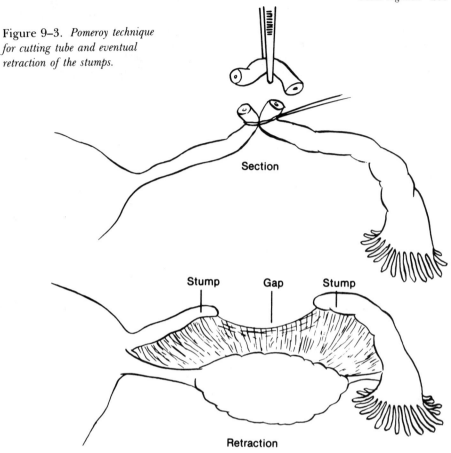

Figure 9–3. *Pomeroy technique for cutting tube and eventual retraction of the stumps.*

Section

Stump   Gap   Stump

Retraction

The loop of tube is then cut off, and by the time the catgut is absorbed several weeks later, the tube stumps will have retracted, leaving between them a scarred gap (figure 9-3). The subsequent pregnancy rate with the Pomeroy technique is 0.3 percent.

Variations used by other doctors have included excision (removal) of the middle portion of the tube, use of different suture material (such as silk), and either excision or suture of the fimbria, which are necessary for picking up the egg as it passes from the ovary (see fimbria).

Several investigators have demonstrated higher subsequent pregnancy rates when tubal ligation is performed at the time of cesarean section or immediately postpartum.

What are the disadvantages of abdominal tubal ligation?

The complication rate following abdominal tubal ligation is 2 to 4 percent, mostly problems such as superficial inflammation of the incision and urinary tract infections caused by bladder catheterization, which precedes the surgery.

Fatal pulmonary embolus (see chapter 2) may occur following any abdominal operation, with a death rate reported at approximately 1 per 100,000 hospital operations. Though this tragic complication is less likely in a young, healthy woman undergoing tubal ligation, it must still be considered a real threat.

Abdominal tubal ligations are usually performed under general anesthesia, so an additional risk is automatically incurred (see general anesthesia, page 225). Hemorrhage from the blood vessels in the *mesosalpinx* (see figure 9-2), undetected at the time of surgery, is a rare cause of postoperative death. Adding all these factors together, the total mortality rate for women undergoing abdominal tubal ligation has been estimated at between 10 and 25 per 100,000 operations performed.

On the practical side, other disadvantages are that the hospital stay following interval abdominal sterilization averages five to six days, at a cost of more than $2,000, and the recovery time following surgery averages six weeks.

What are the advantages and disadvantages of postpartum abdominal sterilization? -

Postpartum abdominal tubal ligation is not as costly as interval sterilization. The incision is smaller and is usually less painful, and the surgery is easier than interval tubal ligation and may even be performed with less difficulty under local anesthesia, though most doctors still prefer general anesthesia. When it is performed immediately after delivery or on the following day, a woman can return home two to four days later. This lengthens her total postpartum hospitalization time an average of only two days.

One disadvantage of immediate postpartum sterilization is that occasionally a congenital or acquired disease or infection is not recognized in the newborn during the first twenty-four hours of life. It is not unusual for a previously healthy baby suddenly to become ill. In some cases, it may turn out that irreversible sterilization has been performed prematurely.

A woman may believe that she wants sterilization following a difficult nine months of pregnancy and a long and grueling labor and delivery, only to regret the decision later. In one study, a significant number of women who requested postpartum sterilization, but had surgery delayed for various reasons, declined to undergo the operation when given the opportunity at a later date.

Finally, pregnancy rates following postpartum abdominal tubal ligation are significantly higher than when the procedure is performed in the interval between pregnancies.

What is a "minilap"?

A "minilap," or *minilaparotomy,* is a relatively new method of interval abdominal tubal ligation. It is gaining great popularity in the United States, as well as in other countries throughout the world. In this procedure, an instrument is inserted through the cervix and into the uterine cavity in order to push the uterus up against the lower abdominal wall. A one-inch skin incision is then made directly over the top of the elevated uterus at a point just above the pubic bone. The tubes are then brought up into the operative field and are either tied, cut, coagulated, clipped, or banded (see Figure 9-4).

A special retractor, resembling a small vaginal speculum, may be inserted through the incision to aid in visualizing both fallopian tubes (figure 9-5).

Though sufficient data has not been accumulated on minilaps, one great advantage is that they may be performed under local, spinal, epidural, dissociative, or general anesthesia as outpatient procedures, so patients can go home several hours later. Because the minilap does not require elaborate surgical equipment, it has been used to great advantage in indigent countries such as India and Thailand, where it is routinely performed by trained technicians rather than doctors. The necessary instruments for minilaparotomy cost about $400.00 and need no extraordinary maintenance. For laparoscopy (see page 214), equipment costs run at least $4,500 and more elaborate maintenance is required. Failure rates as evidenced by subsequent pregnancy have been reported as between 1 to 4 cases per 1,000 operations.

In 1982, the World Health Organization Task Force on female sterilization compared the results of sterilization with 800 minilaparotomies and an equal number of laparoscopic procedures. Major complications occurred at a rate of 1.5 percent in the former group and 0.9 percent in the latter. Minor complaints and minor complications were also slightly more frequent among women undergoing minilap. When thousands

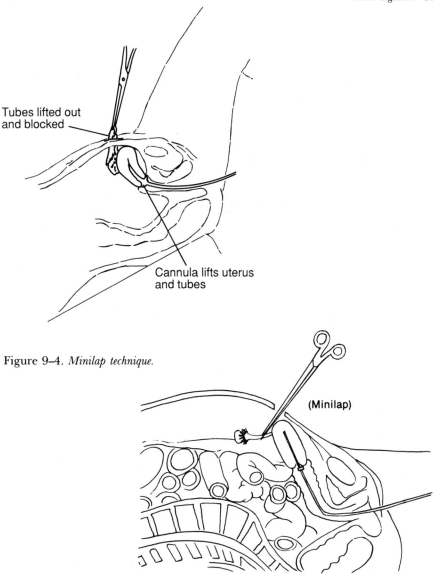

Tubes lifted out
and blocked

Cannula lifts uterus
and tubes

Figure 9–4. *Minilap technique.*

(Minilap)

of Falope ring laparoscopies (see page 224) were compared with Falope ring minilaps in a 1981 study, doctors found that more surgical difficulties were encountered with the minilap, but the total number of complications and the severity of complications were greater in the laparoscopy group.

One potential disadvantage of minilap surgery is perforation of the uterus with the elevating instrument. In a 1986 review of almost 5,000 women undergoing minilaparotomy, uterine perforation occurred at a rate of 2.1 per 1,000 procedures. Difficulties may also be encountered with obese women, and the possibility of intestinal or bladder injury is always present if either of these organs happens to lie between the skin and the top of the uterus when the incision is made. In studies to date, total complication rates with minilap have ranged between 0.4 and 1.5 percent. Chronic pelvic infection, endometriosis, and previous extensive intestinal or urinary bladder surgery appear to be contraindications to using a minilap.

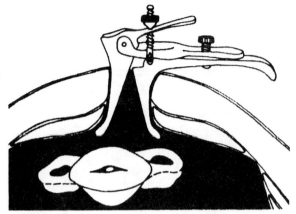

Figure 9–5. *Special retractor for minilap*

What is laparoscopy?

A laparoscope is an instrument with a diameter slightly larger than a pencil. It contains a powerful light source, which, when inserted through the navel, allows visualization of the abdominal and pelvic contents. The injection of two or more liters of carbon dioxide or nitrous oxide gas into the abdomen will move the intestine out of the lower pelvis, making it easier for the physician to view the pelvic organs. Specially designed instruments can then be passed through the laparoscope to accomplish such procedures as tubal sterilization; biopsy of the ovary, liver, or intestinal wall; removal of misplaced IUDs; diagnosis and treatment of ectopic pregnancy; and evaluation and treatment of infertility, pelvic pain, and endometriosis (see chapter 2).

When the laparoscopic procedure is completed, the carbon dioxide is removed from the abdomen and the tiny incision in the navel is closed with one absorbable suture. The suture is then covered with a Band-Aid, hence its nickname "Band-Aid surgery." Another synonym for laparoscopy is "belly-button surgery."

Though newspaper and television coverage of laparoscopic surgery during the past fifteen years has been spectacular, few people realize that the first laparoscopy was actually performed in 1806, by Philip Brozzini. His light source was a candle and his laparoscope was a urological cystoscope. Throughout the years others have attempted laparoscopy, but only the recent refinement of the optical equipment and fiberoptic light source have allowed its popular use today.

How does laparoscopy compare with other methods of tubal sterilization?

Compared with all other forms of tubal sterilization, laparoscopy's total complication rates of under 3 percent are unmatched. Based on the latest statistics, major complications following laparoscopic sterilization will occur at a rate of 1.8 per 1,000 cases performed, with deaths reported at 2 per 100,000 operations. In addition, the pregnancy rate following laparoscopy is less than 1 per 1,000 women. Postoperative hospitalization is usually less one day, and total recovery time ranges from 0 to 5 days. Hospital costs are thus at least one-third less than for traditional abdominal tubal ligation.

What are the details of the laparoscopic sterilization procedure?

Often doctors simply don't take the time to explain the details of laparoscopic procedures to their patients. Consequently, you may be uninformed about and unprepared for some of the events that take place before, during, and after surgery. This may be particularly upsetting for those women having laparoscopy performed under local anesthesia.

As with all abdominal surgical techniques, eating and drinking are prohibited for eight hours prior to laparoscopy. Intramuscular medication is given one hour before surgery, usually a tranquilizer, perhaps in combination with atropine. The latter drug is used to dry up excessive secretions in the mouth and throat which could cause breathing problems when general anesthesia is used. Atropine is also given to women who are having local anesthesia, so that in an emergency the anesthesiologist can switch to general anesthesia without delay. In many centers, however, doctors find that atropine is not necessary for safe and effective anesthesia.

Some doctors instruct their patients to take an enema at home, and others have one administered to their patients in the hospital prior to surgery. Personally, I have found no difference in the degree of surgical difficulty between women who have had an enema and those who have not. Another point of minor controversy is whether to empty the urinary bladder with a rubber catheter immediately prior to surgery. An empty bladder is essential for adequate visualization of the uterus, but many doctors believe it can be achieved simply by instructing the patient to urinate immediately prior to the operation. A good laparoscopist should easily complete the procedure long before the bladder fills with urine again. For women with a history of recurrent urinary tract infections, avoiding catheter use prevents the reintroduction of potentially infectious bacteria into the bladder.

The position you assume on the operating table is similar to that of a vaginal examination, except that your legs rest in stirrups that are far more comfortable than those found in most doctors' offices. The table is tilted at an angle so that your head is lower than the rest of your body. Your abdomen, especially the navel, is thoroughly cleansed with an antiseptic solution.

An instrument is then attached to the cervix which, when moved in different directions during laparoscopy, allows the surgeon to see the uterus, tubes, and ovaries. Though several instruments have been devised for this purpose, the Semm cannula, which creates a suction cup on the cervix, appears to be the safest and least likely to traumatize the cervix or to perforate the uterus (see figure 9-6). The Hulka tenaculum and HUMI device are also popular cannulas with some doctors. Unexplained light vaginal bleeding following laparoscopy is almost always due to the use of the cervical cannula and shouldn't alarm you.

The next step is the injection of Nesacaine or Xylocaine, if local anesthesia is used. Liberal amounts are injected around the skin of the navel and the underlying tissues. The first prick of the needle will usually hurt, but you will not feel the subsequent ones. If general anesthesia is preferred, an intravenous barbiturate rapidly puts you

Figure 9–6. *Semm cannula.*

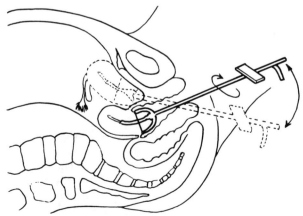

to sleep, and then the anesthesiologist administers a light anesthetic gas by mask. For maximum safety, a flexible plastic tube must be inserted into the trachea (windpipe) after sleep is induced, in order to allow the anesthesiologist to control your respiration. The anesthesiologist can now be totally prepared to handle any heart or respiratory irregularities, which have in rare instances been reported when the abdomen is filled with the carbon dioxide gas. Because of this possibility, it is imperative to have an anesthesiologist standing nearby even when laparoscopy is performed under local anesthesia.

You may experience a slight sore throat postoperatively when general anesthesia is given. This is due to the irritation of the tube placed in the trachea, and it usually subsides within two days. Though there are several reports in the medical literature claiming success with the use of epidural and spinal anesthesia for laparoscopic surgical procedures, the majority of physicians have rejected these methods because of the fear that a woman may be unable to breathe and expand her lungs adequately once the gas is injected into her abdominal cavity.

Once the anesthesia has taken effect, a tiny incision is made at the lower border of the navel. Through it, a long, thin needle, called a Verres, is inserted into the abdominal cavity while the skin is elevated with pinpoint-ended instruments called towel clips. Elevating the skin in this manner prevents the Verres needle from injuring the intestine. The two towel clips will temporarily leave four tiny holes around the navel following laparoscopy. Some doctors report equally good results by elevating the skin of the abdominal wall with their hands, thereby avoiding the towel clip marks.

The Verres needle is then attached to a tube, which in turn is connected to a machine containing either carbon dioxide or nitrous oxide. The gas is then run through the tubing and into the abdomen at a rate of one liter per minute. As the abdomen fills with gas, it becomes firm and tense and will actually sound like a drum if tapped. For a woman of average build, one and one-half to two liters is usually all that is required. A third liter might be needed for an obese woman. If you are awake during laparoscopy, you are likely to experience mild to moderate discomfort and bloating as the gas fills the abdomen. In rare cases, the abdominal discomfort may be bothersome.

Following the injection of the gas, a large, sharp metal instrument called a trocar, encased in an electrically nonconductive sleeve, is inserted through the umbilicus and into the abdominal cavity. Its successful placement will be confirmed by an audible rush of the previously injected gas when the trocar is removed and the sleeve is left in the abdominal cavity.

The laparoscope, which contains an electrocoagulating forceps, is then inserted through the sleeve. The light source is attached to the laparoscope, as is the tubing, which provides a constant flow of carbon dioxide or nitrous oxide from the machine (figure 9-7).

Many doctors prefer the older, two-incision technique in which the second incision is made in the lower abdomen with a smaller trocar and sleeve. The electrocoagulator is then inserted through the second incision (figure 9-8).

If the two-incision technique is used with local anesthesia, Xylocaine or Nesacaine must first be injected into the second site. Even with adequate local anesthesia, the second incision is often responsible for more discomfort than the first. The majority of doctors in the United States prefer the single-incision technique.

The fallopian tube is then grasped with the coagulation forceps. After the surgeon makes sure that no piece of intestine is near enough to the tube to be in danger of accidentally burning, she or he presses a foot pedal which activates an electrical current from the bipolar cautery machine. The current passes through the coagulation forceps and to the fallopian tube. Repeated short bursts of electricity, initiated with each push of the foot pedal, cause the tube to burn and to turn white. A small number of doctors still use the unipolar cautery device in which the current passes through

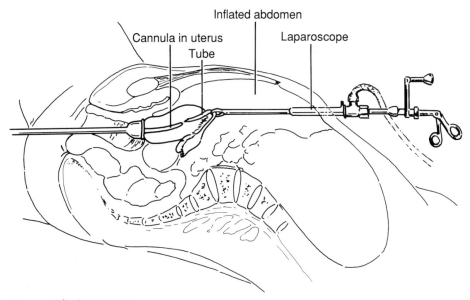

Figure 9–7. *Laparoscopy.*

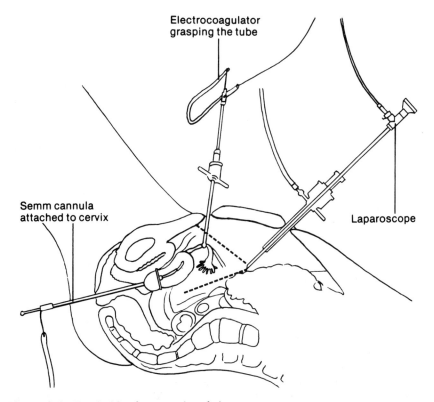

Figure 9–8. *Two-incision laparoscopic technique.*

a ground plate which would be placed on your thigh prior to surgery. This technique is far more dangerous and is not recommended.

Most doctors prefer to burn the tubes at the utero-tubal junction, or the point where they join the uterus. Others prefer the midpoint of the tube. Some preliminary data suggest that subsequent pregnancy rates will be lowest if the tube is coagulated at least 4 centimeters from the point at which it enters the uterus. Regardless of which location is chosen, best results are obtained by burning at three adjacent locations along the tube—the "three-burn technique." Though a minority of doctors still believe that breaking the tube or removing a segment of it through the laparoscope will further reduce the risk of future pregnancy, just the opposite is true. In fact, the more the tube is destroyed after it has coagulated, the greater will be the risk of subsequent intrauterine and ectopic pregnancy. This is because the breakage or removal of a segment of the tube often creates a fistula, or opening, in the separated ends. Sperm can then pass from the uterus to the tube and out into the abdominal cavity. Amazingly, sperm do find their way into the fimbria, or outer fingerlike projections, at the end of the tube where the recently ovulated egg is situated. Fertilization of the egg in this "distal" segment of the tube often leads to ectopic pregnancy.

After the tubes are coagulated, the surgeon checks that there is no bleeding from the arteries or veins in the mesosalpinx (see page 219). He or she then releases as much gas as possible from the abdomen by opening a valve on the sleeve and manually compressing the abdomen. The instruments are removed, and the incision or incisions are closed with a chromic catgut absorbable suture and covered with one or two Band-Aids.

Regardless of the type of anesthesia used, nearly all women can leave the hospital within eight hours. The Band-Aid may be removed the next day. Occasionally, there will be a slight tenderness, redness, or leakage of fluid from the incision. Hot water soaks applied three times a day almost always clear up this minor infection.

What are the potential complications of laparoscopic sterilization?

Nearly all the complications associated with the procedure can be avoided if the anesthesiologist and the surgeon are skilled, experienced, and conscientious individuals. A doctor with inadequate training, or one who performs laparoscopy only on rare occasions, will never develop the facility for the procedure. Statistically, surgeons who perform fewer than 100 cases a year have a complication rate four times greater than more experienced surgeons. For the best possible results, one also needs optimum surgical conditions: the best equipment and experienced nursing personnel.

Drs. Franklin D. Loffer and David Pent, in their excellent review of over 32,000 laparoscopies, have analyzed possible complications of the operation in detail. The most common complication that they noted was cardiac irregularity resulting from the injection of gas into the abdomen. A total of 242 women, or 7.4 per 1,000 laparoscopies, had variations of this problem. Of this group, 85 women experienced changes in their pulse rate, 50 had alterations in their blood pressure, and 10 suffered cardiac arrest. Three of the 10 women died. All of these complications occurred more often with carbon dioxide than with nitrous oxide and are believed to be due to excessive amounts of the gas accumulating within the body and not being eliminated by the usual mechanism of rapid breathing.

Cardiac arrest caused by carbon dioxide accumulation can be prevented if a doctor takes some very simple precautions. The first is not to instill excessive amounts of carbon dioxide into the abdomen. Two liters is usually sufficient, and anything more than three liters is excessive. Second, all patients should have their heartbeats monitored by the anesthesiologist throughout the procedure. This is an indispensable way of detecting early pulse irregularities, which occur long before cardiac arrest. It is interesting to note that in one survey of gynecologists performing laparoscopy, cardiac monitors were present in 91 percent of the operating rooms but a shocking 29 percent of these doctors did not make use of the monitor.

When an irregularity of the pulse is noted in a patient under general anesthesia, the anesthesiologist can usually correct the problem by increasing the respiratory rate, thus enabling the patient to breathe off the excessive amounts of carbon dioxide. The laparoscopist can also help by releasing some of the carbon dioxide from the abdomen. In a 1983 report from the Centers for Disease Control, doctors found that six of the eleven anesthetic deaths associated with laparoscopic sterilization between 1977 and 1981 were the result of lack of adequate ventilation. In all cases, the anesthesiologist had failed to insert prior to the sterilization an endotracheal tube to facilitate carbon dioxide release and oxygen intake.

A fairly common and usually harmless complication may occur when the Verres needle is not placed correctly. If it lies above, rather than in, the abdominal cavity, the carbon dioxide may accidentally enter the area above the abdomen. This problem is more likely to happen in obese women, and can be corrected simply by removing the needle and waiting a few minutes for the gas to be absorbed before trying again.

Very rarely, even with the needle in the correct location, the gas may dissect from the abdominal cavity into the chest cavity near the heart, resulting in an acute emergency. Gas may find its way to the outside of the lung, causing it to collapse. Even rarer is the inadvertent injection of gas into a blood vessel. The gas may then be carried to the heart and lung as an embolus (see page 211), causing instant death. If your doctor adheres to the simple precautions, the likelihood of serious complications will be remote.

What is the incidence of bleeding complications?

Bleeding from a blood vessel in the mesosalpinx is the most common bleeding complication of laparoscopic sterilization. In most cases, it is easily treated by coagulating the bleeding site. Uncontrollable mesosalpinx bleeding requiring exploratory surgery occurs in approximately 2 out of every 1,000 women undergoing laparoscopy. This number can be further reduced if doctors coagulate the tubes without trying to separate or break them.

Bleeding from the navel rarely occurs and is never a serious complication. It is easily controlled with a pressure bandage or a single suture. Fatal or near-fatal bleeding, due to perforation of a major blood vessel with a trocar or Verres needle, is fortunately very rare. Case studies show that this complication is far more likely to occur when the procedure is performed by an inexperienced surgeon.

Can the trocar ever cause perforation of the stomach or intestine?

Perforation may occur with both the Verres needle and the large trocar. Dr. Franklin D. Loffer and Dr. David Pent report that it happens less than 3 times per 1,000 operations. The stomach is usually the most common site of injury, followed by the large and then the small intestine. Perforation of the stomach may occur when it is distended with swallowed air, or filled with gas breathed into it by the anesthesiologist when a tracheal tube is not inserted beforehand.

If the Verres needle perforates the stomach, and carbon dioxide or nitrous oxide is then injected, the elevated pressures on the gas gauge should arouse the doctor's suspicions that the needle is incorrectly placed. Often the anesthesiologist notes that the patient is passing tremendous amounts of gas out through her mouth. If perforation is suspected, the Verres needle should be removed and the procedure attempted again with a new sterile needle. Often the anesthesiologist can help by first emptying the stomach and intestine of gas with a stomach tube.

A hole created in the stomach or intestine with a Verres needle will usually seal itself off and need not be sutured. When the larger trocar accidentally perforates, however, exploratory surgery is mandatory because a hole that size is far too big to close by itself. It is a good idea for the doctor to leave the trocar in place rather than remove it prior to surgery. In this way, she or he can readily identify the exact perforation site as well as the extent of the damage.

Is there any way to avoid needle and trocar injuries associated with laparoscopy?

"Open" laparoscopy uses all of the usual laparoscopy equipment with the exception of the Verres needle and the sharp trocar. Instead, the abdominal cavity is opened under direct visualization with a scalpel or a specially designed, blunt Hasson cannula, named after its designer (figure 9-9).

Purportedly, the main advantage of open laparoscopy over the conventional closed or "blind" technique is the elimination of the risk of injury to the intestine and major blood vessels. This is especially advantageous for women with a history of previous abdominal surgery, pelvic infections, or adhesions, who are at greater risk of injuring an adherent loop of bowel with a sharp trocar or Verres needle. Another advantage of open laparoscopy over the standard closed technique is that the carbon dioxide runs directly into the abdominal cavity through the Hasson cannula, eliminating the risk of its being accidentally injected into the subcutaneous tissues and muscles of the abdominal wall as occasionally happens with the Verres needle and the closed technique.

While proponents of open laparoscopy claim that there is little justification for continuing to use the more hazardous closed technique, their view is not supported by the available scientific data. Though open laparoscopy sounds ideal, it does have its distinct drawbacks. For example, the incision used is at least 2 centimeters (1 inch) long, and in obese women it often has to be extended to twice that length. Because of the larger incision, carbon dioxide gas is more likely to leak out of the abdominal cavity, thereby making visualization more difficult. The larger incision also increases the risk of wound infection. And, unlike closed laparoscopy, open laparoscopy requires an assistant surgeon and a longer operating time, thereby raising the cost of the surgery.

Despite proponents of open laparoscopy's elimination of intestinal injuries, data collected to date shows that it does not have this advantage. In a 1984 survey of over 10,000 open laparoscopies, doctors reported six cases of bowel laceration and eighteen instances of wound infection. In one of the few studies of its kind, Pouru P. Bhiwandivala, M.D., and her associates at Family Health International presented a comparison on the safety of open versus closed laparoscopy sterilization in their 1985 report. Among the 14,000 women studied, surgical difficulties were encountered in 2.9 percent of the open laparoscopies and 2.1 percent of the closed procedures, while surgical complication rates were equal in the two groups. Based on these findings, most gynecologists rightfully believe that there is no compelling need at the present time to abandon standard laparoscopic sterilization for the theoretical and still unproven advantages of a new technique.

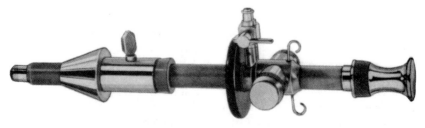

Figure 9–9. *Hasson cannula for open laparoscopy.*

How common are accidental electrical burns during laparoscopic sterilization, and how can their incidence be reduced?

Unipolar instruments burn the fallopian tubes by applying a powerful high-voltage electric current which passes from the operating instruments to the forceps that grasp the fallopian tube (figure 9-10). The current coagulates the tube and must then travel and exit through the patient's body via a ground plate attached to the thigh. The obvious danger of this system is that it makes the patient an integral part of the electrical circuit. Consequently, use of unipolar electrocoagulation has resulted in over 200 cases of serious burn injuries to the bowel as well as in several deaths. Burns resulting from unipolar cauterization usually damage either the skin of the abdomen or the lining of the small or large intestine. A high percentage of intestinal burns has been noted with the single-incision technique, while burns of the skin occur almost exclusively with the two-incision unipolar method. A doctor who performs unipolar sterilization is not immune from injury, and serious burns of the hands, nose, and eyes have been reported among laparoscopists.

Drs. Jacques-E. Rioux and Diogène Cloutier of Quebec devised a safer coagulation system, named bipolar cautery (figure 9-11). With this method, the current travels from one prong of the coagulating forceps to the other, and the only tissue destroyed is that which lies between the two prongs. Since the current does not pass through the patient's body, a ground plate is not required. With bipolar electrocautery, the risk of a spark causing injury to surrounding tissue is entirely eliminated.

In some bipolar models the control switch is in the handle of the forceps, and in others it is in a foot pedal. The amount of current needed to achieve coagulation is only a fraction of what the old-fashioned unipolar method needs, and therefore the bipolar cautery is a safe device. At the present time, bipolar cautery is available for both the one- and the two-incision laparoscopes. I know of only one case in the medical literature in which a bowel burn occurred with the use of a bipolar cautery. But believe it or not, there are still many doctors in the United States who are using the more hazardous unipolar method. If your doctor still uses this technique, it might be time to find another doctor.

In every operating room one nurse or instrument technician must be assigned the important function of maintaining the electrical cauterization and laparoscopy equipment in excellent working condition. A burn caused by worn-out or faulty equipment is inexcusable.

Dr. Clifford Wheeless of Johns Hopkins University Medical School noted in his 1973 study no increased incidence of intestinal injury with local anesthesia, but many doctors believe that a woman's slightest movement at the time of tubal coagulation may increase her chances of such an injury. Aside from careful choice of the anesthetic to be used, the best way to prevent burn injury is to retain an experienced and skilled laparoscopist.

Skin burns are usually noted immediately at the time of surgery. Most burns of the intestine, however, are not detected until symptoms of bowel perforation appear, which may take anywhere from eighteen hours to fourteen days. Early symptoms are vague lower abdominal pain and a low-grade fever, often misdiagnosed as tubal infection. Treatment consists of exploratory surgery and the removal of the damaged segment of intestine. The one common thread linking deaths associated with inadvertent bowel injuries is physician delay in diagnosing and appreciating the severity of symptoms suggesting bowel perforation.

Dr. Barbara S. Levy and her associates at the Mason Clinic in Seattle, Washington, dispute the currently held opinion concerning the dangers of unipolar sterilization. In their research, published in 1985 in *The Journal of Reproductive Medicine,* they created simulated bowel injuries to the intestines of rabbits, using unipolar cautery, bipolar cautery, Verres needle, or laparoscopic trocar. Microscopic analysis of the damaged

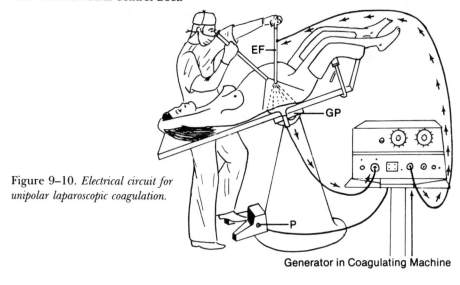

Figure 9–10. *Electrical circuit for unipolar laparoscopic coagulation.*

Generator in Coagulating Machine

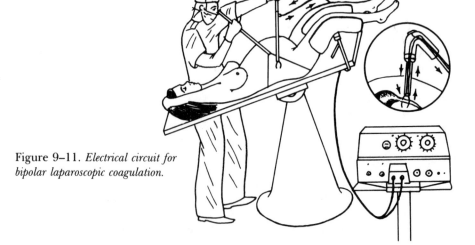

Figure 9–11. *Electrical circuit for bipolar laparoscopic coagulation.*

tissues twenty-four to ninety-six hours later led these investigators to believe that burn and trocar injuries to the bowel each have their own distinct microscopic appearance, and that many reports of intestinal injuries attributed to unipolar electrocoagulation were probably caused by the laparoscopic trocar and not the cautery. In conclusion they stated that "unipolar techniques with appropriate low-voltage generators should be reconsidered as acceptable methods of female sterilization."

Are there any other methods for safe cauterization of the tubes?

Dr. Kurt Semm, a German physician, has devised a laparoscope that uses an electric current from a low-voltage battery to heat forceps at the end of the laparoscope. This so-called thermocoagulation method "cooks" the tube without any of the dangers associated with unipolar electrocoagulation. The great safety feature of thermocoagulation is that the current is reduced markedly after it exits from the standard wall outlet. The apparatus requires only 4 to 5 volts to produce the desired effect.

The newer, more sophisticated thermocoagulation generators are automated, allowing preselection of temperature as well as of length of time the current is to be applied. Included in these devices are ingenious signals, so that the surgeon hears different sounds as the tissue in the tube is heated or cooled. The surgeon will thus know immediately if the tissue is getting too much heat for too long.

Based on the principles described by Dr. Semm, doctors in California have developed a thermocoagulation device containing a small metallic hook heated by a current produced by a battery. The fallopian tube is grasped with the hook and pulled into a protective sheath which provides insulation to surrounding structures. Following isolation of the tube in this fashion, the hook coagulates and cuts it with a minimal amount of tissue damage. One drawback of this device is that the sectioned ends of the tube remain in close proximity, and the complete and spontaneous *reanastomosis,* or rejoining between the two sectioned ends of the tube, has been reported to occur.

While electrocoagulation appears to be far less dangerous than unipolar electrocoagulation, it has not been proven superior to the bipolar device. As a result, American gynecologists are not rushing to trade in their expensive bipolar instruments for thermocoagulation (see chapter 11, "The Future").

Is there a laparoscope that can avoid all hazards of heat injury?

In 1974, Dr. In Bae Yoon of Johns Hopkins University introduced the Falope Ring technique of tubal sterilization as a means of eliminating the hazards of electrocoagulation. The Falope Ring is actually a tiny silicone rubber band which is fitted over a special laparoscope. The forceps of this laparoscope grasp a segment of the tube and pull it up. The Falope Ring is then pushed down over the segment of the tube, causing occlusion (see figure 9-12). Sterilization with use of spring clips is another method of avoiding electrocoagulation burns (see page 224).

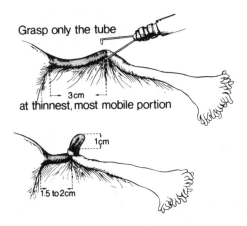

Grasp only the tube

← 3cm →

at thinnest, most mobile portion

1cm

1.5 to 2cm

Ring or Band. A knuckle is formed and a silicone band—similar to a small rubber band—is placed around the base.

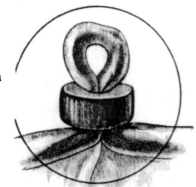

Figure 9–12. *Falope ring technique.*

In addition to eliminating the thermal hazards, the Falope Ring also has the advantage over the electrocoagulator of destroying less tubal tissue. For women who decide at a later date to have more children, there is no doubt that this method has a greater reversibility rate than electrocoagulation.

Many women erroneously believe that Falope Ring sterilization is definitely reversible. Never undergo the operation under this false assumption.

Are there any complications of Falope Ring surgery?

Three complications appear to be directly related to the procedure. One is that 15 to 20 percent of women report a significant degree of lower abdominal cramping for twenty-four to forty-eight hours after the operation, a rare complaint following cauterization. In one large comparison study, Falope Ring patients were about four times more likely than electrocoagulation patients to report postoperative pelvic or abdominal pain. When compared to the Hulka clip sterilization procedure (see following question), pelvic pain is significantly greater with the Falope Ring. The cramping is probably due to the cutting off of the blood supply at the site of the Ring and can be reduced if your doctor dips each Falope Ring in an anesthetic such as Xylocaine (lidocaine) before putting it on the tubes. Another technique is to inject a local anesthetic directly into the occluded loop of the fallopian tube following the ring application.

Another more serious problem related to the technique is bleeding in the mesosalpinx if the doctor inadvertently cuts the tube while trying to pull it up with the forceps. There have been occasions when the tube has been pulled free from the mesosalpinx while the surgeon was trying to slide the Falope Ring into the correct position. Bleeding from such an accident can be serious but can usually be controlled with cauterization—ironically, the one method that users of the Falope Ring are trying to avoid. To date, the frequency of these complications has not been determined, but in one large study conducted by the American Association of Gynecologic Laparoscopists, the incidence of hemorrhage was 24 women per 1,000 sterilizations. Of these, 5 required exploratory surgery to control the bleeding. Comparison figures noted with standard tubal ligation in this study were 4 per 1,000 for tubal hemorrhage, of which only 0.5 necessitated exploratory surgery.

Though subsequent uterine pregnancy does not appear to be a serious complication following Falope Ring sterilization, it has been noted that the incidence of ectopic pregnancy in the fallopian tube (see page 226) may be significantly higher than with other tubal sterilization methods. The incidence of this potentially serious complication among women undergoing Falope Ring surgery has been reported at 2.3 per 1,000.

Though the Falope Ring was introduced only in 1974, it has gained great popularity in the United States, presently accounting for approximately 24 percent of laparoscopic sterilizations.

How successful is the use of plastic clips for tubal occlusion?

Jaroslav F. Hulka, M.D., of the University of North Carolina, first introduced his spring-loaded clip in 1973. Since then it has been redesigned and improved for use with both the one-incision and two-incision laparoscopic techniques (figure 9-13). Several other occlusive clips have been designed, but the Hulka spring-loaded clip remains the most popular. However, because of poor publicity associated with high pregnancy rates using the early defective prototypes of this device, it is currently used in only 3 percent of tubal sterilization procedures performed in the United States. This is unfortunate in view of the fact that the clip causes less tubal damage than cauterization, increasing a woman's chances of success if future reversal surgery is desired. In one comparative study of 103 Hulka clip sterilizations and 97 Falope Ring

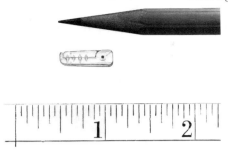

Figure 9–13. *Hulka clip.*

procedures, there was less operative bleeding and pain associated with the clip. In another study, however, in which 108 women received a Hulka clip on one tube and a Falope Ring on the other, no differences in pain were noted between the two devices.

What is the chance of postoperative infection following laparoscopy?

Infection following laparoscopy is extremely rare, affecting only 0.4 to 1.4 of every 1,000 women. Most often it is only a minor inflammation at the navel where the suture was placed. Successful treatment consists of hot, wet compresses applied three times a day. Occasionally, antibiotics are also necessary.

Pelvic infections are even rarer and usually occur as a flare-up of an old infection already present in the tubes at the time of laparoscopy. Many doctors prescribe postoperative antibiotics to those women who have evidence of chronic pelvic inflammation.

Is local or general anesthesia preferred for laparoscopic sterilization?

Though the number of doctors using local anesthesia has increased slightly over the past few years, at least 90 percent of all laparoscopic sterilizations are still performed under general anesthesia. Some doctors have reported success with epidural, spinal, and dissociative anesthesia as well, as previously mentioned, but these methods have not been endorsed by the majority of experts in this field (see page 214, anesthesia).

The reason why most doctors prefer general anesthesia is that in the event of a rare cardiac or respiratory catastrophe, respiration can be more easily controlled when an endotracheal tube is already in place. Second, there will be no delay if emergency surgery is needed because of a problem such as hemorrhge. Many doctors fear that a woman may move when the fallopian tubes are grasped and coagulated under local anesthesia, endangering the procedure. Another advantage of general anesthesia—rarely mentioned by doctors, including myself—is that the doctor avoids the possibility of a distracting conversation with an inquisitive or apprehensive patient while the laparoscopy is being performed.

The one definite advantage of local anesthesia is the avoidance of the rare but definite risk of death that may be encountered with general anesthesia (see chapter 7).

How often does a doctor's attempt at laparoscopic sterilization fail?

For a variety of reasons, a doctor may be unable to accomplish the operation successfully in 2 to 3 cases per 1,000. According to a 1986 review, if a woman has had previous abdominal surgery the chances of failure may be as high as 1 in 100. The failed-laparoscopy rate depends primarily on the skill of the doctor in addition to the presence or absence of conditions such as infection, endometriosis, extreme obesity, and adhesions secondary to previous surgery, any of which may prevent safe visualization and isolation of the tubes for coagulation. If there is even the slightest risk of an intestinal burn, the procedure should be abandoned.

Though the likelihood of failure is minimal, you and your doctor must fully agree beforehand on the course of action to be taken in the event that it becomes a reality. Some women may want the doctor to proceed with the standard abdominal tubal ligation, but others may elect not to undergo so formidable an operation, requiring several days of hospitalization and discomfort as well as added expense.

How common is pregnancy following tubal ligation?

Regardless of the method used, there is always the possibility of pregnancy weeks or even years later, and it may occur after anywhere from 0.1 to 3 percent of all sterilization procedures. Any future pregnancy has a significant risk of being ectopic (see page 224). It is interesting to note that the techniques that destroy a larger section of tube, such as coagulation or burning, lead to higher ectopic pregnancy rates. The reason is that these procedures leave fistulas, or openings, from the uterus to the abdominal cavity through which sperm can find their way to the end of the tube and fertilize an egg.

Preliminary data suggest that fistula formation is less likely to occur if the tube is cauterized at least 4 centimeters from the point where it enters the uterus. In addition, it is best that your doctor not break, separate, or remove a segment from the tube after it has been cauterized. This will only increase the risk of fistula formation (see page 214, laparoscopic technique). In general, fistula formation and accidental pregnancy take at least two years to develop. In contrast, you can bet that a pregnancy occurring within three months of sterilization is the result of a doctor's inadequate attempt at occluding the tubes at the time of surgery.

Most mechanical methods of sterilization, such as tying of the tubes, elastic rings, and plastic spring clips, are associated with remarkably low ectopic pregnancy rates but with higher numbers of intrauterine pregnancies. Statistics suggest that if pregnancy does occur following the standard tying or ligation of the tubes, it is seven times more likely to be an ectopic pregnancy if the procedure was performed abdominally rather than vaginally (see page 229, vaginal tubal ligation). In a 1981 survey, almost 50 percent of total pregnancies following laparoscopic coagulation were ectopic, compared with only 15 percent with Falope Rings and 4 percent with Hulka clips. However, the advantage of extremely low ectopic pregnancy rates following sterilization with Hulka clips is offset by greater numbers of intrauterine pregnancies. In one 1981 evaluation of several sterilization techniques, a disproportionately high intrauterine pregnancy rate of 2.3 percent was associated with the use of plastic spring clips, compared with only 0.8 percent with the coagulation method. For this reason, plastic spring clips such as the Hulka clip have not gained great popularity and are currently used by only 3 percent of American gynecologists. In contrast, 72 percent of doctors prefer coagulation, while 24 percent use elastic bands. The effectiveness of some of the newer techniques is not yet completely known since the true pregnancy rates often take years to determine.

How can I determine whether a doctor is a good laparoscopist?

The most accurate sources of information are recommendations from an operating room nurse, a resident in obstetrics and gynecology at that hospital, or an anesthesiologist who works with each of the gynecologists on a daily basis. Unfortunately, not all women are lucky enough to have access to this inside information.

As in the case of selecting a doctor to perform an abortion, certification by the American Board of Obstetrics and Gynecology is no assurance of one's manual dexterity. The certificate does demonstrate a certain amount of interest and determination on the part of the doctor in mastering the academic side of the specialty, though. There are surgeons and family practitioners who perform laparoscopy, but it is wise to find out how often they do it. As with most surgical techniques, the experience of the operator is reflected in the ease with which the procedure is performed. A doctor who has performed several hundred laparoscopies at a rate of two or more a week is far more likely to be proficient than is an occasional operator. As previously noted, it has been demonstrated that surgeons who perform fewer than 100 cases a year have complication rates four times greater than those of more experienced surgeons. The only way to find out is to ask your doctor how much experience he or she has had.

The American Association of Gynecologic Laparoscopists (AAGL) is a medical organization of physicians interested in laparoscopy. Members of AAGL receive periodic reprints of current literature in the area of laparoscopy, including case reports of serious laparoscopic complications, which are discussed at periodic meetings. Though the aims of this organization are admirable, membership is based not on ability but only on the completion of a short application form and a membership check. Following acceptance into AAGL the performance of a member is not monitored, and there is no disciplining of doctors whose performance is less than adequate. Members are given a very impressive diploma, however, which might give a patient the impression that the doctor can do open heart and brain surgery as well.

The Directory of Medical Specialists is available at most local libraries and is a valuable source of information, listing doctors who are Board-certified in all the various medical specialties and also providing the doctor's age, previous medical training, and present hospital affiliations.

Are there any women who should not undergo laparoscopy?

Commonly listed contraindications to laparoscopy include intestinal obstruction, extensive abdominal malignancy or tuberculosis, previous extensive abdominal surgery, cardiac and respiratory disease, marked obesity, and peritonitis (inflammation of the abdominal cavity). With the exception of the first two, the contraindications are relative rather than absolute, depending on the severity of the disease and the expertise of the laparoscopist.

For example, 11 to 33 percent of all women requesting sterilization have had previous abdominal surgery for cesarean section, ovarian cyst, appendectomy, or ectopic pregnancy. Adhesions or scar tissue from such surgery usually should not discourage a doctor from successfully performing laparoscopy. However, if the previous surgery was for a ruptured appendix or extensive intestinal disease, such as advanced ulcerative colitis or regional ileitis, laparoscopy is best avoided.

If you have heart or respiratory disease that doesn't severely limit your activity, you'll usually tolerate laparoscopy well. Obviously, consultation with a cardiologist should precede all such laparoscopies. Personally, I believe that if you have a severe cardiac condition, laparoscopy is just too dangerous because of the potentially harmful effects of carbon dioxide on your heart and because of the restricted ability to breathe with your feet raised higher than your head and your abdomen filled with gas.

Obesity is often listed as a contraindication to laparoscopy, but quite often doctors are pleasantly surprised at the ease with which it may be accomplished on an obese woman. Actually, the total weight is of less significance than the distribution of body fat, and the doctor may encounter more difficulty operating on a 180-pound woman with excess abdominal fat than on a 230-pound woman of the same height whose weight is more evenly distributed. An obese woman may wish to explore the possibility of laparoscopy when considering methods of tubal sterilization. Although massive obesity sometimes makes laparoscopy more difficult to perform, it remains a safe and effective procedure in the hands of a skilled and experienced gynecologist. This was proved in a 1987 report from the Medical University of South Carolina, by Dr. Gary Holtz. He reported the results of fifteen successful laparoscopies performed on women weighing more than 250 pounds. The open technique was favored in eleven of these women, while four underwent the closed method. All operations were performed under general anesthesia with endotracheal intubation, and the only complication reported was one case of an easily treated wound infection.

Several reports from Scandinavia initially confirmed that laparoscopy can be safely performed on women with peritonitis confined to the lower abdomen. This may be helpful in differentiating between acute inflammation of the tubes and appendicitis. The former condition is best treated with antibiotics, and exploratory surgery for a mistaken diagnosis of appendicitis may thus be avoided. When peritonitis is more extensive and involves the upper abdomen, laparoscopy is contraindicated.

Can laparoscopic tubal coagulation be performed instead of traditional abdominal tubal ligation in the days immediately following childbirth?

Despite some impressive statistics from Cook County Hospital in Chicago and several other institutions indicating success with postpartum laparoscopy, most doctors have never performed this operation at that time. Some doctors even claim that it is hazardous. My personal experience with the technique on over 100 postpartum women at Norwalk Hospital in Connecticut has been excellent. There have been no complications, and all patients have experienced significantly less discomfort and a shorter hospitalization than those undergoing the abdominal procedure. There is also the added benefit of no visible scar. One great advantage of the procedure over the abdominal postpartum operation is that it may be performed on the second or third day following delivery rather than immediately after, allowing a woman more time to decide whether she really wants the operation. Furthermore, if the newborn appears healthy at birth but develops serious complications after the first twenty-four hours, a hasty and tragic decision can be averted. With abdominal tubal ligation, both you and your doctor are rushed into performing the surgery immediately following delivery in order to shorten your total hospital stay.

Can laparoscopic sterilization be performed at the time of an abortion?

Several studies have demonstrated that combining these two procedures does not increase the risk over that present when each is done separately. In fact, a 1985 study from the Centers for Disease Control showed that the risk of complications for women having concurrent tubal sterilization and induced abortion is similar to that for women having tubal sterilization alone.

Are there any disadvantages to performing postpartum and postabortal laparoscopic sterilizations?

Women who have either postpartum or postabortal laparoscopic sterilizations are more likely to have a subsequent unplanned pregnancy than are women who are sterilized at other times. This increased risk of pregnancy appears to be unrelated to whether the tubes are coagulated or closed with rings or clips.

In a study published in *The Journal of Reproductive Medicine* in 1981, doctors found an overall pregnancy rate of 6 per 1,000 sterilization procedures among nonpregnant women, compared with 26.4 per 1,000 among postabortal women and 43.5 per 1,000 among postpartum women. Shockingly high pregnancy rates were noted for women sterilized with the Hulka clip: 19 per 1,000 among nonpregnant women; 85.6 per 1,000 among postabortal sterilization; and 135.8 per 1,000 women who underwent the operation during the immediate postpartum period. Comparison figures for the Falope Ring were 4.3, 7.5, and 20.5 per 1,000 procedures, respectively, while electrocoagulation had the best results with 2.7 (nonpregnant), 8.5 (postabortal), and a surprisingly low 4.7 per 1,000 for women sterilized postpartum.

It has been theorized that the main reason for poor results during the postabortal and postpartum periods are that the anatomical changes and greater vascularity of the tubes at these times create more technical difficulties for the surgeon.

Is it necessary to discontinue other methods of birth control prior to laparoscopic sterilization?

Since oral contraceptives increase the concentration of clotting factors in the blood, many doctors recommend that they be discontinued at least four weeks before tubal ligation, or any major surgery, is performed. This is because postoperative bedrest and inactivity combined with greater blood-clotting potential can increase the risk of deep vein thrombosis and pulmonary embolus (see chapter 2). Other doctors claim that this precaution is unnecessary for laparoscopic sterilization, since recovery and ambulation take place within hours of surgery. Furthermore, stopping birth-control pills for a month or more prior to sterilization can leave a woman vulnerable to the threat of pregnancy.

Based on only one limited study, many doctors recommend that IUDs be removed several days prior to laparoscopic sterilization in order to decrease the risk of postoperative tubal infection. My practice has been to remove the IUD while the patient is under anesthesia, just prior to performing the surgery. I have noted no higher incidence of infection, and my patients have been spared the discomfort of having their IUDs removed while they are awake.

How soon after laparoscopic tubal sterilization can I resume intercourse?

Following an uncomplicated laparoscopic sterilization, you may have intercourse the very same day, but chest and shoulder pain may limit your enthusiasm for such activity. The pain is caused by the presence of a small pocket of gas which remains in the abdomen following laparoscopy. It usually dissolves within two days, but can last for six or seven days. When the gas lies under the abdominal diaphragm, it stimulates a nerve that carries pain messages from the diaphragm to the chest and shoulders. This "referred" pain can be bothersome and may limit activity for as long as one week.

In their enthusiasm to "sell" this operation, some gynecologists often minimize the degree of postoperative discomfort. Though I have known patients who have actually played tennis or worked a full eight hours on the day following surgery, such rapid recovery is unusual. For the vast majority of women, some residual discomfort remains in the navel, shoulders, or chest for three to five days.

After what age should laparoscopic tubal sterilization no longer be performed?

Fertility greatly diminishes after the age of forty-seven, even if menses remain fairly normal. For this reason, I prefer not to perform laparoscopic sterilization on women who are beyond this age. Instead I encourage use of safe contraceptive measures such as the diaphragm, TODAY sponge, condom, and foam. Though laparoscopy is a relatively safe procedure, I still believe that the risk is just too great for a woman older than forty-seven, who most probably is unable to conceive anyway.

VAGINAL TUBAL LIGATION

How is a vaginal tubal ligation performed?

Colpotomy refers to an incision made in the vagina at a point just behind the cervix (see figure 9-14). The lower part of the abdominal cavity, called the *cul-de-sac,* can then be easily entered. When colpotomy is performed by a skilled gynecologist, the tubes may be easily brought out through the incision and tied. The incision is then closed with absorbable sutures.

The advantages of vaginal tubal ligation are that it may be performed under either local, spinal, epidural, dissociative, or general anesthesia, and it leaves no abdominal scar. Postoperatively, the time spent in the hospital may be as little as less than one

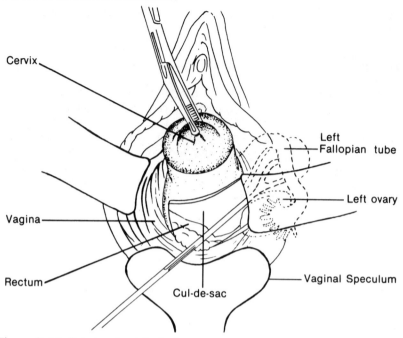

Figure 9-14. *Entering the abdominal cavity through the vagina (colpotomy).*

day, though the average stay is four days. Because the total hospital stay is shorter, the expense is less than that of the standard abdominal tubal ligation method. The postoperative time away from work has been reported as two to four weeks by some researchers, though as many as 50 percent of women undergoing the operation take longer to recover, as demonstrated in figure 9-15.

Are there certain women who should not undergo vaginal tubal ligation?

This operation is contraindicated for women who have an enlarged uterus, because the tubes will be too far away from the vaginal incision. For the same reason, vaginal tubal ligation is never performed immediately postpartum. If you have had previous pelvic or abdominal surgery, scarring or adhesions may prevent easy entry into the cul-de-sac and adequate visualization of the tubes. A history of chronic and acute pelvic infection, as well as severe endometriosis (see chapter 2), also increase the dangers of colpotomy. Colpotomy is easier if you have experienced childbirth, because the ligaments supporting the uterus may be somewhat relaxed. This allows for easier manipulation of the uterus during the operation. For the woman who has never borne children, the operation will often be more technically difficult due to the lack of uterine relaxation and movement.

What are the complications of vaginal tubal ligation via colpotomy?

Several studies have demonstrated a significant number of serious postoperative pelvic infections and hemorrhage, even when colpotomy is performed by a skilled gynecological surgeon. In the hands of a novice, the complication rate may be extremely high.

In one study of 500 vaginal tubal ligations, twenty-six women had complications in the immediate postoperative period. Of these twenty-six women, thirteen required hospitalization for pelvic pain, vaginal bleeding, or pelvic infection. Late complications were present in a total of twenty-eight women, including eighteen with chronic pelvic infection and five with chronic pelvic pain and pain with intercourse.

In another study of 800 women at the University of North Carolina, 4.9 percent experienced complications, while at the University of Michigan an alarming 20.9 percent of 340 women suffered immediate operative and postoperative complications such as excessive bleeding, bowel and bladder lacerations, hematoma at the operative site, and pelvic abscess. Two of the patients with pelvic abscess required hysterectomy and removal of both ovaries. Other investigators have reported similar complications with this procedure.

The point should be obvious: vaginal tubal ligation via colpotomy may seem like an attractive operation, but it often isn't. Complications may develop 3 to 13 percent of the time, and when they do occur they are potentially far more serious than those encountered with abdominal tubal ligation.

Finally, postoperative pregnancy rates of between 0.5 and 2.9 percent for vaginal tubal ligation are slightly higher than those for the abdominal approach. Based on this data, and the availability of so many other techniques, it would appear foolhardy for a doctor to perform vaginal tubal ligation in the face of its potentially serious complications.

What is a culdoscopy?

A *culdoscope* is an instrument used for viewing the contents of the cul-de-sac. Vaginal tubal ligation may be performed using this instrument. The culdoscope is inserted in the same vaginal location used for colpotomy, but the incision is much smaller. In addition, culdoscopy is performed with the patient in a kneeling position, with the shoulders and head on the operating table and the buttocks in the air.

Tubal sterilization via culdoscopy may be performed under either local or general anesthesia. Women are usually able to go home within six hours and can return to work within one week following surgery. When performed by a skilled culdoscopist, the risks of infection, hemorrhage, and rectal and intestinal injury are far fewer than with colpotomy.

Figure 9–15. *Length of hospital stay and time taken to resume work for different methods of sterilization.*

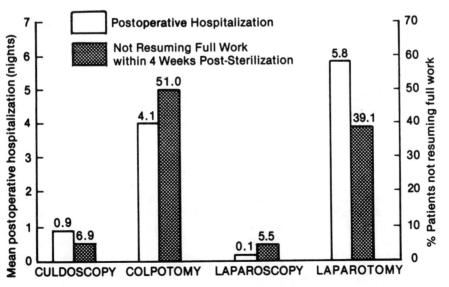

Though it sounds like an ideal method of surgical sterilization, very few doctors are skilled at performing culdoscopy. Because of the ease in performing laparoscopy and minilap surgery, most residency programs no longer teach resident physicians the necessary techniques for culdoscopy.

Is it true that some women experience irregular periods and abnormal vaginal bleeding following tubal ligation?

The terms *post-tubal ligation syndrome* (PTLS), *post-sterilization syndrome,* and *post-tubal sterilization syndrome* (PTSS) have been used interchangeably to describe the presence of menstrual disorders—including irregular cycles, dysmenorrhea (painful periods), heavy menstrual flow, bleeding between periods, and pelvic discomfort—occurring months or years following tubal sterilization. Despite thirty years of study by highly respected researchers, it is still not known whether there is a cause-and-effect relationship between sterilization and subsequent menstrual abnormalities.

Those who believe in the existence of this controversial syndrome theorize that it is caused by excessive destruction of the ovarian blood supply at the time that the tubes are tied. This in turn leads to a diminished output of ovarian hormones, faulty ovulation, and impaired corpus luteum function. It is their contention that sterilization procedures that cause a relatively large degree of tissue destruction, such as the Pomeroy technique (see page 210) and unipolar coagulation (see page 221), may be associated with a higher risk of PTLS than are methods of occlusion causing minimal tubal destruction, such as Hulka spring clips, Falope Rings, and bipolar coagulation. Other equally respectable investigators have reached just the opposite conclusion: that PTLS is nonexistent and that menstrual patterns remain essentially unchanged before and after surgery, regardless of the method used to occlude the tubes.

CREST is the name of a toothpaste and is also the acronym for Collaborative Review of Sterilization—a project, under the direction of the Centers for Disease Control, involved in studying the results of sterilization procedures from twelve participating medical centers. To date, their findings suggest that PTLS is more likely to occur when tubal ligation is performed at the time of cesarean section or in the immediate postpartum period. In 1985, Frank DeStefano, M.D., and his associates at the National Institute of Health analyzed the CREST data as it related to 719 women who underwent tubal sterilization in the early 1970s. For controls they used 1,083 fertile women whose partners had had vasectomies. Some women were followed for seven or more years. The NIH investigators found that abnormal menstrual cycles were three times more prevalent in women who had previously undergone sterilization, and the differences were of greatest significance when the follow-up period exceeded two years. Similarly, the likelihood of worsening menstrual cramps from none or mild to moderate or severe began to achieve significance only two years or more after surgery.

Pouru B. Bhiwandiwala, M.D., and her associates for the International Fertility Research Program in North Carolina, have accumulated statistics on over 25,000 sterilized women from sixty-four institutions and twenty-three countries throughout the world and have reached far more favorable conclusions. In articles published in 1982 and 1983, they interviewed women concerning six different menstruation characteristics before, and six months after, tubal sterilization via clips, Falope Rings, or cauterization. The six parameters measured were cycle regularity, length of cycle, duration of period, amount of menstrual flow, dysmenorrhea (menstrual pain), and intermenstrual bleeding (bleeding between periods). In all of their studies, Dr. Bhiwandiwala and her colleagues found that the overwhelming majority of women noted no menstrual changes postoperatively regardless of the method used to occlude the fallopian tubes. When changes did occur, as many menstrual patterns improved as worsened. Changes were more often associated with discontinuation of the Pill or of an IUD—heavier periods after stopping the Pill and lighter ones after the removal of an IUD. Women using the diaphragm or withdrawal methods were less likely to note postoperative menstrual changes.

The claim of reduced ovarian hormone production following sterilization has also been questioned by researchers. Stephen L. Corson, M.D., and his associates at the University of Pennsylvania School of Medicine measured progesterone levels during the second half of the menstrual cycle among women sterilized with either the Falope Ring or bipolar cautery, and found no differences when compared to controls.

If all of this data appear contradictory and confusing, it is not surprising. One can generalize only to the point that for the vast majority of women, tubal sterilization should not adversely affect the menstrual cycle. To further ensure that there will be no postoperative problems, you should choose a doctor who will use Falope Rings, Hulka clips, or bipolar cautery, rather than the more destructive and dangerous techniques of unipolar cauterization.

Postoperatively, is there any way to be absolutely sure that the tubes have been successfully blocked?

Twelve or more weeks following the procedure a *hysterosalpingogram* may be taken. This is an X ray of the uterus and fallopian tubes following the injection of a special dye through the cervix. Prior to surgery, the dye passes through the cervix, into the uterine cavity, and out through the ends of the tubes and into the abdominal cavity. If the surgery has been successful, the dye will fill the endometrial cavity postoperatively and may pass a short distance up the tube. It should never pass to the end of the tube or into the abdominal cavity. A hysterosalpingogram is never performed routinely, but only on rare occasions when the laparoscopic sterilization procedure was difficult to perform and the surgeon is not completely sure whether both tubes were adequately occluded. Some doctors believe that the procedure is of little aid in determining whether the tubes are open, and others are of the opinion that forcing dye through the occluded segments of the tubes can have the adverse effect of reopening them.

If I later decide I would like to have more children, what are my chances of success following reconstructive surgery on the fallopian tubes?

Based on the latest statistics, it is estimated that as many as 1 to 2 percent of all women who undergo tubal sterilization will seek reversal at a later date, and as many as 15 percent regret the decision without going so far as trying to reverse the procedure. The enormity of the problem is evidenced by the statistic that almost 6,000 American women undergo tubal reversal surgery annually, at an average cost of $10,000.

Until recently, the success rate for reversal surgery was no higher than 40 percent. New techniques such as microsurgery and laser are now achieving overall successful pregnancy rates of 70 percent. This figure is a bit inflated, however, since a conscientious physician will decline to perform surgery on a substantial number of women whose preoperative evaluation indicates excessive tubal destruction from the previous operation. Success rates will depend on several factors, including the skill of the physician performing the operation, the technique previously used to occlude the tubes, the amount of tube previously destroyed, and the location along the tube where the previous surgery was performed.

Too many physicians delude themselves into believing that they are capable of performing tubal reconstructive surgery when these operations really require a skilled microsurgeon with expertise in the use of the operative microscope and laser. Such specialists are very few in number, and are usually found in large medical centers rather than in neighborhood hospitals. All too often, a referral to a trained specialist occurs only after a local physician has failed to perform adequate initial surgery. This is unfortunate because the best chance of successful reversal is always on the first surgical attempt.

The success of reconstructive tubal surgery often depends on what sterilization technique was used. Methods in which there is minimal tubal destruction, such as the Hulka spring-loaded clip and the Falope Ring, are associated with the greatest number of reversal successes. In contrast, women who have had a previous unipolar cauterization, Pomeroy tubal ligation, or *fimbriectomy* (removal of the fimbriated or outer portion of the tube), fare the worst. Though statistics vary from one surgeon to another, the approximate percentage of successful full-term pregnancies following the various techniques are as follows: Hulka clip, 80 to 85 percent; Falope Ring, 70 to 80 percent; bipolar cauterization, 60 to 70 percent; Pomeroy tubal ligation, 50 to 60 percent; unipolar cauterization, 40 to 50 percent; and fimbriectomy, 20 to 40 percent.

To reopen the tubes, a microsurgeon has to excise, or cut out, the closed and damaged portion and then reanastomose (rejoin) the two open ends on either side. When the damaged segment of tube is immediately adjacent to the uterus, it is best to remove it and then implant the remaining healthy part of the tube directly into the uterine cavity. Both anastomosis and implantation of the fallopian tubes require meticulous and painstaking microscopic techniques.

As noted in chapter 1, the fallopian tube increases progressively in diameter as it passes from its *proximal* (near the uterus) to its *distal* (outer) end. The progressively widening segments are named the interstitial, isthmic, ampullary, and fimbriated portions. The poor results associated with trying to restore fertility following fimbriectomy are not surprising in view of the fact that the fimbria, the fingerlike projections at the end of the tube, serve the vital function of catching a newly ovulated egg each month (see fimbriae, chapter 1). In contrast, the greatest microsurgical reversal successes occur following the anastomosis of two adjacent isthmic portions of tube (see the figure in Chapter 1). Under these ideal circumstances, success can occur in more than 80 percent of all cases, possibly as high as a startling 90 percent if the isthmic-isthmic reanastomosis follows sterilization with a relatively atraumatic Hulka spring-clip technique. Ampullary-ampullary reanastomosis has the second highest success rate, but procedures such as ampullary-isthmic and ampullary-interstitial are more likely to fail because of the technical difficulties of joining two segments of tube with such different diameters. Though the overall risk of an ectopic pregnancy following tubal reversal surgery is quoted at approximately 5 percent, it increases to nearly 10 percent when tubal segments of significantly different diameters are joined. Based on this information, many microsurgical specialists recommend that all tubal sterilizations be performed in the isthmus portion of the tube using Hulka clips.

Several studies have indicated that the success of reanastomosis is also dependent upon the length of fallopian tube remaining following the corrective surgery. In a 1986 article published in *The American Journal of Obstetrics and Gynecology,* Manuel M. Spivak, M.D., and his associates at the University of Toronto reported a pregnancy rate of only 20 percent when the final tube length was less than 4 centimeters. With a tubal length of 4 to 6 centimeters, the pregnancy rate rose to 55 percent, increasing to 73 percent with a length greater than 6 centimeters. In a 1985 study from Queen Victoria Medical Centre in Melbourne, Australia, doctors reported no successful pregnancies when the tubal length was less than 3 centimeters. Some clever physician has determined that the approximate chance of a successful pregnancy following tubal reconstructive surgery is equal to the longest remaining tubal length in centimeters multiplied by ten.

The interval between surgical sterilization and attempted reanastomosis may also play an important role. In one report, doctors noted a 30 percent subsequent pregnancy rate after an interval of five years. Doctors have theorized that this may be because the tubal lining continues to atrophy over a period of several years following the initial surgery. Others hypothesize that destruction of blood vessels near the tube compromises ovarian function and ovulation over a period of time (see post-tubal ligation syndrome). In a 1986 article published in *The British Journal of Obstetrics and Gynecology,* doctors reported a 9 percent greater success rate when reversal tubal surgery was performed on women between the ages of twenty-five and twenty-nine, as compared with those aged thirty-five to thirty-nine.

Why do many women request tubal sterilization reversal at a later date?

With the soaring divorce rate in the United States, it is no wonder that women who were previously involved in an unhappy marriage may seek sterilization reversal when they remarry. In a 1986 study published in *The American Journal of Obstetrics and Gynecology,* researchers found that 66 percent of all requests for surgery reversal came from women with new husbands. Another 30 percent of the women expressed regrets, religious guilt, and depression about their original decision. Other reasons cited for requesting reversal of sterilization included the loss of a child through crib death, or death from other diseases or accidents.

Sometimes it is easier to understand why a woman seeks sterilization reversal in light of her original decision to undergo tubal ligation. For example, in one report, women named financial and social reasons as the second most important determinant of their sterilization decision. Later reversal of their economic fortunes could clearly alter their decision to limit their family size. Other factors listed for the decision to be sterilized included contraceptive failure with other methods, an unhappy marriage, insistence of a husband to limit family size, and medical conditions making pregnancy complicated or difficult.

Even if a general psychiatric assessment is obtained before sterilization, there is never a guarantee of subsequent satisfaction. In a 1984 study, published in *Fertility and Sterility,* doctors tried to determine whether any particular psychological characteristics could help identify those women who would be most likely to experience dissatisfaction at a later date. They interviewed 180 women requesting reversal, and an equal number of women who were content with their decision to undergo sterilization. Though both groups were similar in the number of children they had, the women who requested reversal were younger than the control group when they were sterilized (average age: twenty-four versus thirty-three), and younger when they had their first and last child (seventeen versus twenty-four, and twenty versus twenty-six, respectively). In addition, more women in the dissatisfied group were divorced and remarried, were of a lower socioeconomic status, and were likely to complain of menstrual disorders associated with the post-tubal ligation syndrome (PTLS). A psychological substudy of thirty-five women from each group revealed that those requesting reversal surgery were more likely to test positive for neurotic complaints, hysteria, and other psychological disorders.

At least two separate reports have confirmed that women are more likely to regret their decision to be sterilized if the operation is performed in the immediate postpartum period or in combination with an abortion. Similarly, if the sterilization operation is done on an emergency basis, a woman is far more likely to be dissatisfied. In one study, over 25 percent of those undergoing cesarean section in combination with tubal ligation were unhappy with their decision. In contrast, dissatisfaction was voiced by only 2 percent of the women who had had only tubal ligation performed. In another report, one-third of the women scheduled for immediate postpartum sterilization changed their minds and decided against the surgery when it had to be delayed by a few weeks. For these reasons, it is probably best for doctors to avoid combining sterilization operations with other procedures whenever possible. Many regrettable decisions can be avoided if a woman is allowed four to six weeks from the time of a delivery or abortion before making the final decision to undergo sterilization. This decision should never be made at a time of emotional distress.

In the next chapter I will discuss the medical and surgical indications for hysterectomy. Emotional factors play an important role in tubal sterilization, but they often pale in comparison to those associated with a woman's loss of her uterus. Unfortunately, hysterectomy continues to be performed in the United States at a rate far higher than is warranted, making it, after knee surgery, the most unnecessarily performed operation in the United States.

10

HYSTERECTOMY

In the first edition of this book, published in 1977, I expressed concern that the number of hysterectomies performed annually in the United States had increased by about 25 percent between 1970 and 1977. Surveys conducted at that time estimated that anywhere from 15 to 40 percent of all hysterectomies were unnecessary. The upward spiraling trend toward more and more surgery seemed inevitable, but I am happy to report that these pessimistic forecasts have not materialized. In fact, the number of hysterectomies performed has actually been reduced, from the 1977 total of 442,000 among women in the reproductive age group of fifteen to forty-four, to 421,000 in 1985.

In his excellent in-depth analysis of obstetric and gynecologic operations performed from 1979 to 1984, Ira M. Rutkow, M.D., noted that the total number of surgical procedures actually declined by 1 percent. This is an amazing statistic in view of the fact that, during that same time period, the number of physicians practicing obstetrics and gynecology increased by 22 percent and the female population rose by 6 percent. Dr. Rutkow explains: "The one inescapable conclusion from this large study is that the numbers of obstetric and gynecologic operations have not increased over the last five to ten years, in spite of constantly increasing numbers of physicians who practice obstetrics and gynecology. The belief that more surgeons means more surgery is not supported by this study."

In commenting on this trend, Dr. Donald A. Grimes of the Centers for Disease Control stated that as the average gynecologist's caseload decreased, more time would be devoted to primary prevention of disease rather than to surgery. His statement that "social gynecology may emerge as a discipline of equal stature as surgical gynecology in the United States" is welcome news to consumer advocates, feminists, and insurance carriers alike.

There are many reasons for this healthy development away from gynecological surgery. Certainly public awareness has been heightened by consumer books and magazine and newspaper articles over the past ten years. In addition, the willingness and insistence of insurance carriers to pay for second and even third opinions has helped reduce the number of unnecessary operations. In one survey, researchers found that in 30 percent of the cases, doctors who gave a second opinion failed to confirm the decision of the first doctor to perform hysterectomy. The old arguments that second opinions are responsible for delaying vital surgery and for raising costs of health care are unfounded and not supported by scientific data. In the most impressive study of its kind, reported in the prestigious *New England Journal of Medicine,* doctors in Saskatchewan, Canada, performed 33 percent fewer hysterectomies when surgical cases were carefully monitored by a surveillance committee.

More stringent government and hospital regulations and stricter medical peer review committees have all played important roles in reducing the incidence of unnecessary hysterectomies. The last ten years have also seen the development of a greater number of prepaid health maintenance organizations, or HMOs. Since the financial incentive to performing surgery is lost when health care is prepaid, one could argue that many HMO doctors are simply unwilling to bother to perform the surgery needed to relieve distressing gynecological conditions.

Though the number of hysterectomies has declined steadily since the peak year 1977, one constant and unexplained phenomenon is that a woman living in the South is 2.5 times more likely to undergo hysterectomy than one who lives in the Northeast. Hysterectomy rates in other geographical areas of the country fall somewhere between these two extremes. Women in the thirty-five-to-forty-four-year age group experience the highest hysterectomy rates. The most encouraging change over the past ten years has been a 34 percent reduction in the rate of hysterectomies for black women, compared to a 14 percent decline for whites. In addition, the year 1982 marked the first time since surveillance began in 1970 that the hysterectomy rate of 6.7 per 1,000 for black women was lower than that of 7.7 per 1,000 for white women in our population.

Despite these gains, hysterectomy remains the most commonly performed major operation for American women of reproductive age. One must never lose sight of the fact that it is a potentially dangerous procedure, responsible for the death of 600 to 1,200 women per million undergoing this operation each year—approximately 1 death per 1,000 operations.

What is a hysterectomy?

Hysterectomies are often incorrectly referred to as *complete* or *incomplete* based on whether the ovaries are removed. Actually, *total hysterectomy* is the surgical removal of the entire uterus, including the cervix. On rare occasions, a surgeon may be unable to remove the cervix, in which case the operation is called a *supracervical hysterectomy.* (Removal of both fallopian tubes and both ovaries is termed *bilateral salpingo-oophorectomy,* and if only the tube and the ovary on one side is removed, it is called a *unilateral salpingo-oophorectomy.*)

Hysterectomy may be accomplished either with an abdominal incision or through the vagina, in which case no incision is required. Based on the latest national statistics, abdominal hysterectomy accounts for 73 percent, and vaginal hysterectomy for 27 percent, of the approximate 600,000 total hysterectomies performed in the United States each year. An abdominal hysterectomy performed at the time of cesarean section is called a *cesarean hysterectomy.* A *postpartum hysterectomy* is one that is performed during the eight weeks following childbirth.

In the absence of gynecological disease, is hysterectomy ever justified as a method of permanent sterilization?

No. The rationale often cited for performing hysterectomy on a young woman is to prevent the 3.5 percent risk of her developing cancer of the cervix or uterus at a later date. Using the same reasoning, removal of the ovaries at the time of hysterectomy will preclude a combined cancer risk of 4.5 percent. If we continue with this deluded thinking, removal of both breasts at the age of thirty-five should prevent practically all cases of breast cancer. One epidemiological study determined that the performance of hysterectomy as a means of preventing future cancer can be expected to increase average life expectancy by approximately two months. Unfortunately, this is achieved at a considerable cost in dollars and postoperative illness. In addition, the two months for the most part amounts to prolongation of life for women in their late sixties and seventies. The estimated 600 women per million who may be expected to die from hysterectomy are for the most part young mothers.

Besides the risk of death, other complications of hysterectomy may be significant, including a major-complication rate estimated as high as 14 percent and a minor-complication rate of approximately 50 percent. In one study at the University of Michigan, it was noted that 16 percent of women undergoing abdominal hysterectomy required a blood transfusion, and almost 50 percent needed antibiotics. Late complications of hysterectomy—such as depression, fatigue, painful intercourse due to scarring of the vaginal tissues, and sexual dysfunction related to emotional factors involved with the loss of the uterus—are rarely mentioned by doctors to their patients prior to surgery, though these problems do occur in a significant number of women. Your doctor's assurance that you will "bounce back" to your normal routine within a couple of weeks following surgery should be taken with a grain of salt. For some women the recuperative period will be two or three months.

Studies by physicians at the Centers for Disease Control reveal that the risk of death from hysterectomy is ten times greater than that for tubal sterilization, and that major complication rates are eight times as high. These statistics should dissuade any doctor from performing hysterectomy rather than tubal ligation as a means of permanent sterilization. Hysterectomy entails a hospital stay of seven to eight days, as well as an average of forty-two days away from work. Not to be forgotten is the doctor's fee, which may range from a low of $1,000 to a high of $3,500.

Is vaginal hysterectomy safer than abdominal hysterectomy?

Because a vaginal hysterectomy produces no visible scar, women are often led to believe that it is a safe, uncomplicated method of sterilization. Nothing could be further from the truth. If anything, for a young woman, the incidence of postoperative hemorrhage, pelvic infection, and urinary tract infection is probably higher than with abdominal hysterectomy. The blood supply to the uterus of a menstruating woman is much greater than it is in a postmenopausal woman. As a result, there is less control of bleeding during surgery, which in turn predisposes the younger patient to secondary infection.

In 1975, Russell K. Laros, Jr., and Bruce A. Work, Jr., from the University of Michigan, reported the results of 111 vaginal hysterectomies performed solely for the purpose of sterilization. When compared with other methods such as laparoscopy, vaginal tubal ligation, and abdominal tubal ligation, the results were dismal. A total of 89 women, or 90 percent of the vaginal hysterectomy group, experienced postoperative fever. In more than 40 percent of these women, the fever persisted for more than two days; 20 women suffered from pelvic infection, while 17 had urinary tract infections. Surgery was significantly prolonged and involved a blood loss greater than 500 cubic centimeters, or one unit of blood, in 18 of these 111 women. Finally, the average length of hospitalization was 9.5 days.

In summary, Laros and Work appropriately conclude: "Vaginal hysterectomy is not an ideal method of female sterilization. It is attended by significant morbidity, prolonged hospitalization, a long operating time, and significant blood loss. We feel that it should be used only in highly selected patients where there is a clear indication for hysterectomy alone and beyond the desire for sterilization."

When should a vaginal hysterectomy be performed?

The prime reason for vaginal hysterectomy should be not sterilization but rather a condition called *uterine prolapse.* Uterine prolapse refers to the dropping of the entire uterus, so that the cervix actually falls into the lower vagina, and occasionally even out of the vagina (see figure 10-1). This condition usually occurs at or after the meno-

Figure 10–1. *Uterus and urinary bladder in normal and prolapsed position.*

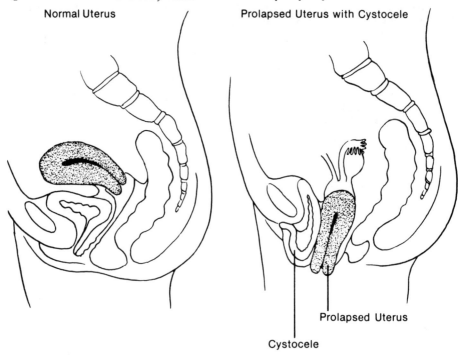

Normal Uterus   Prolapsed Uterus with Cystocele

Prolapsed Uterus

Cystocele

pause, but milder degrees of prolapse are not uncommon in young women who have borne two or more children.

The cause of uterine prolapse is a loosening of the ligaments and muscles supporting the uterus. Symptoms may include pelvic pressure or heaviness, especially when standing; low backache; and the feeling that "something is falling out."

What is a cystocele?

A *cystocele* is a relaxation and bulging of the urinary bladder that often accompanies uterine prolapse. Women with cystocele may experience recurrent urinary tract infections and frequent loss of urine while coughing, sneezing, and bearing down, such as with defecation. The loss of urine with such stress is called *stress incontinence.* Occasionally, a cystocele may be accompanied by a slight bulge below the urethral opening. This is called a *urethrocele* (figure 10-2).

A *rectocele* is a bulge at the back wall of the vagina near the rectum. It is also due to a weakening of the supportive tissues. A woman may easily detect the presence of a cystocele or rectocele with a hand mirror, simply by bearing down while in a squatting position.

If I notice that I have a cystocele and experience rare episodes of stress incontinence, what should I do?

Many women who have given birth experience a slight degree of prolapse, cystocele, stress incontinence, or rectocele. It is rarely a sign that they need vaginal hysterectomy or urinary bladder and rectocele repair. Rather, steps can be taken to prevent the condition from becoming progressively worse. Obese women benefit greatly from weight reduction, while the heavy smoker who quits will cough less and thereby lose less urine. Muscle setting, or Kegel's exercises, is very useful in overcoming mild or moderate stress incontinence. These exercises are designed to strengthen and reeducate the muscles around the bladder and rectum. The simplest method is to tighten the muscles of the buttocks as though trying to prevent the escape of feces from the anus. The same group of muscles is also used in trying to stop the flow of urine in midstream. After learning Kegel's exercises, you must practice them at least 100 times per day for a minimum of six months. In addition, each time you pass urine, voluntarily interrupt the flow several times. If these exercises are diligently performed, you will note improvement in mild cases of stress incontinence within two months. For more severe cases, it may take six months or more—a small price to pay for avoiding major surgery.

What ulterior motives could lead doctors to prefer vaginal hysterectomy to abdominal hysterectomy?

One reason may involve the fact that all reputable hospitals have pathology departments and tissue committees which study the specimens removed during a surgical procedure. When an abdominal hysterectomy is performed, it is required that the uterus contain at least a minimal degree of pathological change to warrant its removal. If not, the physician who removed it must explain his reasons for having performed the surgery to both the tissue committee and the members of his department. Repeated violations may cause a doctor to lose hospital and operating room privileges. A uterus that is removed vaginally is not reviewed by tissue committees because the presumed diagnosis is always uterine prolapse. Sadly, it is for this reason that some doctors might attempt a difficult vaginal hysterectomy, rather than the more simple abdominal approach, when the amount of disease present is questionable.

If a woman requesting sterilization has a disease of the uterus, tubes, or ovaries, would hysterectomy then be indicated for sterilization?

That would depend on the disease and its severity. In the presence of severe and incapacitating conditions such as endometriosis (see chapter 2) or chronic pelvic infection, hysterectomy certainly would appear to be indicated. Preinvasive cancer of the cervix, or carcinoma-in-situ, has a good chance of becoming the more dangerous invasive carcinoma at a later date and might therefore also make a woman a candidate for hysterectomy as a sterilization technique. If she has completed her childbearing, it would probably be better for such a woman to have her uterus removed than to have the tubes tied and leave the cervix in place.

Figure 10–2. *Cystocele and urethrocele.*

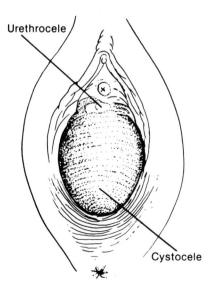

Doctors too often use the diagnosis of an ovarian cyst as an indication for removal of the ovary containing the cyst, the other normal ovary, or even the uterus. Though there are many types of ovarian cysts, the overwhelming majority of those that develop in menstruating women are not cancerous. In fact, the large percentage of those benign cysts form within the ovarian follicle or within the corpus luteum (see chapter 1), and are usually not larger than 5 centimeters (2 inches) in diameter. These cysts always disappear within one or two months. In the absence of symptoms such as severe abdominal pain, surgery is not indicated. Instead, a menstruating woman with a cyst should be reexamined after one month. If the cyst appears smaller, the chances are that it will be gone by the next month. If it is the same size or larger after one month, it usually means that it is not a follicle or corpus luteum cyst, and surgery is indicated. The one-month delay causes no harm, since almost all cysts in young women are benign. And it avoids many unnecessary operations. Beware of the doctor who rushes to put you on his operative schedule for an ovarian cyst after only one vaginal examination.

What are fibroids?

By far the most common reason for hysterectomy in the United States is the presence of fibroid tumors of the uterus. Many of these operations could and should be avoided. *Fibroids,* or *leiomyomas,* are benign tumors of the uterus which have a firm to rock-hard consistency. They are found in as many as 40 percent of all women over the age of thirty-five, and their size ranges from that of a pea to that of a large grapefruit (see figure 10-3). More often than not, a woman with fibroids will have several of them.

Figure 10–3. *Fibroid tumors in the uterus.*

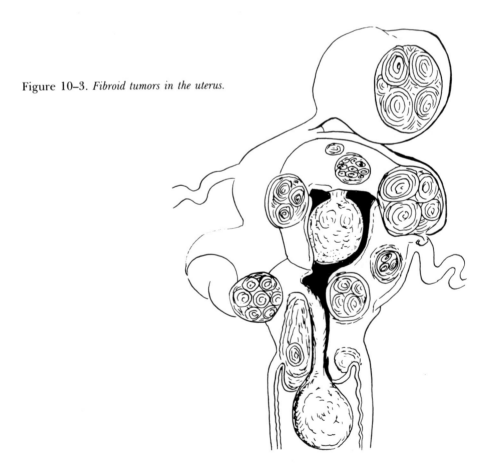

More important than the size of these tumors is their location. A very small fibroid located below the surface of the endometrium, known as a *submucous fibroid,* will often cause profuse bleeding at the time of the menses, while a large one in the uterine muscle, called an *intramural fibroid,* may produce no symptoms at all.

The size of fibroids decreases, and the symptoms they may produce disappear, after the menopause, since these tumors are hormonally dependent. Birth-control pills that contain high doses of estrogen are best avoided in a woman with a uterus enlarged with fibroids. But recent statistics demonstrate that newer formulations of birth-control pills can be used safely in women with fibroids (see chapter 2).

When fibroids cause symptoms, the most common one is heavy and prolonged menses with passage of blood clots. When the bleeding is severe and the symptoms last for several cycles, you may become anemic. Pain may accompany menstruation, along with a feeling of heaviness in the pelvis which may be present throughout the entire month. Rectal pressure and urinary frequency and urgency may be caused by large fibroids pressing on the rectum and urinary bladder.

When hysterectomy is performed for fibroids that produce no symptoms, the requirements of the hospital's tissue committee will be met, though your best interests may not be served. For this reason, you should have one or two outside consultations before you undergo hysterectomy for so-called asymptomatic fibroids. Happily, many insurance companies will pay for such consultations. In the absence of symptoms, most authorities agree that hysterectomy is indicated when the size of the uterus equals or exceeds the size of a twelve-week pregnancy. With such an enlarged uterus, symptoms are usually inevitable—unless, of course, the menopause is imminent.

It is easy enough to determine whether the size of your uterus is that of a twelve-week pregnancy or greater. When the urinary bladder empties, a uterus of twelve weeks' size should be palpable above the pubic symphysis bone (see figure 4-3). Fibroid tumors of this size feel like hard, irregular bumps above the symphysis. If you can't feel them, ask your doctor to demonstrate them by pressing your hand on them during the examination. A good rule of thumb is that if you can't feel your fibroids, your doctor can't take them!

If a fibroid suddenly grows rapidly in a young woman, what does it mean?

Assuming that you're not using high-estrogen birth-control pills, the sudden increase in size of a fibroid may mean that you're pregnant. During pregnancy both the uterus and the fibroid grow substantially, though it is rare for a fibroid to interfere with the pregnancy or with labor.

A second possibility for a rapid fibroid growth may be that it has degenerated into a cancer. Some doctors have been known to use this argument as a scare tactic for performing hysterectomy. Actually, malignant change in a fibroid is extremely rare, occurring in less than one-half of 1 percent of all women with fibroids. Characteristically, it occurs in the postmenopausal years and is so rare that most busy gynecologists have never seen a single patient with this type of malignancy.

Is there an alternative to hysterectomy for the young woman with fibroids who may want to have children?

Myomectomy—removing the fibroids but preserving the uterus—can usually be accomplished by making an incision over the fibroid, dissecting it out of the surrounding muscle, and then closing the defect.

Prior to myomectomy, you must be informed that there is a fibroid recurrence rate necessitating repeat surgery in 10 to 20 percent of cases. Furthermore, despite the fact that the uterus is not removed, the amount of bleeding at the time of surgery and the postoperative complication rate may be as high for myomectomy as for hysterectomy, or higher. Subsequent pregnancies must usually be delivered by cesarean section, due to weakening of the uterine wall following myomectomy.

Though only 5 percent of all fibroids are submucous (located below the endometrial surface), they are responsible for an inordinate number of hysterectomies because of the heavy periods they produce. A doctor can easily diagnosis the presence of submucous fibroids at the time of a D and C, because they give the endometrial cavity an irregular and distorted shape.

Other successful techniques for making the diagnosis include ultrasound, hysterogram (X ray of the uterine cavity after injection of a dye solution), and *hysteroscopy*, which is the most exciting and potentially most useful of these methods. The viewing instrument, or hysteroscope, has a high-powered fiberoptic light source and a diameter no wider than a pencil. By passing it through the cervix, a doctor is able to visualize the entire endometrium and may perform various procedures (see chapter 3 and chapter 11). Though many gynecologists use the hysteroscope in their practice, few are skilled at resecting (cutting out) submucous fibroids with specially designed instruments placed through the hysteroscope. One such expert, Robert S. Neuwirth, M.D., of St. Luke's Hospital Center in New York City, estimates that as many as 70,000 to 80,000 women could be treated in this manner each year, thereby avoiding the more traumatic abdominal myomectomy or hysterectomy.

Is there any other method of using the hysteroscope to treat uterine bleeding?

In an effort to reduce the number of hysterectomies performed because of abnormally heavy periods, clinical studies are being conducted in several centers throughout the United States to determine the feasibility of a procedure known as *laser ablation of the endometrium*. With this technique, a powerful neodymium-YAG laser, or Nd: YAG, is introduced through a hysteroscope, and its beam used to destroy permanently as much of the endometrium as possible. This creates permanent scarring and sterility without causing menopausal symptoms, since the ovaries are uninvolved. Without build-up and shedding of the endometrium each month, menstruation and abnormal uterine bleeding of any type will no longer occur in 50 percent of the women treated. Those who do continue to menstruate will usually need no more than one sanitary napkin per day for no more than three days. The amount of bleeding depends on how much functioning endometrium remains following the laser ablation.

Though results are only preliminary, authorities believe that laser ablation will significantly reduce the number of hysterectomies performed each year for uterine hemorrhage. Compared to hysterectomy, laser ablation is simpler, safer, less painful, and less expensive. Postoperatively, hysterectomy often requires a week in the hospital followed by a recuperative period of several weeks. In contrast, laser ablation can be performed as a forty-minute outpatient procedure at a fraction of the medical cost. Postoperatively, there is minimal if any discomfort and a blood-tinged watery discharge which may last as long as one month. The greatest potential application for the Nd:YAG laser is in avoiding the major surgery of hysterectomy for high-risk women with diabetes, hypertension, kidney disease, heart disease, and bleeding disorders.

Milton Goldrath, M.D., chairman of the department of obstetrics and gynecology at Sinai Hospital in Detroit, is credited with developing the technique of using the Nd:YAG laser through a hysteroscope. In his 1986 review of 300 patients treated with laser ablation, Dr. Goldrath showed a 97 percent success rate, with only one woman later requiring hysterectomy. Though these early results are encouraging, it will take several years for this sophisticated and expensive instrument to reach more than the handful of gynecologists presently using it.

How can LH-RH agonists be used to treat fibroid and abnormal uterine bleeding?

Luteinizing hormone-releasing hormone LH-RH (GnRH) is produced by the hypothalamus and stimulates the pituitary gland to release LH (see chapter 1 and chapter 5). It is the sudden surge of LH that triggers ovulation each month. Laboratory-developed LH-RH compounds, or analogs, were originally introduced as a means of stimulating fertility among women with ovulation dysfunction. It is now apparent that they do exactly the opposite. When given as an injection or inhaled as a nasal spray every few days over a period of weeks or months, LH-RH analogs will lower LH, FSH, and estrogen levels and disrupt or stop the menstrual cycle completely (see chapter 11).

The growth of fibroids is directly related to estrogen hormone levels in a woman's body, and experimental studies to date have confirmed that use of the LH-RH analog buserelin (trade name: Suprefact) for a period of at least eight to ten weeks will cause fibroids to shrink in size. In a 1986 report of twenty-five young women given buserelin by either injection or nasal spray, researchers found that the average reduction in fibroid volume, as measured by ultrasound, was 71 percent among those using the spray and 55 percent for women given injections. Serious complications were nonexistent, though several women complained of hot flashes, probably secondary to their low estrogen levels. This problem is much more common with injections than it is with nasal spray. In a 1977 multicenter study in which forty women received the LH-RH analog leuprolide (trade name: Lupron), doctors were encouraged by the findings of very light periods and a significant decrease in fibroid size in at least 28 percent of the women treated. Following daily subcutaneous (below the skin) injections for six or more months, ultrasound examinations confirmed that the average tumor volume decreased by 50 percent among the forty women studied. To avoid the inconvenience of this daily routine, researchers are trying to develop a once-a-month intramuscular injection of leuprolide.

Both an advantage and a disadvantage of LH-RH analog therapy is that the therapeutic effects last only as long as the medication is administered. Several women have experienced heavy periods and fibroid growth soon after stopping the medication.

LH-RH has also undergone experimental trials as a contraceptive (see chapter 11, "The Future"), and as a method of treating endometriosis, prostate cancer, premenstrual syndrome (PMS; see chapter 2), and precocious sexual development of children and teenagers.

Aside from fibroids, what other benign gynecological condition of the uterus is most likely to necessitate hysterectomy rather than tubal sterilization?

Adenomyosis is a benign, though progressively disabling, condition caused by endometrial glandular tissue being displaced into the muscle of the uterus. Unlike endometriosis, which is also caused by displaced endometrial glands, adenomyosis usually occurs in women who have given birth several times, with the onset of symptoms beginning in their late thirties or beyond the age of forty. Though many women have never heard of the condition, adenomyosis is almost as common as are fibroids, and is present in approximately 20 percent of all hysterectomy specimens. The incidence of adenomyosis at autopsy in women who have died of other causes has been reported to be as high as 50 percent, and 50 percent of all women with adenomyosis also have fibroids.

The most common symptoms of the disorder are very heavy and frequent periods which become progressively more painful. Intercourse may also cause deep pelvic pain. On vaginal examination the findings may be variable, but usually the uterus is tender and slightly or moderately enlarged, with a globular shape. Characteristically, when hormones such as birth-control pills and progesterone are given to relieve the pain, the stimulation to the displaced endometrial glands actually intensifies the discomfort.

The diagnosis of adenomyosis is often extremely difficult to make, because a D and C removes tissue from only the endometrium and not from the muscle of the uterus. Study of the hysterectomy specimen by a pathologist is the only way to confirm a doctor's suspicion that adenomyosis exists. Like fibroids, it causes no further difficulties after the menopause. For this reason, a woman in her late forties with tolerable symptoms may best be left alone rather than treated in a surgical manner. If pain medication is required for this condition, some of the newer antiprostaglandin preparations may be tried.

If the ovaries are not removed at the time of hysterectomy, will ovarian hormonal function be altered?

In the not too distant past, doctors, including myself, often reassured concerned patients that their ovaries would continue to function normally if left intact at the time of hysterectomy. Sadly, too often the recommendation to women who suffered from postoperative hot flashes, vaginal dryness, painful intercourse, nervousness, and depression was psychotherapy rather than estrogen hormone replacement therapy. More recent studies have shown that as many as 30 to 50 percent of women will experience premature ovarian failure following hysterectomy. It is now believed that circulation in the ovaries and uterus shows great variability from one woman to the next. For some, surgery to the uterus has the effect of compromising the ovarian blood supply and adversely affecting subsequent ovarian function.

In a 1986 report, published in *The Journal of Reproductive Medicine,* doctors at the University of Kiel in West Germany sent questionnaires to 164 women between the ages of twenty-seven and forty-two who had had a hysterectomy without oophorectomy (removal of an ovary) during the preceding ten years. Thirty-nine percent of the women reported menopausal symptoms, while others who were asymptomatic still demonstrated lower than normal concentrations of estrogen and progesterone. In another 1986 study, doctors from Sao Paulo University Medical School in Brazil found no change in ovarian hormone levels among twenty-five women tested before, and one year after, hysterectomy. Comparison biopsies of the ovaries taken at these times, however, showed microscopic evidence of fewer follicles and more connective tissue postoperatively. Though the significance of these changes remains unknown, it is a certainty that hysterectomy alters the ovarian function of a significant number of women.

What are some of the possible psychological problems associated with hysterectomy?

Regardless of whether a woman's ovarian function is compromised after hysterectomy, the postoperative days and months may be complicated by a significant likelihood of psychological problems. High levels of anxiety and emotional reactions related to the stress of surgery are associated with all operations, but there is no doubt that special factors are at work when a woman has her uterus removed. The statistic that mental illness following hysterectomy is almost three times more likely than after gallbladder surgery should dispel the myth that hysterectomy is just another operation. In one survey from the University of California, forty women between the ages of eighteen and forty underwent hysterectomy; 43 percent reported some emotional problems immediately after surgery, while 18 percent had more serious difficulties. One year later, 29 percent still reported psychological problems related to the surgery. Other investigators have observed that women who undergo hysterectomy are twice as likely to be readmitted to the hospital for psychiatric difficulties than they are following any other surgery. These and other statistics should convince even the most jaded gynecologist that the uterus is a special organ which carries powerful emotional significance to women—and to many men as well. Some women's femininity, sexuality, self-image, and self-worth are intimately tied up with their cyclic menstrual changes and their capacity to bear children. Studies have demonstrated that women who perceive themselves as living within the confines of raising children and taking care of a husband will be more likely to suffer postoperative psychological problems than those who have no wish for future children and are committed to interests and achievements outside the home.

Nancy C. A. Roeske, M.D., of the University of Indiana, has researched the many psychosocial factors that can influence a woman's response to hysterectomy. One of the key determinants is the circumstances surrounding the decision to operate. There is significantly less depression when symptoms such as incapacitating uterine bleeding or severe pelvic pain are present. Similarly, it is easier for a woman to accept the lifesaving quality of surgery performed to eradicate precancerous or cancerous disease of the cervix, uterus, or ovaries. In trying to anticipate which women will be more likely to fare poorly following hysterectomy, Dr. Roeske lists several prognostic signs that should alert a conscientious gynecologist to consider preoperative psychiatric evaluation: previous history of adverse reactions to stress; younger than thirty-five years old; the desire to have more children; a history of multiple complaints, especially low back pain; numerous hospitalizations and surgeries; marital dissatisfaction and instability; disapproving cultural and religious attitudes of family and friends; lack of outside interests; fear that surgery will diminish sexual interest and decrease satisfaction in the relationship; and negative attitudes of a husband or other significant person toward the operation.

In no other area of surgery is the preoperative evaluation as important as it is with hysterectomy. Though a gynecologist must carefully answer the obvious questions, it is probably more important that he or she anticipate concerns and initiate discussions about matters that are not verbalized. For example, many women are embarrassed to confess the fear that following removal of the uterus their sexuality will no longer be the same and that they will "never again function like a whole woman." Only a careful explanation of the reasons for recommending surgery as well as a description of the operation and anatomic results will clarify such misconceptions. A doctor must use language that the woman can understand, not medical doubletalk. It is important to emphasize that since the external genital organs and vagina will be left intact, the experience of intercourse and orgasm should remain unchanged postoperatively. It is also comforting for a woman to know that many individuals have an increase in sexual desire after a hysterectomy, because they no longer have a fear of pregnancy or of long, painful periods. A doctor must never minimize or be insensitive to a woman's pain and sense of loss often associated with hysterectomy.

Too often, husbands or mates are omitted from preoperative discussions, when they should instead be strongly encouraged to attend and participate. The value of their participation cannot be overstated, in view of the fact that research suggests a higher incidence of impotence in men whose wives have undergone hysterectomy. The question most often asked by men is whether intercourse will "feel different" after hysterectomy. The answer to this should be an emphatic *no.*

Postoperatively, it is important that a doctor help a woman recognize any depression she might have and offer reassurance that it is a normal and temporary reaction to stress and surgery. As previously stated, it is important to determine whether psychological problems and depression following hysterectomy are the result of an estrogen deficiency caused by interference with the ovarian blood supply. Often, a simple blood test measuring the levels of the pituitary hormones FSH and LH will supply the answer, and hormone replacement therapy will ameliorate the symptoms.

A doctor is well advised to keep in mind the results of a survey to determine the qualities women most wanted in their surgeons: gentleness, kindness, thoughtfulness, and understanding. An even greater attribute may be the commitment to avoid surgery unless it is absolutely necessary.

If hysterectomy is performed for a benign disease of the uterus, should a woman's healthy ovaries be removed?

The proper decision about whether to retain normal-appearing ovaries at hysterectomy has concerned physicians for many years. If you were to ask ten gynecologists at what age they think normal ovaries should be removed at the time of hysterectomy, undoubtedly ten different answers would be received, ranging from "age thirty-five" to "never." Past practice had been to remove normal-appearing ovaries in women between the ages of forty and forty-five when hysterectomy was performed. Recently, there has been a distinct shift of opinion in favor of retaining the ovaries in women as high as fifty years of age. One of the reasons for this shift is the realization by the medical community of the importance of ovarian function in preventing osteoporosis (loss of calcium from the bones), premature heart disease, and vaginal atrophy (vaginal aging and thinning of the tissues). In addition, the average age of the menopause for this generation has advanced to fifty-one.

What are the facts? For one thing, of all malignancies that strike the genital tract, cancer of the ovary is the leading cause of death, killing approximately 10,000 women in the United States each year. Though it is less common than cancer of the cervix and the endometrium, at the present time there are no adequate screening methods for detecting it, such as the Pap smear for cervical cancer. In addition, there are not usually any early symptoms. By the time symptoms do appear, the cancer has usually reached the incurable stage. For those two reasons, 6 out of every 10 women afflicted with ovarian cancer will die from it.

Statistically, more than 90 percent of ovarian tumors discovered in women between the ages of twenty and thirty are benign. Between the ages of fifty and seventy, however, the ratio of malignant to benign tumors is approximately even. Based on these statistics, and prejudiced by the fact that I have known several wonderful women who have been afflicted with this terrible disorder, it is my policy to encourage women aged forty-five and over to have their ovaries removed when surgery is performed for benign disease of the uterus. I have even made this suggestion to younger women who are at especially high risk of developing ovarian cancer—that is, who have never borne children. Statistically, such women are 2.5 times more likely to develop ovarian cancer than a woman with a history of three or more pregnancies. In addition, a woman with a history of breast, endometrial, or colon cancer is known to be at greater risk for developing ovarian cancer. If you have a family history of ovarian cancer, your likelihood of contracting this disease is also significantly greater.

Several studies have been conducted to determine whether an ovary retained at hysterectomy carries with it a greater potential for recurrent pelvic pain and both malignant and nonmalignant disease at a later date. Such problems are referred to medically as the "residual ovary syndrome." It may occur in approximately 1 to 3 percent of all women undergoing hysterectomy and retaining either one or both ovaries.

A review of the residual ovary syndrome was published in 1975 by J. E. Christ and E. C. Lotze from Baylor College of Medicine. Their findings are based on a study of 202 women who required repeat surgery due to problems associated with retained ovaries. Of the group, almost 54 percent required repeat surgery within five years of the hysterectomy. The most common complaint leading to reoperation was chronic pelvic and lower abdominal pain, affecting 77 percent of the women, and pain with intercourse, in 67 percent. Benign tumors were found in 23 percent, and malignancy was present in a surprisingly high 3 percent. Since the chance of developing cancer of the ovary is approximately 1 percent in women more than forty who have never undergone hysterectomy, 3 percent represents a significant increase.

Cancer of the retained ovary following hysterectomy has been studied by other groups, and many have found a significant potential for malignant change ranging from a fraction of a percent to as high as 11 percent. In a statistical analysis of ovarian cancer rates, one researcher calculated that prophylactic removal of the ovaries at the time of hysterectomy may save 3 patients from ovarian cancer out of every 10,000 hysterectomies performed. Dr. Larry McGowan of the George Washington University Medical Center reviewed the histories of forty-one women with ovarian cancer who had undergone previous hysterectomy. In his report, published in the March 1987 issue of *Obstetrics and Gynecology,* Dr. McGowan found that the interval between surgery and discovery of ovarian cancer was ten years for women with a previous vaginal hysterectomy and eighteen years if the procedure was performed abdominally. The most frightening statistic was that women who had retained their ovaries at hysterectomy had an 80 percent death rate if they developed cancer. This is far greater than the usually quoted rate of 50 to 60 percent for women without a previous hysterectomy.

Unfortunately, many women are fearful of taking hormonal replacement therapy postoperatively. The overwhelming evidence convincingly demonstrates that this form of therapy is a safe and efficient method of controlling premature menopausal symptoms. In the absence of the uterus, you need not fear the only potentially serious problem associated with this medication: cancer of the endometrium. Continuous use of estrogen without the balance of progesterone can cause cancerous endometrial changes. Estrogens taken either daily or cyclically, combined with medroxyprogesterone acetate (Provera) tablets for ten to twelve days each month should provide protection against osteoporosis, vaginal atrophy, and probably cardiovascular disease as well. The reason why Provera is given with the estrogen is that it is believed to eliminate totally any risk of breast cancer.

Can hysterectomy be performed for the combined purpose of abortion and sterilization?

I am both amazed and appalled by the number of gynecologists who recommend this hazardous combined procedure. One study of 200 women who underwent vaginal hysterectomy for the purpose of abortion clearly demonstrated the hazards inherent in the procedure. A significant postoperative temperature elevation was noted in 18 percent of the patients over a period of two days. If one includes those women with a temperature higher than 100.4°F for one day, then the number with postoperative fever soars to ninety-five, or almost half of the women in the study. In addition, three women required exploratory surgery, two suffered injury to the urinary bladder, and six experienced a significant blood loss of more than one and one-half units.

Dr. Harold Schulman of the Albert Einstein College of Medicine has stated: "It is difficult to understand extending minor procedures [suction abortion and laparoscopic tubal sterilization] into major operative procedures. If a physician's guiding principle is to do no harm, then the reason for this conversion from a minor procedure should be compelling." Dr. Schulman goes on to say that when a hysterectomy is substituted for a simple procedure, a doctor must inform you that he or she is recommending a procedure that increases your risk of dying at least twenty times.

Is hysterectomy at the time of cesarean section ever indicated?

Cesarean hysterectomy in the presence of an acute obstetrical emergency, such as uncontrolled hemorrhage or severe infection, is a valuable, life-saving procedure. However, when used as a means of sterilization at the time of a routine cesarean section, it is unwarranted. Several studies have demonstrated that tubal ligation is a far safer procedure. Even in the presence of coexisting conditions such as a fibroid uterus or carcinoma-in-situ of the cervix, many gynecologists prefer to delay hysterectomy until at least eight weeks after childbirth, when the uterus and its blood vessels are more normal in size.

As with vaginal hysterectomy, however, the advocates of cesarean hysterectomy continue to perform surgery in the face of overwhelming evidence demonstrating its hazards. Even in the best of hands, 20 percent of such patients will need a blood transfusion. In one study from Columbia-Prebysterian Medical Center, 116 of 165 women undergoing cesarean hysterectomy were transfused. Allergic reactions to transfused blood have in the past been responsible for the deaths of several patients, while the risk of hepatitis and AIDS from a contaminated unit of blood is always a threat.

A postoperative complication rate of 30 to 50 percent is not uncommon. Some of these complications are quite serious, such as damage to the urinary bladder and ureter, which carries urine from the kidney to the bladder. Severe pelvic infections have caused death in a small but significant number of women.

As Dr. Schulman says, the physician's guiding principle is to do no harm, but not all doctors seem to be aware of that very simple message. Otherwise, how could they in good conscience continue to use vaginal and cesarean hysterectomy as a method of sterilization? You must approach health care with the same "buyer beware" skepticism you display when obtaining other goods and services. As a consumer of health care services, you must educate yourself to be able to distinguish between treatment that is good, not good, and just plain deplorable.

11

THE FUTURE

While the lay public may envision scientists busily at work in their laboratories developing the perfect method of birth control, the sad truth is that a steady decline in funds spent worldwide for contraceptive and reproductive research since 1972 has made this scene all but imaginary. The lack of interest and financial support for contraceptive research projects in the United States has been attributed to a host of factors, including costly and time-consuming stringent government regulations, failure to offer attractive financial incentives for private investors and pharmaceutical companies to invest in research, and the difficulties of obtaining product liability insurance. Carl Djerassi, Ph.D., professor of chemistry at Stanford University and developer of the first oral contraceptive, decries the lack of progress in the field of contraceptive research as a "global tragedy," while Jeannie I. Rosoff, president of the Alan Guttmacher Institute, states that "none of the breakthroughs in contraceptive technology that seemed tantalizingly close a decade or more ago have come to market."

Of the many promising contraceptive ideas that I discussed in the first edition of *The Birth Control Book* in 1977, most have failed to achieve even a modicum of success and others have proven to be either impractical, inefficient, or too costly. Several pages of the last chapter of that book were devoted to discussing new, longer-lasting copper devices and other IUDs with exotic names like Ypsilon, Antigon-F, and Anderson Leaf. Since then, enthusiasm for IUD research has been dampened by the great number of lawsuits which have forced all but one manufacturer to withdraw their products from the market. Given the potential for lawsuits, it is unlikely that any manufacturer will be interested in marketing a new IUD in the United States in the near future.

In 1977 I wrote about the controversy surrounding the use of intramuscular injections of medroxyprogesterone acetate, or Depo-Provera, as a contraceptive. Today, the controversy is even more intense than it was in 1977. It is still prohibited in the United States to use Depo-Provera for this purpose, despite the fact that it enjoys great success in more than eighty countries throughout the world. Unfortunately, political rather than medical considerations have determined the fate of this excellent contraceptive.

Unfortunately, none of the projects on male contraception that I described in 1977 have reached fruition today. Despite previous optimistic predictions by scientists, safe and reversible oral contraception for men continues to be an elusive goal of researchers. A breakthrough may come through studies of drugs such as gossypol, LH agonists, and the recently isolated protein named inhibin. Even if these methods are developed satisfactorily, the most optimistic assessment is that it will take at least fifteen years before they will be widely available.

The definition of "the perfect contraceptive" is one that is 100 percent effective, reversible, free from side effects, and completely safe. The discovery of such a magic bullet remains as elusive today as it was ten and even twenty years ago. If funds available for contraceptive research continue their downward spiral, the next ten years may prove as fruitless as the past ten.

Though it seemed unlikely ten years ago, several European countries are now making significantly more rapid advances in contraceptive research than the United States. According to Dr. Djerassi, this is not surprising because "our emphasis on safety and avoidance of risk, coupled with the compulsively litigious character of American society, has had an enormous impact on the nature and scale of clinical work." If our policies remain unchanged, I would not be surprised to find financially able American women traveling abroad to receive the newest in contraceptive technology which will be unavailable in the United States.

Despite these drawbacks, there have been some exciting contraceptive breakthroughs. While the Depo-Provera battle rages, other highly effective long-acting progestational agents, such as the NORPLANT system, are being more favorably received. Compounds described as LH agonists and progesterone antagonists have become an integral part of the new contraceptive research vocabulary. In this chapter I will review some of the more ingenious and promising contraceptive projects.

BIRTH-CONTROL PILLS AND OTHER HORMONES FOR WOMEN

Are there any new and improved estrogens and progestins that will be available in the Pill in the future?

It is unlikely that we will see many new revelations concerning the currently available oral contraceptives over the next ten years. Most authorities believe that any further lowering of the ethinyl estradiol dose in today's birth-control pills below 0.025 to 0.030 milligrams will result in an unacceptably high frequency of breakthrough bleeding. Similar problems can also be anticipated if the total amount of progestin in each cycle is reduced any more than that contained in the new triphasic pills (see chapter 2). As scientists have learned more about oral contraceptives, they have become increasingly concerned about the progestins' capability of disturbing glucose tolerance and lipid metabolism and increasing a woman's risk of atherosclerosis and heart disease. For this reason, researchers are working to develop a safer progestin. Among the new progestins expected to have a salutory effect on serum lipids is *gestodene.* Scientists are impressed by the fact that gestodene's pharmacologic and biochemical characteristics are more similar to the natural hormone progesterone than to other progestins. In early clinical trials, gestodene has been found to increase levels of high-density lipoprotein cholesterol, or HDL-C, without changing those of low-density lipoprotein cholesterol (LDL-C; see chapter 2). This is an especially important benefit since low HDL-C concentrations and high LDL-C levels are associated with an increased risk of atherosclerosis and heart disease.

In other clinical studies of gestodene-containing triphasic birth-control pills, alterations in glucose and insulin metabolism have been either nonexistent or minimal. One study from Ireland compared concentrations of various clotting factors in the blood of women using a birth-control pill containing either gestodene or levonorgestrel. Researchers found that both progestins adversely altered the levels of several coagulation factors to a slight degree, but that one factor (VII) was more likely to be higher in the gestodene-treated group.

Since gestodene behaves as a more estrogen-dominant preparation than does levonorgestrel, it is less likely to cause other undesirable progestin side effects such as acne, weight gain, abnormal liver function, and hypertension. In one clinical trial of 700 women using a birth-control pill containing gestodene and ethinyl estradiol, there were no pregnancies and less than a 1 percent incidence of spotting or absence of mestrual flow while taking the Pill.

Cyproterone acetate is a new synthetic progestin that is closer in structure and function to natural progesterone than to the progestins in all currently available birth-control pills. Researchers believe that it will be less likely to be associated with unpleasant side effects, such as facial hair, acne, and oily skin. In a preliminary study reported in *Obstetrics and Gynecology* in 1987, researchers demonstrated that cyproterone acetate significantly lowered free testosterone levels in women with higher than normal amounts of this hormone in their body. As previously noted (see chapters 1 and 2), the male hormone testosterone is similar in structure to the progestins that are present in all currently available birth-control pills. It is these progestins that are responsible for some of the above-mentioned unpleasant side effects.

Attempts have been made to substitute the body's natural estrogens, estradiol and estriol, for the synthetic ethinyl estradiol found in most of today's birth-control pills. Estradiol is the most potent natural estrogen produced by the ovary, and it can also be extracted from soybeans. Though available for many years only as an injection, scientists have recently developed a method allowing it to be taken in pill form as well. Theoretically, use of pure estradiol in birth-control pills should almost completely eliminate the risk of abnormal clotting and thromboembolism and changes in liver function (see chapter 2). In a Swedish study of more than 200 women treated with either standard birth-control pills or ones with estradiol, doctors found them to be equal in contraceptive efficacy. The main reason cited for stopping the estradiol-containing pill was breakthrough bleeding.

Is there any other oral contraceptive research that appears promising?

Doctors in Edinburgh, Scotland, have studied the effects of administering a standard combination birth-control pill in cycles of eighty-four consecutive days followed by six days off to allow withdrawal bleeding. The obvious advantage of this method is to reduce the number of periods to four per year. In their report, published in *The British Medical Journal,* they treated 200 volunteers in this manner and noted that the overwhelming majority were enthusiastic in their response. The less frequent periods, fewer menstrual problems, and easier pill-taking regimen were cited as the most appealing aspects of taking birth-control pills in this manner. On the negative side, the main objection was excessive weight gain, with ninety women, or 45 percent, reporting a weight gain of over four pounds. Though breakthrough bleeding was the second most common complaint, it tended to improve after the first cycle of pills.

In research sponsored by the Center for Population Research, doctors are trying to perfect a birth-control pill containing a slow-release estrogen-progestin combination that can be taken less often than once a day. Much research remains before such a pill will become a reality.

What is Depo-Provera and how effective is it as a contraceptive?

Provera is the popular trade name for a synthetic derivative of progesterone named medroxyprogesterone acetate. It is hormonally active when given orally or intramuscularly, but when used as an intramuscular injection it is called *Depo-Provera.* Innumerable studies and worldwide clinical experience since 1963 has demonstrated that Depo-Provera is a potent, safe, and extremely effective contraceptive. When 150 milligrams is injected intramuscularly every three months, it successfully prevents pregnancy in 99.5 to 100 percent of all women who use it. It has also been demonstrated that a 300-milligram dose, given every six months, is capable of keeping a pregnancy rate down to 1.73 per 100 woman-years.

Depo-Provera is similar in chemical structure to progesterone and therefore produces very few of the unpleasant side effects associated with the estrogens and progestins found in birth-control pills (see chapter 2). Contraception is achieved by Depo-Provera's effect on the hypothalamus, preventing its release of those factors necessary for stimulating ovulation. In addition, medroxyprogesterone acetate alters the cervical mucus and inactivates the glands of the endometrium so that they are incapable of receiving an egg. Unfortunately, these beneficial effects are also its major drawbacks, since prolonged absence of ovulation and menstruation may occur in as many as 70 percent of women who use Depo-Provera. One year after the injections are stopped, 25 percent of previously fertile women remain infertile, and many women do not experience a return of menses for a year or more. Though it is believed that these effects are not permanent, Depo-Provera is far too powerful a drug to use on individuals who may want to conceive at a later date. For the woman who has completed her childbearing, however, it is unmatched for safety and efficacy.

Why isn't Depo-Provera approved for use by the FDA?

Though the drug is currently being used as an effective contraceptive by 2 million women in more than eighty countries throughout the world, including Sweden, the United Kingdom, and Canada, at the present time it is not approved by the FDA for this purpose. Despite scientific evidence attesting to its safety, powerful lobbying groups have successfully kept it off the market while less promising hormonal preparations have been enthusiastically supported. Over the past ten years, whenever the FDA has appeared ready to signal its approval for Depo-Provera, another baseless and unscientific claim has hindered its progress. Even though millions of women have taken Depo-Provera over the past twenty years, no deaths have ever been attributed to its use. This undoubtedly makes it safer than either the Pill or the IUD.

Dr. Elizabeth B. Connell, former head of Planned Parenthood and professor of gynecology at Emory University School of Medicine, has probably said it best: "It's a national disgrace that we don't have [Depo-Provera] here. The Food and Drug Administration has bowed to political pressures and has not given sufficient credence to the scientific information."

Is there a relationship between Depo-Provera and cancer?

In the past, the FDA reversed its decision to approve Depo-Provera because of claims that women who were treated with it had a higher incidence of cervical cancer. Based on current knowledge about cervical cancer (see chapter 2), most authorities agree that Depo-Provera does not adversely influence this disease. Epidemiologists have amassed convincing evidence that cancer of the cervix is truly a venereal condition related to both early age of first coitus and exposure to multiple sexual partners. The most likely culprit is a strain of the human papilloma virus (HPV; see chapter 2). The invasive, potentially deadly, form of cervical cancer does not suddenly appear, but progresses slowly over several years from a microscopic precancerous condition called *dysplasia* to a harmless form of cancer limited to the upper layers of the cells within the cervix and known as *carcinoma-in-situ.* Often there is a ten-year hiatus between the development of carcinoma-in-situ and invasive cancer, though in many cases the disease never progresses beyond the in-situ stage. Doctors who criticize the Depo-Provera–cervical cancer link point out that in the study influencing the FDA to reject the drug, it was given for so brief a period of time that it would be impossible for it to have produced the spectrum of change from dysplasia to cancer, which usually takes several years. In addition, women have been treated with a host of other progestins and birth-control pills for many years without any apparent epidemic of cervical cancer.

It has also been stated that Depo-Provera may cause endometrial cancer. The basis for this statement is one flawed study involving ten monkeys who were given fifty times the normal human dose of Depo-Provera over a period of ten years. Two of these animals developed cancer. But twenty other monkeys who had received lower doses of the drug experienced no evidence of malignancy. A subsequent review found no relationship between Depo-Provera and endometrial cancer, and indeed any claim to the contrary seems ludicrous in view of the fact that Depo-Provera has been approved by the FDA as *treatment* for advanced stages of endometrial cancer, a disease known to be estrogen-dependent. Very high doses decrease the size of these cancers in as many as one out of every three patients with advanced disease. When Depo-Provera is given as a monthly intramuscular injection over a period of six months to a woman with precancerous, microscopic overgrowth of the endometrial glands (hyperplasia), the disease process can be totally reversed. This hardly speaks in favor of the theory that Depo-Provera is an endometrial cancer–causing agent. Depo-Provera has also been used extensively in treating a variety of medical and hormonal conditions in both very young and old women without any reported increase in cervical cancer rates.

Beagle dogs treated with very high doses of Depo-Provera have had an increased incidence of benign and malignant breast tumors. This bit of information has been one of the leading arguments against its approval by the FDA as a contraceptive agent, despite the fact that several studies in humans have not confirmed such a relationship. Depo-Provera opponents neglect to point out that all beagles are unusually susceptible to breast tumors.

Epidemiologists at the Centers for Disease Control studied the rate of occurrence of breast, uterine, and ovarian cancer among 5,000 women who received Depo-Provera injections for contraception between 1967 and 1976. They were followed from four to thirteen years for a total of 40,000 woman-years of observation. Compared with a control group, the Depo-Provera users actually experienced a lower incidence of breast cancer and an equal risk of uterine and ovarian cancer.

Which women could benefit from using Depo-Provera?

Depo-Provera appears to be an excellent contraceptive for most women who have completed their childbearing and are unable or unwilling to use birth-control pills or to undergo permanent sterilization. Mentally handicapped women and women who are forgetful or unmotivated to use birth control conscientiously are ideal Depo-Provera candidates.

In addition to treating cancer of the endometrium, Depo-Provera has been successfully used in treating kidney cancer and endometriosis. It is also used to control heavy periods, often eliminating the need for hysterectomy. For some reason, Depo-Provera works remarkably well in relieving the hot flashes of the menopause, and, unlike estrogen, it is beneficial rather than harmful to the endometrium. Depo-Provera has also been used to halt premature breast development and menstruation in physically precocious young girls who would otherwise experience these phenomena prior to the age of eight. It has been used with limited success in preventing the premature closure of the long bones of young girls destined to be abnormally short. If given before the adolescent growth spurt, it may affect the ultimate adult height by as much as two inches.

What are the disadvantages of using Depo-Provera?

During the three months after the first injection, the majority of women experience bleeding between eight and thirty days of each thirty-day period. Thereafter, the incidence decreases significantly, so that most women experience no periods at all after the first twelve months. Following repeated injections, amenorrhea (the absence of periods) and infertility may remain up to eighteen months and occasionally longer. By eighteen months after the last Depo-Provera injection is given, the ability to achieve pregnancy is equal to that of former IUD and oral contraceptive users.

The absence of menses for prolonged periods of time affects individuals differently.

For those women with previously heavy and prolonged menses accompanied by painful cramps, their absence provides welcome relief. Many women who view the monthly menses as a sign that their reproductive system is healthy may understandably be concerned by the absence of periods. Others express concern that potentially harmful menstrual products are being retained in the uterus. It is important that those individuals be reassured that Depo-Provera prevents the formation of menstrual products by its action on the hypothalamus and endometrium. It is also comforting to know that normal menstrual function eventually returns in practically all women after stopping the Depo-Provera injections.

Some evidence suggests that Depo-Provera may alter results of a glucose tolerance test and also cause abnormalities in plasma insulin levels. In one study, 15 percent of women with a previously normal glucose tolerance test converted to an abnormal test after taking Depo-Provera. In addition, a significant number of diabetics need more insulin while they are using this medication. Though this would not contraindicate the use of Depo-Provera in women with a family or personal history of diabetes, such individuals would certainly have to be watched more closely for any changes in their insulin requirements.

Despite the fact that Depo-Provera does not contain estrogen, it is best not taken by individuals with a previous history of thrombophlebitis or thromboembolism (see chapter 2). Some evidence suggests that Depo-Provera causes a slowing or stagnation of blood flow to the extremities which makes thrombophlebitis more likely to occur.

Women who have a history of depression may sometimes have a recurrence of this problem when taking Depo-Provera. For a small number of women, the first signs of depression may occur while using this drug and it is best for them to discontinue its use. Loss of libido has also been reported with Depo-Provera.

Finally, practically all clinical studies to date have demonstrated a gradual increase in body weight among the majority of individuals who receive Depo-Provera injections. The weight gain may vary from two to twenty pounds, and tends to increase with longer use.

What is the NORPLANT system of birth control?

The NORPLANT subdermal implant system consists of six Silastic rod-shaped capsules, each a little more than 1 inch in length and 0.1 inch in diameter, containing 36 milligrams of the synthetic progestin levonorgestrel (see figure 11-1). The rods are implanted just under the skin of the upper arm under local anesthesia, and the total of 216 milligrams is slowly released in daily increments of 30 micrograms over a period of approximately five years. This daily dose is significantly less than the 50 to 100 micrograms released from levonorgestrel-containing birth-control pills such as Levlen and Nordette. Consequently, it causes no adverse effects on lipoproteins, glucose tolerance, or blood pressure.

Another NORPLANT prototype, named NORPLANT-2, contains two slightly larger subdermal rods, each containing greater amounts of levonorgestrel. Both NORPLANT systems are undergoing clinical testing by the Population Council. Of all reversible hormonal contraceptives presently being studied, the NORPLANT system is deemed the most likely to succeed and to be available to American women within the next two to three years. It is currently being marketed in several countries, including China, Finland, Sweden, Great Britain, and Thailand. To date, the NORPLANT system has been tested successfully in more than 15,000 women worldwide.

The levonorgestrel released from the NORPLANT capsule prevents ovulation in 60 percent of all menstrual cycles. Even when ovulation does occur, pregnancy is highly unlikely because levonorgestrel also thickens the cervical mucus, making it impenetrable to sperm, and alters the endometrium so that a fertilized egg is incapable of implanting. In fact, NORPLANT's pregnancy-preventing capability is better than that of the IUD, and probably more effective than birth-control pills because it

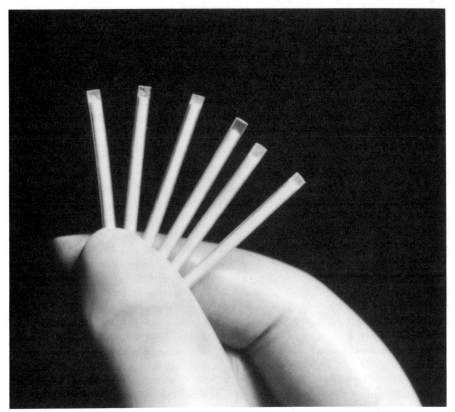

Figure 11–1. *NORPLANT subdermal implant system.*

eliminates the occasional pregnancy resulting from forgetting to take the Pill. In studies of women using the NORPLANT system for five years, pregnancy rates have been an impressive 0.2 to 0.5 per 100 woman-years for the first three years, and 1 to 2 per 100 woman-years during the fourth and fifth years of use. Unlike Depo-Provera, restoration of fertility is rapidly achieved once the capsules are removed. It should be noted that this minor surgical procedure is more difficult than the insertion, because scar tissue often forms around the capsules after they have been below the skin for a period of time.

The NORPLANT system has been particularly well received by women seeking an effective, reversible, long-term method of contraception. It is an excellent alternative to permanent sterilization. Unlike the birth-control pill, it can be used by women over thirty-five years of age, smokers, and those unable to tolerate the side effects and complications associated with the estrogen and progestin in combination birth-control pills. NORPLANT's advantage over the progestin-only Minipill is its significantly lower pregnancy rate (see Minipill, page 31). Though the cost of the NORPLANT device itself and for its insertion and removal every five years has not been determined, it will probably cost significantly less than the monthly use of birth-control pills over this period of time.

The main disadvantage of the NORPLANT system is the high incidence of menstrual irregularities and the persistent spotting it produces. About 60 percent of women report irregular bleeding, characterized by longer periods and longer intervals between periods. During the first year, 44 percent experience at least one episode of bleeding lasting eight or more days, and 15 percent report at least one of fifteen or more days. By the third year these percentages fall to 24 percent and 7 percent, respectively. Approximately 25 percent of NORPLANT users report at least one episode of going for three months or more without bleeding. Of those who elect to discontinue this method of contraception, 90 percent do so because of some derangement in their menstrual cycles, and another 10 percent because of complaints concerning progestin-related side effects such as changes in libido, weight gain, acne, depression, headache, and nausea. The incidence of infection at the implantation site has been reported to occur at a rate of 0.5 percent, though some studies have noted it to be as high as 1.3 percent or as low as 0.1 percent.

What are vaginal contraceptive rings and how effective are they in preventing pregnancy?

A Silastic vaginal ring, to which a variety of long-acting progestins either alone or in combination with estrogens has been added, has achieved encouraging results. It is inserted into the vagina on the fifth day of the menstrual cycle and removed on the twenty-sixth day. Following removal of the ring, menstruation will occur within a few days and the ring can be used for up to six months before needing to be replaced. The experimental rings used to date have had a diameter ranging between 50 and 58 millimeters, slightly smaller than the average diaphragm size of 70 millimeters. Insertion is identical to that of the diaphragm (see chapter 4), though the technique does not have to be as precise. Contraception is achieved by slow release of the hormones through the vaginal wall directly into the bloodstream. When estrogens and progestins are combined in the ring, ovulation is more likely to be inhibited. When progestins are used alone, contraception is achieved by retarding endometrial development, thereby preventing implantation of the fertilized egg. In addition, the progestin thickens the cervical mucus and makes it impenetrable to sperm. One great advantage of the contraceptive ring over the diaphragm is that if it is uncomfortable, it can be removed before intercourse without any loss of protection, provided it is replaced soon afterward.

Worldwide clinical trials with the vaginal contraceptive ring over the past fifteen years have demonstrated that the greatest contraceptive efficacy and the least likelihood of side effects are achieved with rings containing the natural estrogen estradiol and the progestin levonorgestrel. Pregnancy rates have been reported at less than 2 percent after two years of use with this device. In addition, the total amount of estrogen and progestin released into the bloodstream each day is less than that of the lowest oral contraceptive formulations. The use of the natural hormone estradiol in the vaginal contraceptive ring, rather than the synthetic ethinyl estradiol and mestranol present in birth-control pills, is believed to have beneficial effects on blood coagulation and hypertension. In addition, the direct absorption of the estrogen from the ring into the bloodstream bypasses the liver and the activation of some of its proteins, globulins, and enzymes which are believed to be responsible for initiating adverse Pill effects such as blood clotting abnormalities, hypertension, stroke, and heart attack. Several clinical trials have found no changes in blood pressure, glucose tolerance, cholesterol, or triglyceride levels in women using the vaginal contraceptive ring over a period of several months.

In a 1980 study from the University of Southern California School of Medicine, Dr. Subir Roy and his associates measured blood levels of angiotensinogen, a substance produced by the liver. It is theorized that the development of hypertension among some Pill users is the result of an estrogen-stimulated increase in angiotensinogen production. Dr. Roy found that even with low-dose estrogen formulation birth-control pills, angiotensinogen levels still increased threefold in some women. In contrast, those wearing vaginal contraceptive rings showed no increase in angiotensinogen and a decrease in triglyceride levels.

The University of Southern California researchers also noted that antithrombin III levels remained within normal limits among women wearing vaginal contraceptive rings. (Antithrombin III is responsible for preventing a rise in blood clotting factors which can precipitate thrombophlebitis and embolus formation; see chapter 2). In contrast, it is known that women using birth-control pills are more likely to demonstrate a decline of antithrombin III.

In addition to these medical benefits, investigators have found that the vaginal contraceptive ring may eliminate some of the side effects associated with oral contraceptive use, such as nausea, dizziness, and headaches.

Despite the many positive aspects of the vaginal contraceptive ring, it does have some serious disadvantages. In all clinical studies to date, menstrual problems have been cited as the main reason why women discontinue this method. Irregular bleeding, bleeding between periods, and failure to bleed during the week the ring is removed have been reported to occur in 7 to 26 percent of vaginal-contraceptive-ring cycles. Some women have also abandoned use of the ring because of levonorgestrel-related side effects such as acne, vaginitis, irritability, depression, increase in body hair, and, in one study, an average weight gain of three pounds.

One potentially serious side effect of the vaginal contraceptive ring is that 3 to 6 percent of wearers show areas of irritation and even ulcerations of their vaginal walls caused by pressure of the ring over a period of many days. In view of the fact that toxic shock syndrome—TSS—has been reported to occur with tampons, diaphragms, and the TODAY contraceptive sponge, which are all left in the vagina for much shorter periods of time, I have serious concerns about the possibility of TSS occurring among vaginal contraceptive ring users. The fact that no statistics have been reported to date may be only because too few women have worn the device for the condition to have become statistically significant.

Are there other promising hormonal contraceptives?

Long-acting intramuscular injections of progestins such as levonorgestrel and deladroxate are being tested in several countries by the World Health Organization. Comparative studies of these hormones with Depo-Provera have shown no great advantages and possibly the disadvantage of a higher pregnancy rate. In an attempt to minimize the problems of breakthrough bleeding and menstrual irregularities, the World Health Organization is testing a new injectable preparation containing the progestin norethindrone enanthate (NET-EN) combined with the synthetic estrogen estradiol valerate. There is not yet enough data available to evaluate completely the effectiveness of this method, but in one clinical trial of 3,500 Mexican women, there were no pregnancies reported after twelve months. Unfortunately, 60 percent of the women discontinued the method mainly because of abnormal bleeding. Other groups have reported discontinuation rates of 70 percent or more.

Doctors in the department of endocrinology at the Medical College of Georgia have reported success with implanting crystalline pellets of estradiol subdermally (below the skin) in over 200 fertile volunteers. Withdrawal bleeding was brought on each month by giving them a progestin such as norethindrone orally for five to seven days. Of the 234 women completing a total of more than 6,000 menstrual cycles, only two pregnancies occurred. This represents a contraceptive effectiveness of 0.37 unintended pregnancies per 100 woman-years. Side effects, which usually subsided after the first cycle, included heavy periods, bleeding between periods, and headache. Unlike the prolonged effects of Depo-Provera, spontaneous ovulation usually returned soon after the estradiol pellets were removed.

While all of these injectable hormone preparations provide excellent contraception, they remain inferior to implant systems such as NORPLANT because they require injections every few months in order to maintain sufficient hormone levels in the bloodstream. In addition, abnormal bleeding patterns continue to be the main deterrent to their continued use.

There is no doubt that the thrust of research efforts over the next decade will be in developing hormone implant systems with the contraceptive efficacy of NOR-PLANT but without its unpleasant side effects and the difficulties associated with its insertion and removal. To avoid the minor surgery involved in inserting and removing progestin rods or capsules, scientists have devised a variety of biodegradable subdermal implants which can release progestins over a specific period of time and then completely dissolve within the body. Currently being evaluated are microcapsules made from biodegradable polymers containing tiny micronized crystals of levonorgestrel and norethisterone. Particle sizes of the hormone are less than 200 micrometers, and the rate and amount of progestin released is determined by the size and number of micronized progestin crystals as well as the size and composition of the polymer that contains them.

To assure complete biodegradability of these systems, the progestins are attached to naturally metabolized substances such as lactic acid and various natural amino acids. Population Council researchers have fused norgestrel and norethindrone with a small amount of pure cholesterol to ensure total biodegradability, while Dynatech Research Corporation has developed a levonorgestrel-containing biodegradable implant that has a release duration of approximately eight years. It contains 90 percent lactide and 10 percent glycolide blended with 50 percent levonorgestrel.

Scientists at the University of Alabama in Birmingham are working on a six-month norethisterone-release system consisting of the biodegradable polymer DL-polylactic acid, in which micronized crystals of norethisterone are dispersed homogeneously. Ninety-day and six-month slow-release systems are now undergoing clinical testing.

Researchers at the Center for Population Research have developed a levonorgestrel implant system similar to NORPLANT but not requiring surgical removal. Instead of silicon rubber containers, tiny crystals of levonorgestrel are placed in polycaprolactone (Capronor) tubes, which are implanted below the skin with a trocar or large needle. Levonorgestrel is then released by membrane diffusion for up to two years. After that time, the polycaprolactone is absorbed over another one to two years, making surgical removal unnecessary. Other formulations containing 30, 90, and 180 days of levonorgestrel release are also being evaluated. Studies suggest that the daily amount of hormone needed to exert a contraceptive effect is only one-tenth that of the levonorgestrel in the currently available birth-control pills.

A third biodegradable system relies on suspending micronized crystals of norethisterone or levonorgestrel in a matrix of a new biodegradable polymer named Alzamer. Developed by the Alza Corporation, which introduced and manufactures the Progestasert IUD (see chapter 3), Alzamer is eroded by the body tissues it comes in contact with at a specific time and at a predictable rate. The most popular prototype currently being tested is composed of 20 percent micronized norethisterone and 10 percent buffer suspended in a matrix of Alzamer in a 14-millimeter by 3-millimeter biodegradable rod. Researchers have found that fairly constant plasma levels of the drug can be maintained for four to six months.

Preliminary testing has been carried out on snugly fitting Silastic contraceptive bracelets. Progestins contained in the bracelet are absorbed directly into the bloodstream through the skin. Experiments have been conducted with three different progestins and two different types of Silastic bracelets. The main problem with this system to date has been in designing a bracelet that can provide a constant rate of progestin release into the body over a prolonged period of time.

How successful is danazol as a contraceptive?

Danazol (trade name: Danocrine) is a synthetic hormonal preparation similar in structure to the progestins. Used with great success in the treatment of endometriosis (see chapter 1) and chronic cystic mastitis of the breasts, preliminary data indicate that danazol may also be an effective contraceptive. It acts by preventing the release of FSH and LH from the pituitary gland, thereby preventing ovulation. Research on female rhesus monkeys at the University of Texas Health Science Center has also demonstrated that danazol decreases progesterone production by the corpus luteum, thereby preventing an adequate hormonal environment for the newly fertilized egg. Its potential for use will be among those women who can't tolerate estrogen-containing contraceptives and those with such conditions as fibrocystic disease of the breasts, varicose veins, and phlebitis.

Danazol is chemically similar to progestins, and thus the side effects it produces are also similar: weight gain, decrease in breast size, and *moniliasis,* an infection caused by a microscopic yeastlike organism. Symptoms of this condition are a white, cheesy vaginal discharge accompanied by severe itching of the external genital area (see chapter 2). Other less common danazol side effects are acne, oily skin, voice changes, decreased libido, an increase of hair growth on the extremities and the face, edema (fluid retention), and breakthrough bleeding. At the present time, danazol has FDA approval only for use in treating endometriosis, not for use as a contraceptive.

What alternatives to the Pill are there for the woman who has difficulty swallowing pills and tablets?

Though oral contraceptives do not come in liquid form, the next best thing is now undergoing clinical trials in England: chewable paper contraceptives, identical in appearance to a sheet of stamps. The stamps are made of cellulose impregnated with estrogen and a progestin, and they have a taste similar to rice. At the present time they are not available in the United States.

Even at the lowest estrogen and progestin concentrations, a significant number of women discontinue oral contraceptive use because of nausea and other gastrointestinal complaints. In a 1982 report, published in *Fertility and Sterility,* doctors in Brazil instructed twelve volunteers to insert vaginally either one or two birth-control pills containing levonorgestrel and ethinyl estradiol (trade names: Levlen, Nordette) for twenty-one days followed by a week without pills. Of the four women who inserted one tablet daily, breakthrough bleeding was a common complaint, but for those using two tablets daily this was not a problem. All twelve women experienced withdrawal bleeding during the week off the Pill. Ovulation was suppressed regardless of whether a woman inserted one or two pills daily, and nausea bothered only one of the six women who had discontinued oral Pill use specifically for that reason. Obviously, the experience of these twelve women would not be sufficient evidence to endorse the vaginal use of oral contraceptives. However, there are currently thousands of women in this country who are using less effective methods of contraception because they are unable to tolerate birth-control pills in their present form. It is likely that further studies will be carried out to confirm or refute the efficacy and safety of the Pill when used in this manner.

What is RU-486 and how does it prevent pregnancy?

Of all the methods of contraception currently being researched, none promises to be as successful as *mifepristone,* or RU-486, named after its developer, the *R*oussel-*U*claf Company of France. This wondrous drug, similar in structure to the progestin norethindrone, can prevent pregnancy when used as a "morning-after pill" (see chapter 6, "Postcoital Contraception"), and can also abort most pregnancies of five weeks or less. Though RU-486 has been studied for only a short time, it has acquired a number of descriptive names such as the month-after pill, the menstrual induction pill, the abortion pill, the last-chance pill, the contragestational pill, and the menstrual regulator.

RU-486 is classified as a progesterone-blocker, meaning that it adheres to receptor cells in the endometrium of the uterus that under normal circumstances accept progesterone, the hormone that prepares the uterine lining each month to receive a fertilized egg. RU-486's affinity for the progesterone receptor is about five to eight times greater than it is for progesterone itself. Because the presence of RU-486 blocks the action of progesterone, the endometrium sloughs off, and the fertilized egg is expelled.

Ideally, in the future RU-486 will be used by women for two to three days during the second half of each menstrual cycle. Those who are not pregnant would simply menstruate normally, and any pregnancy that might have developed during the cycle will be unable to implant and will be passed out with the menstrual blood. Developers of RU-486 hope that if it is used conscientiously, it will make surgical abortion obsolete and will eliminate the need for currently used birth-control pills.

In one study, published in *The New England Journal of Medicine* in 1986, 100 women were treated with 400 to 800 milligrams of RU-486 for two to four days. All were within ten days of having missed their period, and sensitive pregnancy tests confirmed that they were pregnant. Within four days of starting the medication, 85 of the women aborted spontaneously while 15 required suction curettage to terminate the pregnancy. Though 18 reported heavy bleeding, none required a transfusion or any medication to stop it. Of those who aborted, 25 percent noted painful uterine contractions, while a similar amount complained of nausea and fatigue. Other clinical studies have concluded that heavy uterine bleeding may be more of a problem than originally anticipated, especially when RU-486 is used to induce abortion rather than early menstruation. In a clinical trial of 700 women treated with RU-486 for pregnancy termination, 7 women required a blood transfusion. This potentially serious side effect would suggest that when RU-486 is used as an abortifacient, rather than as a morning-after pill, careful medical supervision and monitoring are necessary. The optimistic prophecy that RU-486 will allow a woman "to have an abortion in the privacy of your own home" appears unlikely at the present time.

In a Scandinavian study in which RU-486 was administered over a period of four days, followed by a "chaser dose" of prostaglandins (see prostaglandins) on the fourth day, the successful abortion rate for pregnancies of six weeks or less was 100 percent. As a result of this report and other similar studies, European researchers are attempting to devise a product that will contain a combination of RU-486 and prostaglandins, in order to more effectively induce early abortion without the unpleasant side effects usually associated with prostaglandins. Other investigators are working with intramuscular injections of RU-486 as well as tampons laced with RU-486. In one study, published in *Fertility and Sterility* in 1985, no pregnancies occurred when tampons containing RU-486 were inserted in eight monkeys postcoitally. In addition, pregnancy was terminated in five other monkeys who were treated within one week of their missed period.

One of the reasons RU-486 appears to cause so few side effects is that it remains in the body for less than forty-eight hours. It is known to block the body's cortisone receptors as well as its progesterone receptors, but no studies to date have noted abnormalities in adrenal gland function among women receiving RU-486. No information is yet available on what effect this drug might have on a fetus were it to fail to induce abortion in a woman and she chose to continue her pregnancy.

RU-486's efficacy is greatest during the first five weeks of pregnancy, because progesterone originates mostly from the corpus luteum of the ovary during this time and its levels are fairly low (see chapter 1). After the sixth week of pregnancy, implantation of the egg is better established and the placenta then starts to produce considerable amounts of its own progesterone. This is more difficult for RU-486 to block effectively. Nevertheless, it does show some promise as an adjunct in midtrimester abortions. When given for two consecutive days to forty-four women with an average pregnancy duration of twenty-three weeks, RU-486 consistently softened and dilated the cervix and produced uterine contractions, thereby facilitating the abortion procedure. Researchers have theorized that, in addition to its progesterone-blocking effect, RU-486 is responsible for the release of natural prostaglandins from the endometrium. It is the prostaglandins that then cause these changes to take place.

Though RU-486 is currently being marketed in France and Scandinavia, the drug's future in the United States is not certain. Anti-abortion activists have labeled it "chemical warfare against the unborn." Pharmaceutical companies are concerned that production of RU-486 may lead to boycotting of their other products. Promotion of RU-486 as a contraceptive rather than as an abortifacient is unlikely to make it acceptable in the eyes of anti-abortionists, since its mode of action is to destroy the fertilized egg. In addition, the painfully slow and conservative process of new drug approval by the FDA makes it highly unlikely that RU-486 will be available to American women within the next five years.

Is there a pregnancy hormone vaccine that can be used as a contraceptive for women?

Vaccination against pregnancy is a concept that has been investigated for more than twenty years. Despite occasional optimistic predictions by scientists that such a vaccine is just around the corner, a more realistic estimate is that, even under the best of circumstances, we are at least ten years away from this concept's becoming a reality.

The most intense laboratory research and clinical trials have involved the development of a vaccine derived from the pregnancy hormone named human chorionic gonadotropin, or HCG. HCG is produced by the placenta and is the most important hormone in early pregnancy. As mentioned in the preceding chapter, it is the elevated levels of this substance that are measured in the commonly performed urinary pregnancy tests. A fraction of HCG, called its beta-subunit, or B-HCG, is the basis for more specific and sensitive pregnancy tests being used by most modern laboratories. To create a pregnancy vaccine, scientists have purified the beta-subunit of HCG and then combined it with tetanus toxoid. When this combination of proteins or antigens is injected into a woman's body, it induces her immune system to form antibodies against it. If pregnancy occurs, the HCG antibodies will attack the B-HCG antigens formed during the first few days of pregnancy and abortion will ensue. To date, four clinical derivatives of B-HCG have been tested on laboratory animals and on a small number of women volunteers without any detectable disturbances in endocrine, metabolic, or organ functions. The researchers' goal is to create a vaccine that will provide effective contraception for one to three years, followed by a return of fertility as B-HCG antibody levels decline. If contraception is requested for longer periods of time, a simple booster vaccination in the final months of the contraceptive period would suffice.

Is it possible to develop a vaccine that would prevent pregnancy by altering the egg or the sperm?

Scientists have attempted to create a vaccine with specific protein antigens derived from a key element in either the female or male reproductive system. Depending on the antigen selected, circulating antibodies against it would then interfere with either ovulation, corpus luteum function, sperm formation or penetration of the egg, early implantation in the uterus, or maintenance of an early pregnancy.

The *zona pellucida* is a transparent glycoprotein protective coating or shell surrounding the follicle (unfertilized egg) that forms in the ovary each month. Under normal conditions, sperm attach to binding sites in the zona pellucida during the early stages of fertilization. Researchers have found that if an extract of zona pellucida is injected into a woman, she will produce antibodies to block fertilization at sperm binding sites by inducing the formation of a precipitate on the outer surface of the zona pellucida. Research on experimental animals has been encouraging, but much more work remains in order to be sure that such a vaccine would not cause irreparable damage to the ovary.

Research to create a vaccine for men or women from one of several sperm proteins remains at the clinical testing stage. New laboratory techniques have enabled scientists to identify proteins or antigens from specific points, or loci, on the sperm. Lactic acid dehydrogenase C4, or LDH-C4, is the most promising sperm antigen isolated to date. Experimental immunization of female mice, rats, and rabbits with LDH-C4 has reduced fertility by as much as 50 to 75 percent in the animals studied. In addition, the circulating LDH-C4 antibodies are capable of reacting with human LDH-C4 antigen. As with the HCG vaccine (see previous question), however, antibody levels remain unpredictable, making immunization of humans only a distant possibility.

Hyaluronidase is a protein enzyme that has been purified from spermatozoa of birds, cattle, and rabbits. Antibodies to rabbit sperm hyaluronidase have been shown to immobilize and destroy sperm. *Acrosin* is another sperm enzyme which, when injected as a foreign protein, has produced successful antibody formation in both sheep and humans. Researchers are encouraged by preliminary experiments on female sheep showing marked reduction in fertility following injection with purified ram acrosin. Numerous other sperm antigens are under investigation. Most of these vaccines have not been shown to be very effective and have not yet approached the stage where they are ready for widespread testing on humans.

What is an intracervical device?

Unlike the intrauterine device, or IUD, which is placed in the uterine cavity, the *intracervical device,* or ICD, is placed inside the cervical canal. Current interest in intracervical devices by scientists has been stimulated by the need to reduce the incidence of heavy uterine bleeding and pelvic infection associated with intrauterine devices.

While the intracervical device is considered a new and experimental method of contraception, it was actually one of the most popular methods of birth control in the United States at the end of the nineteenth century. At that time, ICDs came in a variety of shapes and were fashioned from wood, leather, glass, metal, and rubber. But by the beginning of the twentieth century, interest in intracervical devices waned because of a high incidence of pelvic infection associated with their use.

Though several Silastic intracervical devices have undergone testing, there is currently no device that appears likely to undergo extensive clinical trials in the near future. Some common problems with ICDs have been difficulty in inserting them, high rates of cramping and discomfort, abnormal bleeding, and unacceptably high expulsion rates.

Most ICDs are designed to block mechanically the ascent of sperm into the endometrial cavity. One device undergoing testing at Wayne State University School of Medicine employs a different concept. It consists of a hollow cylinder filled with a progestin and attached to a pair of plastic horns which extend upward into the endometrium to hold it in place. Though the cylinder fits snugly into the cervix, it is not designed to block the ascent of sperm. Instead, the slowly released progestin thickens the cervical mucus (see chapters 1, 2, and 5), making it impenetrable to sperm. To date, the main problems encountered with this ICD have been spotting, breakthrough bleeding, and expulsion of the device.

An even more ingenious ICD has been designed by a team of researchers at the Women's Medical Pavilion in Dobbs Ferry, New York. It consists of a cylindrical intracervical implant three-quarters of an inch long and one-quarter of an inch in diameter connected by wires to a tiny three-volt lithium carbon monofluoride coin cell. This creates a weak electrical field in the cervical mucus which immobilizes sperm by generating a weak current across the cervical canal. The charge created is imperceptible to the woman using the device. The mechanism by which the electricity immobilizes the sperm remains a puzzle, but the inventors of the device theorize that the weak electric field interferes with the normal electrical polarity of the sperm tails. Even after the electric field is turned off, the sperm remain immobile once they have been electrically charged. This gynecological equivalent of an electrified contraceptive fence has been tested successfully in laboratory monkeys and on semen specimens in the laboratory, but must undergo redesign and extensive investigation before it will be ready for testing in humans. One obstacle to its success is that the lifetime of the coin battery used in this preliminary testing is only forty-eight hours. A battery capable of lasting several months must be developed if the device is to be successful. The electricity used in the device is at an extremely safe level, and the current generated is considerably less than a person would experience when wearing a pacemaker.

IUDS

Are there any new methods of prolonging the contraceptive effectiveness of IUDs?

Despite the fear and reluctance of manufacturers to introduce new IUDs (see chapter 3), some interesting improvements in design and function should make future devices more effective and acceptable. Even though there have been recent setbacks for all IUDs except the Progestasert, the appeal continues to be strong for this unique method of contraception that requires one simple insertion procedure and subsequently provides years of relatively safe protection from pregnancy.

Much of the current IUD research has centered around prolonging the amount of time that the device can safely be left in the uterine cavity while effectively preventing pregnancy. The Population Council is now testing two IUDs that contain copper in the form of sleeves, rather than as wound wire as in the Copper-7 and Tatum-T (see chapter 3). These new devices are more solid and less subject to erosion. It is estimated that they may be left in the uterus for at least six years, possibly as long as ten to fifteen years, and they are superior to the Copper-7 and Tatum-T devices in effectiveness, expulsion rates, and other characteristics. The more promising of these two new IUDs—the Copper-T 380, or TCu380-A—has a copper sleeve on each of the transverse arms of the T and a copper wire wrapped around the vertical arm. The other device, the Copper-T220, has five copper sleeves on the vertical arm of the T and one on each of the transverse arms. During one four-year study, the TCu380-A was found to yield a pregnancy rate about one-fourth that of the Tatum-T copper device, amounting to 0.5 to 1 pregnancy per 100 woman-years. Although this excellent device is available throughout the world, it cannot be obtained in the United States.

Another IUD, named the Multiload Copper 250, has been used successfully in many countries throughout the world. Developed in the Netherlands, the Multiload Copper 250 is a polyethylene device with flexible arms and a central stem wound with copper wire. The device conforms to the shape of the uterus and flexes with uterine contractions. In addition, it comes in three sizes: "short," for a uterus with a length on uterine sounding (see chapter 3) of less than 6 centimeters; "mini," for a length from 6 to 7 centimeters; and "standard," for more than a 7-centimeter uterine cavity length. This device contains more copper than the older IUDs and provides better rates of contraceptive effectiveness. Extensive studies indicate that, despite the dissolution and the fragmentation of the copper wire after a period of time, the Multiload Copper 250 continues to maintain the same contraceptive efficacy even after five years of continuous use.

A significant amount of research has centered around prolonging the time that progesterone-containing IUDs can be left in the uterine cavity free of the risk of pregnancy. The present twelve-month limit of efficacy with the Progestasert device is its main drawback. A three-year version of this device is currently undergoing clinical trials. Scientists at the Population Council have evaluated several T-shaped Silastic IUDs that slowly release progestins and retain contraceptive effectiveness for up to seven years. Though the progestins d-norgestrel and norethisterone have been tested, levonorgestrel (see chapter 2 and NORPLANT, this chapter) appears to be the most promising. In addition to its contraceptive efficacy, the levonorgestrel-containing device is associated with less uterine bleeding problems and may also afford some protection against PID (pelvic inflammatory disease; see chapter 2) by its hormonal effect of thickening the cervical secretions and making them less permeable to pathologic bacteria that cause gonorrhea and chlamydia. The most popular levonorgestrel-containing IUD tested to date releases 30 micrograms of the hormone every twenty-four hours from the vertical arm of a Silastic T-shaped device. In studies involving thousands of women, results have been no less than sensational, as demonstrated in the following table.

CLINICAL PERFORMANCE OF THE
LEVONORGESTREL-RELEASING IUD

Reasons for Discontinuing Use	*Net Rates for Two Years of Use (Based on 2,685 Woman-Years of Use)*
Pregnancy	0.0
Expulsions	3.1
Complaints of pain or bleeding	10.4
Amenorrhea (cessation of menses)	13.8
Pelvic infections	0.0

SOURCE: *Compiled by the author.*

What research efforts have been made to reduce the incidence of tubal infection and PID associated with IUD use?

The threat of tubal infection, pelvic inflammatory disease, and subsequent infertility has been the main deterrent to the success of the IUD (see chapter 3). Most studies indicate that PID occurs in approximately 1 to 3 percent of women wearing IUDs, with higher rates for those who have never borne children and those with more than one sexual partner.

As discussed in the last question, the newer progestin-releasing IUDs offer protection against the ascent of pathologic bacteria into the cervical canal by thickening the cervical mucus. Some epidemiologists have theorized that the tail or strings of an IUD act as a mechanism for the transport of infectious organisms from the vagina and cervix to the endometrial cavity and fallopian tubes. This is especially likely during the first three to four months following insertion. To correct this problem, scientists are testing an iodine-treated fiber to replace the nylon tail string of current IUDs. The fiber, which can be made of either biodegradable or nonbiodegradable material, slowly releases iodine over a period of several months. Theoretically, the iodine would inhibit the growth and ascent of bacteria present in the cervix at the time of insertion. Extensive clinical trials are being carried out to determine whether this iodine-fiber combination reduces the incidence of infections.

Researchers in Japan have developed a tailless IUD, which is actually a newer version of an old stainless-steel device named the Grafenberg Ring. Though results are preliminary, it does not appear that the absence of an IUD tail will totally eliminate the risk of infection. In addition, tailless IUDs are more difficult and more painful to remove because they require the insertion of special instruments into the endometrium. Scientists have tried to develop a tailless device that can still be located and removed easily. One such effort, developed by gynecologists and engineers at Georgia Technical Institute in Atlanta, has resulted in a copper IUD with a magnetized cobalt component. The device permits precise location of the device within the uterus, and removal is accomplished with a specially designed viewing instrument placed into the cervix.

Even if the cervix is antiseptically prepared prior to insertion of an IUD, bacteria from within the cervix will always pass into the endometrium when the device is inserted. This was convincingly demonstrated in a 1986 research project published in *The American Journal of Obstetrics and Gynecology.* Doctors at the University of Calgary inserted both tailed and tailless IUDs into the uteri of experimental rabbits. Some of the IUDs were inserted in the standard fashion, through the cervix, while others were surgically placed directly into the uterine cavity via an abdominal incision. When the devices were removed one to eight weeks later, all of the vaginally inserted IUDs had been colonized with bacteria while none of those inserted abdominally contained bacteria. The scientists concluded that it is the method in which an IUD is inserted rather than the presence or absence of a tail that determines whether bacteria will invade the surface of an IUD. Though this study does not suggest that IUDs should be inserted abdominally, it does emphasize the difficulty in keeping them free of bacteria at the time they are inserted. The endometrium of most women is usually able to control bacterial reproduction and ward off infection, but a small percentage will continue to become infected. Scientists have suggested that these few individuals may be more susceptible than other women to endometrial and cervical immunologic deficiencies.

In laboratory studies, the copper in IUDs has been found to inhibit the growth of certain potentially harmful bacteria (see chapter 3). However, in actual practice, this effect is of no significance in reducing the incidence of PID associated with IUD use. Zinc can also stop bacterial growth, and has the additional advantage of inactivating the herpes virus. Scientists have proposed the development of a zinc-containing IUD as a possible method of reducing the number of infections associated with other devices.

Is it possible to design an IUD that can be inserted minutes after a woman gives birth?

Providing intrauterine contraception immediately following delivery is an extremely appealing concept; however, in actual practice it is difficult to accomplish. The main problem associated with insertion of an IUD in the immediate postpartum period has been unacceptably high expulsion rates, reported to be three times more frequent than when the device is inserted during the menstrual cycle. In a 1980 World Health Organization study in which a variety of IUDs were inserted immediately postpartum, expulsion rates by six months after insertion ranged from 31 to 41 per 100 women. This is not surprising in view of the fact that the uterine muscles contract and the size of the endometrial cavity is drastically reduced in the eight weeks following childbirth.

To improve these statistics, doctors at Family Health International have created the Delta Loop and Delta T IUDs. These are actually modifications of the Lippes Loop D and Tatum-T devices, with the addition of biodegradable catgut suture knots to the superior loop and the horizontal arm of the respective devices. The Delta Loop has three knots while the Delta T has two; their purpose is to allow the device to adhere to the walls of the endometrium in an enlarged postpartum uterus (see figures 11-2).

Developers of these two devices had hoped that by the time the catgut disintegrated, the uterus would have decreased in size and would be less likely to expel the IUD—but this has not been the case. Other investigators have fashioned a T-shaped device with molded plastic projections with the hope of bracing the IUD against the walls of the endometrium to hold it in place. Once again, this has proved less than ideal. While these devices are theoretically sound in concept and design, they have performed disappointingly in clinical practice. Among over 1,200 women who had the Delta Loop inserted within ten minutes after delivery of the placenta, expulsion rates after six months were an unacceptably high 23 per 100 devices. Delaying insertion of the device from ten minutes to thirty-six hours following delivery only increased expulsion rates at six months to 37 per 100. The Delta T did not fare much better among the 438 women tested with it. When inserted within ten minutes of delivery, expulsion rates were 17 per 100, rising to 31 per 100 when insertion was delayed for longer than ten minutes. Unfortunately, when expulsion rates for the Delta Loop and Delta T were compared with those of the standard Lippes Loop and Tatum-T, there were no differences noted.

The most important factor in determining the likelihood of expulsion of an IUD is whether the device is placed high enough into the enlarged postpartum endometrial cavity. Special long IUD inserters have been designed in an attempt to accomplish this more easily (see figure 11-2).

The insertion of an IUD increases endometrial production and release of prostaglandins (see prostaglandins). The effect of prostaglandins on uterine contraction and IUD expulsion remains unknown, but it appears that the cramping some women experience is directly related to attempts by the uterus to expel the IUD. Clinical studies are now under way to determine whether postpartum IUD expulsion rates can be reduced by treating women with prostaglandin inhibitors, such as ibuprofen (Motrin) and naproxen (Naprosyn and Anaprox), before and after an IUD is inserted. Scientists have also been exploring the possibility of attaching prostaglandin inhibitors to an IUD to be slowly released over a period of time and to keep endometrial prostaglandins at low levels.

What other IUD innovations can we expect to see in the future?

Approximately 15 percent of all IUD users have their devices removed because of heavy uterine bleeding. Various researchers have attempted to solve this problem by equipping IUDs with Silastic capsules that release *antifibrinolytic* agents, which are chemicals that prevent the rapid breakdown of blood clotting products and subsequent hemorrhage. The most frequently tested of these products has been ethylene aminocaproic acid (EACA) and tranexamic acid (AMCA). Although the majority of reports conclude that these substances do reduce excessive menstrual bleeding, it is difficult to produce a capsule or an IUD that can contain sufficient quantities of the drug to allow months or years of antifibrinolytic activity.

As noted in chapter 3 and earlier in this chapter, prostaglandin inhibitors help to decrease the incidence of uterine cramps associated with use of the IUD. Several studies have demonstrated their value in decreasing menstrual blood loss as well. In one study, women wearing IUDs were given mefenamic acid (trade name: Ponstel) at a dose of 500 milligrams three times a day for seven to ten days, beginning on the first day of menstruation. The blood loss of the women studied fell from an average of 162 and 128 millimeters in the two pre-drug cycles, to 49 and 80 milliliters during the treatment cycles. Other antiprostaglandins have produced similarly impressive results. Scientists are thus exploring the possibility of introducing antiprostaglandins into or alongside IUDs. If successful, this would allow continuous, slow release of these medications over a period of months or years and obviate the need for oral antiprostaglandin medications with each period.

Other treatments to reduce blood loss attributed to the IUD have included high doses of vitamin C and the intrauterine instillation of coagulants. In one study of fifty-four women complaining of heavy uterine bleeding with the Copper-7, the length

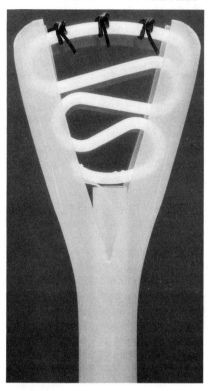

Figure 11–2. *Delta loop in special inserter.*

of periods was reduced by 50 percent following two instillations of coagulants such as tranexamic acid and apotinin.

Scientists are also working to develop more effective IUD contraception by incorporating chemical agents that interfere with specific sperm enzymes such as acrosin and hyaluronidase (see vaccines). IUDs with antibodies to progesterone receptors and to the pregnancy hormone HCG have also been suggested as possibilities.

One T-shaped IUD being studied contains pellets of quinacrine hydrochloride attached to its transverse arms. This drug, once used to treat malaria, is released from the IUD over a period of several days and promotes the formation of scar tissue and permanent closure of the tubes and their site of entry into the uterine cavity. In a recent clinical study, seventeen of twenty-three women volunteers experienced total closure of the tubes three weeks after receiving a quinacrine-releasing IUD. Quinacrine hydrochloride and other similar drugs are called *sclerosing agents* because of their ability to form scar tissue.

Following exposure to a sclerosing agent, the tubes can be examined with a hysteroscope, a viewing instrument inserted through the cervix (see hysteroscopy), to be sure that they are totally occluded. If complete tubal occlusion has not been accomplished, the IUD still provides contraception until another quinacrine-containing device can be inserted. Currently, this method has been 90 to 95 percent effective, but there are concerns that incomplete tubal closure could increase the risk of a life-threatening ectopic pregnancy. Another concern to be resolved before the method can become widely available is the safety of quinacrine hydrochloride used in this fashion. Adverse central nervous system reactions have been reported when large amounts of the drug have inadvertently entered the general circulation. Though much research remains to be done, there are potentially great advantages to perfecting this nonsurgical, relatively painless, and inexpensive method of tubal occlusion.

BARRIER CONTRACEPTION

Are there any new and improved methods of barrier contraception?

Clinical trials on several new spermicidal agents, notably benzalkonium chloride and menfegol, are under way. *Menfegol* is manufactured in Japan and Europe as a foaming vaginal tablet named Neo Sampoon. Extensive experience with this agent has shown pregnancy rates equal to the popular spermicide nonoxynol-9, but it is believed to be less irritating to vaginal and penile tissues. *Gossypol* is a promising male oral contraceptive developed in China (see gossypol, this chapter) which has recently received great publicity in the United States. Scientists have found that gossypol has a direct sperm-inactivating effect on contact, suggesting future use as a vaginal spermicide. Other researchers are attempting to develop a spermicide consisting of agents that attack sperm enzymes and proteins (see vaccines, this chapter). Other spermicides with chemicals capable of killing the bacteria that cause gonorrhea and chlamydia are also being tested.

Propranolol hydrochloride (trade name: Inderol) is an extremely popular drug used in the treatment of hypertension, cardiac arrhythmias, and migraine. In a 1983 article, published in *The British Medical Journal,* doctors at Family Health International in North Carolina reported that propranolol appears to be an effective vaginal contraceptive. They instructed 198 fertile women to insert one 80-milligram propranolol tablet into the vagina every evening from the last day of menstruation until the first day of the next menstrual period, over a span of eleven months. Five women conceived, giving a pregnancy rate of 3.4 per 100 woman-years. This success rate is equal to if not better than that achieved with standard vaginal spermicides. Tests indicated that sperm movement was inhibited up to ten hours after insertion of the tablet. All five women who conceived underwent abortion, and no fetal abnormalities were detected as a result of propranolol exposure. Women using propranolol were also noted to have a small but significant reduction in their blood pressure and pulse. On the negative side, thirty-three women discontinued propranolol use because of vaginal itching or discomfort.

The feasibility of manufacturing nonprescription disposable latex diaphragms is also being explored. These would be available in two to four different sizes and could be packaged with a small supply of spermicidal gel or cream. An even more appealing product under consideration for future marketing is a disposable diaphragm that would release its own supply of spermicide after insertion.

THE RHYTHM METHOD

Despite extensive research aimed at improving the accuracy of the rhythm method, none of the newer and often elaborate devices and tests have proven as effective as the basic techniques described in chapter 5. To pinpoint more accurately the day of ovulation and to determine a woman's "safe" and "unsafe" days, most current research has centered on studying the cyclic changes in chemical, hormonal, and enzyme concentrations at different times of the month. These changes are often reflected in temperature shifts (see chapter 5) and fluctuations in the composition of a woman's cervical mucus, urine, blood, and saliva.

What are some of the more promising methods for evaluating the cervical mucus?

As previously noted, the increase in concentrations of sodium, potassium, and chloride in the cervical mucus at ovulation is the basis of the vaginal readings obtained by the CUE Ovulation Predictor (see chapter 5). The study of other cervical components also appears promising.

Most enzymes found in cervical mucus show a cyclic pattern throughout the month. This determination may prove to be of value in assessing ovulation. The enzymes named esterase, alkaline phosphatase, aminopeptidase, and lactate dehydrogenase all show a precipitous decrease in concentration in the cervical mucus immediately prior to ovulation, followed by a return to normal values after ovulation. Development of a dipstick-type measure to detect these enzymes in a home test is a distinct possibility for the future. Doctors at Wayne State University School of Medicine used a modified tampon to collect and test cervical mucus specimens for alkaline phosphatase concentrations. After being inserted in the vagina for ten to fifteen minutes, the tampon was dipped in a solution that would allow development of a color. Four colors were used to determine the concentration of alkaline phosphatase. In 77 percent of the cycles studied, it was possible to detect ovulation one to three days in advance. Researchers at Howard University have reported similar success in measuring peroxidase levels in cervical mucus.

Though the levels of glucose in the cervical mucus usually reach maximum concentrations on the day of ovulation, use of Tes-Tape in so-called fertility test kits has proven unreliable for practical use in determining the time of ovulation.

Sialic acid is a chemical that decreases in cervical mucus concentration as ovulation approaches. It reaches its nadir precisely at ovulation and then rises again until the time of the period. Determination of the sialic acid content of cervical mucus, though promising, is not yet suitable for clinical application.

How can a woman's saliva and urine be tested in the future to improve the efficacy of the rhythm method?

The concentration of hormones and enzymes in a woman's saliva and urine often mirror those in her bloodstream. For example, the serum and salivary peaks of one estrogen named estradiol are similar at ovulation, while progesterone levels in the saliva rise soon after and correlate with those in the bloodstream. Pregnanediol is the major urinary metabolite of progesterone. Urinary concentrations are usually less than 1 milligram per day prior to ovulation, and levels rise sharply just after ovulation. Scientists have developed a test kit for measuring pregnanediol concentrations in the urine. The kit can be set at a level of 2 milligrams per day, and when it rises above this level it means that ovulation has occurred. Peak progesterone concentrations are usually recorded between the eighteenth and twenty-second day of the typical twenty-eight day cycle.

The urinary concentrations of luteinizing hormone, or LH, can be determined with a variety of test kits (see chapter 5). Less expensive and more specific kits may be available in the near future to pinpoint the LH surge, which occurs just prior to ovulation.

One new, simple, and inexpensive salivary method of predicting ovulation is now undergoing investigation. It is based on the principle that the concentration of alkaline phosphatase in the saliva, unlike that in cervical mucus, is greatest at ovulation. In this test, a woman chews a small piece of paraffin in order to stimulate saliva production. She then puts in her mouth a filter-paper test strip saturated with material that will show a color change from white to blue in the presence of alkaline phosphatase. At the present time, this method has been able to predict ovulation within a period of one to seven days, which still makes it too inaccurate for widespread use.

Another salivary constituent, named salivary phosphate, has been studied in volunteer women and found to rise precipitously on the day of ovulation. In contrast, sialic acid concentrations begin to decrease one to two days prior to ovulation and reach their lowest levels at the time of ovulation. Development of a simple salivary test to anticipate impending ovulation would be a great benefit for couples using rhythm.

What are some of the newer devices and instruments for improving the accuracy of the rhythm method?

Periodically we read optimistic news releases touting new and exotic instruments for those trying to perfect the rhythm method. Some of these devices have measured the consistency and stretchability of cervical mucus, while others have concentrated on more accurately assessing body temperature and electrical potential changes on the skin surface which occur at ovulation. In the original edition of this book, published in 1977, I spoke enthusiastically of instruments with names such as Tachmeter, Ovu-timer, and Ovulometer. Now I must note that they have all been relegated to a place in the attic.

The newest addition to this list of gadgets is named the Ovix Fertility Computer. This contraption contains a microcomputer and a temperature probe. Upon awaken-ing, a woman takes her temperature with the probe, and after three minutes a sound signal and a screen light up to tell her to give the machine certain information via six special buttons. Included in this input of facts are the presence or absence of illness, changes noted in the cervical mucus, and the presence of any bleeding. The device digests this material and is programmed to record one of four red display buttons: fertile, infertile, pregnant, and postovulation. The Ovix Fertility Computer costs $250.00—for this price, it should have another button that says, "Do not pass go, do not collect $250."

Are there new ways to improve the temperature method of rhythm?

Yes, if your partner is willing to take *his* daily temperature! Dr. Margaret Henderson of Australia reported findings to the Royal Australian College of Physicians from a study of the daily basal body and evening temperatures of twenty-five healthy men between the ages of twenty and fifty-six. She found that ten of these men, who had each been living with a woman for a prolonged period of time, had temperature cycles synchronous with those of the women with whom they lived. They actually ex-perienced a midcycle temperature drop just prior to the woman's ovulation. Even more amazing, the men experienced a two-to-five-day temperature elevation coinci-ding with the woman's ovulation and the subsequent rise in her body temperature.

Another recent development that may improve the temperature method is a special heat-sensitive transmitter that has been developed by the National Aeronautics and Space Administration. This device can measure with great accuracy the intravaginal temperature prior to and after ovulation. Though it is not currently available, such a sensitive device may have a great future in pinpointing more subtle temperature changes during the menstrual cycle.

FEMALE STERILIZATION

What are some of the newest abdominal sterilization techniques?

As I mentioned in the discussion of tubal sterilization in chapter 9, the goal of future sterilization techniques will be to destroy as small a segment of fallopian tube and surrounding tissue as possible. Though a woman must never undergo sterilization with the thought of later having it reversed, unpredictable events occurring months or years later often prompt such requests. The success of microsurgery often depends on the degree of damage incurred during the sterilization procedure. While bipolar electrocoagulation is less damaging to the fallopian tube and ovarian blood supply than unipolar techniques, both are inferior to the endocoagulation methods devel-oped in Germany over the past fifteen years (see chapter 9). Microscopic studies have shown that the blood vessels and nerves in the mesosalpinx (the tissue below the tube) are not damaged with endocoagulation, and therefore no disruption of the blood supply to the remainder of the tube or ovary occurs. Future research in this field will deal with the refinement of endocoagulation instruments and the far more extensive use of this technique.

In addition to endocoagulation, we can anticipate further development and refinement of various clips for occluding the tubes. Clips offer a high rate of microsurgical reversibility, since they destroy only a 4-millimeter portion of tube. One new clip developed in England is made of titanium and silicone rubber, and is designed to avoid tears and bleeding in the mesosalpinx. In addition, it has the flexibility to accommodate and fit securely on thickened as well as normal tubes.

Modern laparoscopes are designed to be used with laser forceps and accessory equipment. A number of surgical procedures that formerly necessitated abdominal surgery can now be performed through the laser laparoscope, and several medical centers have reported excellent results in using it for tubal sterilization. Since the laser beam can be focused to a diameter of 1 millimeter or less, the amount of tissue destruction is usually minimal. The design of the laser laparoscope forceps is such that the laser beams are always directed between the two arms of the forceps grasping the fallopian tube, precluding burn injuries to the surrounding tissues.

The development of a totally reversible sterilization technique has eluded researchers for years. One new method has shown promise in animal experiments and is expected to be tested clinically on women in the near future. It consists of suturing a Silastic hood over the fimbria of each tube to prevent them from picking up the egg as it is extruded from the ovary each month (see chapter 1). The hoods can be removed whenever pregnancy is desired. To date, preliminary studies in rabbits and monkeys have shown that the Silastic hood produces no adhesions or tubal damage after one year of use.

What are some of the simpler experimental methods of occluding the fallopian tubes?

In an attempt to simplify tubal sterilization, doctors have instilled various caustic solutions and pastes through the cervix and into the uterine cavity. These substances create inflammatory scar tissue in the endometrium and at the point where the tube enters the uterine cavity, thereby occluding or blocking it. Chemicals used for this purpose have included silver nitrate, zinc chloride, phenol, plastic occlusives, tissue adhesives, methyl cyanoacrylate (MCA), and quinacrine. This last drug, formerly used in the treatment of malaria, has also been incorporated into experimental IUDs, so that its slow release could accomplish this same goal of blocking and scarring the tubes. Though it is the goal of scientists to develop these methods to a point where tubal sterilization can be performed as a safe, effective, and simple office procedure, this ideal is still far from being realized. It is estimated that it will be at least ten years before chemical occlusion techniques are widely available in the United States.

The greatest number of chemical occlusion procedures have been performed in the People's Republic of China. The method, which requires no anesthesia, involves instilling a dye visualized on X ray, phenol, and mucilage paste mixture into the tubes. A thin metal instrument is passed through the cervix and into each local area where the tubes enter the uterine cavity. A polyethylene tube is then advanced into the tubal opening. Amazingly, the Chinese physicians are able to accomplish this "blindly"—by touch, without the aid of a hysteroscope, or viewing instrument. The radiopaque paste containing 35 percent phenol is injected into each fallopian tube, rapidly causing extensive damage to the lining tissues. After extended exposure to the phenol, the tubes eventually become completely filled with scar tissue. Experience with more than 30,000 Chinese women has shown a remarkable 98 percent rate of bilateral tubal occlusion three months after the procedure is performed. Overall, some 4,000 women have been followed for as long as five to ten years with a subsequent pregnancy rate of only 1.6 percent. No major complications have been reported, and side effects have been limited to mild abdominal discomfort for several days in 30 percent of the women studied.

Methyl cyanoacrylate (MCA, trade name: Femcept) is a clear liquid form of instant glue which solidifies upon contact with moist body tissues. When MCA is injected into the uterine cavity, some of it enters the fallopian tubes and occludes, then destroys their epithelium, or lining. In this procedure, a premeasured amount of MCA is pumped into the uterus through a special cannula. The MCA is propelled 2 to 3 centimeters into the tubes by a small balloon at the top of the cannula which is inflated an instant after injection. The rapid filling of the balloon drives the MCA into both tubes before it solidifies. Once in the tubes, the MCA forms a solid plug which eventually biodegrades, leaving behind scar tissue that permanently closes the tubes. In clinical studies conducted throughout the world, 70 to 78 percent of the volunteers treated have had initial successful tubal closure proven by X ray. Reinjection of MCA one or more months later has increased this rate to a still unacceptable 85 to 90 percent. Side effects have included abdominal pain for one month or more in over 20 percent of those treated, fever in 7 percent, and hospitalization for PID in another 1 percent.

After more than fifteen years of research, the mechanism by which quinacrine closes the fallopian tubes is not yet understood. Use of liquid quinacrine requires great care since it may cause severe pain and injury to intra-abdominal tissues. To prevent this danger, scientists have developed a pellet that slowly releases quinacrine into the tubes. Three types of pellets have been produced: one releases its entire dose of quinacrine in ten minutes; another does so in a hundred minutes; and the third in sixteen hours. Studies have been carried out on hundreds of women given three quinacrine instillations in either liquid or pellet form over a period of three months. Ten percent of the women receiving liquid quinacrine became pregnant within one year of the last instillation procedure, compared with 3 to 5 percent of those who were treated with pellets. As previously mentioned, the safety of using quinacrine has been questioned since adverse central nervous system reactions have been noted in some women.

Though these methods appear promising, none has reached the ideal of a totally effective, safe, and simple nonsurgical method of sterilization.

How can sterilization be performed through the hysteroscope?

A hysteroscope is a viewing instrument with a powerful fiberoptic light source which is used to look into the uterus ("hystero"), through the cervix. A separate operating channel is provided for introducing a variety of instruments and for injecting substances such as silicone to occlude the tubes (see figure 11-3). Doctors have also attempted hysteroscopic tubal sterilization by cauterization, laser, and cryosurgical techniques. Obvious advantages of hysteroscopic sterilization are that it can be performed safely and inexpensively in a doctor's office, with paracervical block anesthesia (see chapter 7).

If hysteroscopic sterilization is perfected, it could be offered to women who would otherwise be denied laparoscopy because of previous extensive abdominal surgery, obesity, or cardiac and respiratory disease. Unlike the so-called blind techniques of chemical installation (see previous question), hysteroscopic visualization and blockage of both tubes at their point of entry into the uterine cavity require a significant degree of experience and surgical skill. Even in the hands of experts, the opening of the fallopian tubes cannot be visualized sufficiently to accomplish the injection in 10 to 15 percent of the women treated. Postoperative pregnancy rates ranging between 5 and 10 percent make hysteroscopic sterilization procedures less than adequate at the present time.

Several thousand women volunteers in the United States have been treated with an injection of foaming silicone through the hysteroscope. Once the tubes have been

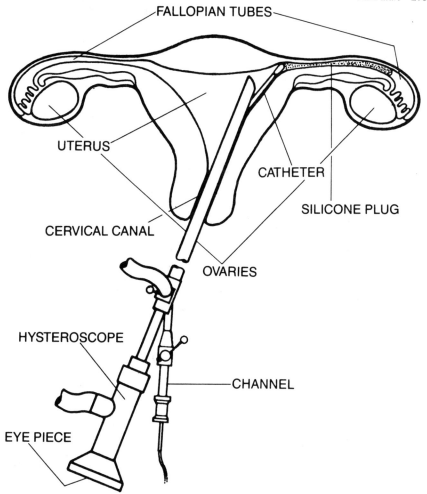

Figure 11–3. *Silicone injection through the hysteroscope.*

located, the silicone, which has the consistency of honey, is injected into the tube. In less than five minutes the silicone hardens into a flexible, solid rubber plug throughout almost the entire length of the tube. The procedure takes an average of thirty-five to forty minutes.

The developers of one silicone device have fashioned four small, fishhook-like metallic attachments to hold the plugs in place at the utero-tubal junction. Another researcher attaches a little retrieval loop to the plug, with the intention of possible removal at a later date in the event that reversal of the procedure is requested. This sounds like a workable idea, but in practice the presence of the plug in the tube has been found to damage its lining, or epithelium, making reversibility unlikely. Of the women tested with this device, approximately 80 percent have had successful occlusion of both fallopian tubes following the initial attempt. If more than one procedure is required, an additional 10 to 12 percent of the women treated can be successfully sterilized. This still represents an unacceptably high number of failures.

French investigators have developed a minihysteroscope which doesn't have a fiberoptic light, so it is smaller in diameter than the standard model. This makes it easier to insert and does not even require a local anesthetic. Under direct visualization, the minihysteroscope allows the doctor to insert a little tubal plug made of a nonbiodegradable polymer. The entire procedure takes about ten minutes. Efficacy rates have been near perfect, but studies on many more women will have to be performed before it can be considered an effective alternative.

Can ablation of the endometrium with laser or cryosurgery be used as a method of sterilization?

As mentioned in chapter 10, *ablation* (destruction) of the entire endometrium with the laser hysteroscope has controlled uterine hemorrhage and averted hysterectomy for a significant number of women. At the present time, this method must still be considered experimental, and its mastery is limited to very few American physicians. Total and permanent destruction of the endometrium with laser should theoretically prevent a fertilized egg from implanting into the endometrium. But many women who have undergone laser ablation continue to have light periods, indicating that a small amount of endometrium continues to function. Whether it is enough to allow implantation of a fertilized egg has not yet been determined.

Attempts at completely ablating the endometrium with cryosurgery (freezing) have been unsuccessful. Scientists continue to be amazed by the capacity of the endometrium to repair itself and regenerate even after extensive exposure to subfreezing temperatures. Not only is the procedure time-consuming, but long-term studies have demonstrated areas of endometrium that are not destroyed even after several cryosurgical applications.

MALE CONTRACEPTION AND STERILIZATION

Isn't there a new birth-control method that can be used by both men and women?

Under normal circumstances, luteinizing hormone-releasing hormone (LH-RH), also known as gonadotropin-releasing hormone (GnRH), is released from the hypothalamus of both men and women in what scientists call a pulsatile rhythm of one-to-two-hour intervals (see chapter 1). From there, LH-RH is carried by veins to the pituitary gland where it binds or attaches itself to specific receptors and stimulates the release of luteinizing hormone (LH) and follicle-stimulating hormone (FSH). LH and FSH are responsible for sperm formation and the production of male sex hormones by the testes as well as for the release of an egg from the ovary each month (see chapters 1 and 5).

LH-RH and chemically similar, but more potent, synthetic compounds called analogs were originally studied by scientists as a method of enhancing both male and female fertility. Much to their surprise, the analogs were found instead to have far greater potential as contraceptives. Paradoxically, it appears that these analogs, which are more than 100 times stronger than LH-RH, totally upset the delicate pulsatile LH-RH release pattern that occurs naturally. Instead of stimulating the pituitary gland, they overwhelm its thermostat with more LH-RH than it can handle. The pituitary then becomes incapable of responding to the body's pulsatile secretions of LH-RH. As a result, LH-RH is not released and the desired contraceptive effect of inhibiting ovulation and sperm formation is achieved.

LH-RH analogs appear to decrease progesterone production by the corpus luteum, and have proven effective in terminating early pregnancies in laboratory animals. Because of this, scientists have theorized that they could be effective morning-after medication, similar to RU-486 and prostaglandins. However, analogs currently under study have not proven powerful enough to terminate progesterone production by the corpus luteum once a woman's pregnancy test is positive. In clinical studies to date,

LH-RH analogs have been administered either in the form of a daily intramuscular or subdermal injection or as a nasal spray sniffed one to three times daily. Extensive trials on Canadian and Swedish women have reported over a 98 percent contraceptive success rate, with almost immediate return of reproductive function when treatment is stopped. Unfortunately, some women have reported distressing menopausal symptoms due to a lack of estrogen production by the ovary secondary to inhibited FSH and LH release. In addition, a smaller number of women have complained of vaginal dryness and breakthrough bleeding or absent periods. Some men given LH-RH have complained of loss of libido and impotence due to the testosterone-inhibiting action of LH-RH. A significant number of men have noted hot flashes such as those experienced by menopausal women.

Though scientists at the National Institute of Health are optimistic that LH-RH analogs will eventually replace birth control pills for women and become the first successful chemical contraceptive for men, some obstacles to this lofty goal remain. In addition to eliminating the above-mentioned side effects, scientists must develop a more convenient form of administration, such as a daily pill, a vaginal or rectal suppository, or a yearly subdermal implant. Though the nasal spray has been well received, the daily intramuscular injections are unacceptable to most people. In order for LH-RH analogs to serve satisfactorily as a male contraceptive, testosterone supplements in the form of subdermal implants or pills would probably be required to maintain libido. Unfortunately, the addition of testosterone in low doses increases the chances of raising the sperm count—the one condition they are trying to avoid. Similarly, those women experiencing hot flashes with LH-RH analogs would require estrogen replacement therapy. The need for supplemental hormones would limit the acceptability of LH-RH as a male or a female contraceptive. Even if the new analogs now undergoing trials prove successful, it would take at least ten years before their safety could be thoroughly evaluated and they could become widely available as a contraceptive for either men or women.

How do LH-RH antagonists differ from other LH-RH analogs?

Scientists have synthesized chemical compounds that are similar in structure to LH-RH, but that antagonize or block it from stimulating the pituitary gland to release its FSH and LH. LH-RH antagonists attach themselves to receptor sites in the pituitary gland which would normally be occupied by the body's own LH-RH. The antagonists thereby prevent the pituitary from secreting amounts of FSH and LH necessary for both normal ovulation and sperm formation. Research on LH-RH antagonists, in the form of nasal sprays and intramuscular injections, is in its preliminary testing stages. When given to laboratory rate, LH-RH antagonists effectively reduce sperm production—but they also decrease the size of the rat testes. Clinical testing on a small number of men resulted in suppression of testosterone levels, the same problem encountered with other LH-RH analogs.

How can the hormone inhibin function as a possible birth-control pill?

After forty years of work, endocrinologists finally isolated inhibin in 1977. The hormone, produced by cells in the testes as well as in the developing follicle in the ovary, may eventually prove to be the perfect male oral contraceptive. Inhibin has the unique ability to suppress FSH levels effectively without altering LH or testosterone release (see chapter 1). Since FSH stimulates the sex glands to produce an egg or a sperm cell, inhibin indirectly prevents this from happening. It is different than all other experimental male contraceptives because it can lower the sperm count without adversely altering a man's libido and sexuality. Since inhibin blocks FSH without upsetting the body's hormonal balance, it may eventually lead to the development of an improved birth-control pill for women as well as for men.

How effective is gossypol as a birth-control pill?

Gossypol is a cottonseed oil impurity which has been used as a male birth-control pill in China since 1972. It was discovered by alert Chinese epidemiologists in Hebei Province in the 1950s after they noted an epidemic of infertility. In tracing the cause of the problem, they found it was the result of a subtle change in the way people were extracting cooking oil from cottonseeds. Instead of first heating the seeds and then pressing the oil out of them, they had changed their technique to pressing the raw cottonseed. As a result, the impurity named gossypol was not destroyed. Research has demonstrated that gossypol exerts its contraceptive effect by inhibiting an enzyme named dehydrogenase X, which is found in the sperm-producing cells of the testes. Without this enzyme, sperm become incapacitated. Gossypol also attacks sperm motility in the epididymis (see chapter 1). Since gossypol does not appear to affect the cells that produce the male sex hormone testosterone, it should not harm a man's libido.

Chinese scientists claim to have administered gossypol to almost 20,000 men, with sterility achieved in greater than 99 percent of those treated. Pills are taken daily for almost two months, until sperm are no longer observed in the ejaculate. After that, they are taken every one to two weeks for as long as contraception is desired. Though restoration of fertility occurs about three months after discontinuing the gossypol, some research shows that 10 to 20 percent of men will experience permanent sterility. Such rates would be acceptable only to couples who do not expect to want children in the future. One great advantage of gossypol as a contraceptive would be its low cost, since it is easily extracted from cottonseed oil and is available in unlimited quantities throughout the world.

Worldwide chemical studies of gossypol are being conducted to determine whether long-term use could prove detrimental. Gossypol may well have some adverse side effects in humans, since it is known to be highly toxic to some animal species. Laboratory studies have shown that high concentrations of gossypol build up in many organs and are slow to disappear from human tissues. In addition, concern has been expressed that a gossypol-damaged sperm cell that fertilizes an egg may be responsible for an abnormal fetus.

Some studies have reported that as many as 10 percent of men using gossypol will have low serum potassium levels. This important mineral element, found in many foods, is essential for the normal functioning of muscles. A smaller percentage of men studied had severe potassium deficiency manifested as temporary muscle weakness, paralysis, and electrocardiogram changes secondary to weakening of the heart muscles. Other reported side effects have included intestinal discomfort, nausea, and poor appetite. Other researchers have found no association between gossypol use and serum potassium deficiencies. In a 1983 report of seventy-five men who had been using gossypol for over one year, doctors found potassium levels to have remained unchanged. They attributed the previous reports of low potassium to the fact that men in certain regions of China have diets that are deficient in this element.

It seems unlikely that gossypol or one of its analogs will be widely available to American men for many years.

How effective is use of the male hormone testosterone as a birth-control method for men?

Doctors at the University of Washington and several other medical centers throughout the world started clinical testing of a synthetic testosterone preparation named *testosterone enanthate* in April 1987. Hundreds of men are being treated with weekly injections of this agent over a period of at least one year. The researchers conducting these studies have found that if testosterone is maintained at high enough levels, it can suppress the release of FSH and LH from the pituitary gland, thereby stopping sperm production. Weekly injections of testosterone are an impractical method of birth control, however, and researchers at the World Health Organization are working on another synthetic testosterone that could be injected every three months. Other investigative teams have been testing a subdermal microencapsulated testosterone preparation which would release the hormone over a period of three to six months. Side effects of this treatment have been nonexistent, and return of fertility has been complete within three months after it is stopped.

One unexpected side effect of using subcutaneous testosterone as a male contraceptive was reported by doctors in France. They found that several of the female sexual partners of the men involved in their study developed an increased amount of hair on the upper lip and the inner thighs after a few months of treatment. It was theorized that the testosterone dissolved in sweat and infiltrated the skin of the women during intercourse. Laboratory testosterone evaluations showed elevated levels in eleven of the twelve women tested.

C. Alvin Paulsen, M.D., and his associates at the University of Washington have combined testosterone with other hormones in an attempt to find the ideal male contraceptive. Best results have been obtained with danazol, a synthetic hormone used in the treatment of endometriosis (see chapter 2). One advantage of this method is that danazol can be administered orally, with testosterone injections given only once a month. To date, this danazol-testosterone combination has produced absent or few sperm in 85 percent of the men tested, with no loss of libido. In addition, fertility returned within five months after the medication was stopped.

What are some of the other promising birth-control methods for men?

Though a host of possible male contraceptives are under consideration, most are more theoretical than applicable at the present time.

FRP, or follicle-stimulating hormone-releasing protein, is a recently discovered substance, chemically similar to inhibin (see inhibin), which affects the gonads in both sexes. Like LH-RH, FRP stimulates the pituitary gland to produce FSH. Unlike LH-RH, it does not stimulate LH release. In women, normal amounts of FRP prevent all but one egg from ripening each month, while higher levels prevent ovulation completely. Though the mechanism is not understood, FRP eliminates sperm production when given to experimental animals. Researchers believe that men will require treatment with FRP only once every two months in order to interrupt the cycle of sperm production. They also theorize that FRP will prove to be a safer form of contraception for women, because, unlike birth control pills, it acts only on the ovary and not on other organs. Clinical testing of FRP appears to be several years away.

Another promising and reversible birth-control pill for men is 5-thio-dextro-glucose. When tested on laboratory animals, it has been found capable of safely inhibiting the sperm count within four weeks. The pill acts by preventing real glucose from being taken up by the sperm cell, thereby inactivating it. Fertility is usually restored within four weeks after the pill is stopped.

Cimetidine, more commonly known by its trade name Tagamet, is one of the most commonly prescribed drugs for ulcer conditions, and researchers in the United States and England have found that it can significantly reduce sperm count in men and cause temporary impotence. This phenomenon has led researchers to explore the possibility of finding a compound chemically similar to cimetidine that can lower sperm count without lowering a man's libido.

In the past, sulfasalazine was the principal drug used for treating ulcerative colitis. However, in the late 1970s, it was found to be associated with a significant incidence of low sperm counts. Fertility was restored soon after sulfasalazine was stopped. Further work is needed to determine whether this medication or one of its metabolites is the cause of the low sperm counts. A chemically similar drug might be able to lower sperm counts without causing unwanted side effects.

What mechanical methods have been devised to reduce fertility in men?

Various researchers have inserted plugs, valves, and clips into the vas deferens of dogs, guinea pigs, and a few men—all with uniformly poor results. The devices have been of various sizes, shapes, and materials. One rather ingenious device contains a magnetic ball which can be moved on or off simply by passing a magnet over the scrotum. (One could envision serious problems with this device if its wearer were to pass through an airport security system!)

The newer valves have been made mainly of gold and plastic. Silicone rubber implants have also been inserted into the vas deferens as a means of reversible sterilization. For now, most investigators agree that these devices are far from being ready for use by the general public. A problem with many of these devices is that the tissues around them react with inflammation and scarring following their insertion. Such reactions prevent reversibility and speak unfavorably for the future of such devices.

A few investigators have attempted vas deferens occlusion by injecting strong chemicals directly into the *lumen,* or cavity, of the vas. The injection is placed through the skin under local anesthesia and avoids the more extensive surgical technique of vasectomy. To date, the most successful solution has been a mixture of 90 percent alcohol and 10 percent formalin. Preliminary studies in rats, dogs, and a small number of male volunteers have been discouraging. In one report, less than 50 percent of men treated became sterile after a single alcohol-formalin injection. This number improved to 70 percent following multiple injections. Other investigators have achieved success rates as high as 80 percent. But these chemicals also produce an inflammatory reaction and the formation of scar tissue within the vas, and will therefore never be practical as a reversible method of sterilization. Another chemical, alpha-chlorohydrin, has been shown to prevent normal maturation of sperm when injected into the epididymis of rats. The immature sperm are incapable of fertilizing an egg.

Occlusion of the vas deferens by electrocoagulation has the advantage of not requiring a surgical incision. This is accomplished by the introduction of special bipolar needles which can be placed directly below the skin of he scrotum. Several prototypes are under study and may become available soon.

One fascinating method of decreasing sperm counts was reported at the University of Missouri School of Medicine, where sperm formation was suppressed in dogs and in a small number of male volunteers by the use of ultrasound. The subjects sat on a special chair with their testes resting in a Plexiglas cup filled with water. The water served as a conductor for the high-frequency sound emanating from the ultrasonic transducer.

Following treatment, both the dogs and the men had suppressed sperm counts. The effect is believed to be reversible, though it may last for one or two years. The advantages of ultrasound are that there are no harmful side effects, it is painless, and the procedure is even reported to be pleasurable. In this study, the libido of the men undergoing treatment actually improved. It will be several years before this method of male contraception could be applied clinically.

AFTERWORD

Though several new and exciting developments have been discussed in this chapter, the search for the magic bullet of perfect contraception remains an elusive goal of researchers throughout the world. It is somewhat discouraging to note that few if any of these promising techniques will reach fruition within the next decade. Many potentially excellent methods appear doomed to failure simply because of the sharp decline in funds allocated to contraceptive research, and of the reluctance of major corporations to risk financial ruin resulting from lawsuits against a new and relatively untested product. Since the litigious climate in the United States is more severe than in any other country, it is not surprising that we are no longer the world leader in contraceptive research. The FDA's painfully slow process for authorizing clinical testing of new methods and techniques has further dampened the enthusiasm of scientists and financial investors in this technology.

Many of the effective contraceptive and sterilization options currently available to men and women are underused because of misinformation and myths surrounding their use. The many years of adverse publicity concerning the Pill have left many women with an inaccurate and exaggerated impression of its supposed dangers. Other misconceptions abound regarding the safety of vasectomy, tubal sterilization, and IUDs and the success rate of natural family planning methods, among a host of other subjects.

In the preceding chapters I have tried to impart my knowledge of contraception, sterilization, and abortion technology in an unbiased way. I have tried to dispel old myths and to explain and evaluate new advances in contraceptive technology. I will have succeeded if I help individuals to select rationally the contraceptive method that is most appropriate for them and to use that method with a maximum degree of efficacy and safety.

SELECTED BIBLIOGRAPHY

CHAPTER 1

Andreyko, J. L. et. al. Therapeutic uses of gonadotropin-releasing hormone analogs. *Obstetrical and Gynecological Survey*, 42 (1987):1–17.

Croxatto, H. B., et. al. Studies on the duration of egg transport by the human oviduct. *American Journal of Obstetrics and Gynecology* 132 (1978):629–34.

Ryan, K. J. Interpreting the controls of the menstrual cycle. *Contemporary OB/GYN*, Vol. 26 (September 1985):107–10.

Schmeck, H. M., Jr. Brain hormone regulating fertility is discovered. *The New York Times* (August 10, 1985), p. 5.

Yen, S. S. C. Neuroendocrine regulation of the menstrual cycle. *Hospital Practice* (March 1979):83–97.

CHAPTER 2

Bennion, L. J., et. al. Effects of oral contraceptives on the gallbladder bile of normal women. *The New England Journal of Medicine* 294 (1976):189–92.

Beral, V., S. Ramcharan, and R. Faris. Malignant melanoma and oral contraceptive use among women in California. *British Journal of Cancer* 36 (1977):804–09.

Blumenstein, B. A., M. B. Douglas, and W. D. Hall. Blood pressure changes and oral contraceptive use: A study of 2,676 black women in the Southeastern United States. *American Journal of Epidemiology* 112 (1980):539.

Bragonier, J. R. Influence of oral contraception on sexual response. *Medical Aspects of Human Sexuality* (October 1976):130–43.

Buehler, J. W., et. al. Maternal mortality in women aged 35 years or older: United States. *Journal of the American Medical Association* 255 (1986):53–57.

Cramer, D. W., et. al. Factors affecting the association of oral contraceptives and ovarian cancer. *The New England Journal of Medicine* 307 (1982):1047–51.

Fasal, P., and R. S. Paffenberger. Oral contraceptives as related to cancer and benign lesions of the breast. *Journal of the National Cancer Institute* 55 (1975):767–73.

Harlap, S., P. H. Shiono, and S. Ramcharan. Congenital abnormalities in the offspring of women who used oral and other contraceptives around the time of conception. *International Journal of Fertility* 30, no. 2 (1985):39–47.

Higgins, J. E., et. al. Hospitalizations among black women using contraceptives. *American Journal of Obstetrics and Gynecology* 153 (1985):280–86.

Janerich, D. T., J. M. Piper, and D. M. Glebatis. Oral contraceptives and congenital limb-reduction defects. *The New England Journal of Medicine* 291 (1974):697–700.

Jick, H., et. al. Oral contraceptives and breast cancer. *American Journal of Epidemiology* 112 (1980):577.

Katz, Z., et. al. Teratogenecity of progestogens given during the first trimester of pregnancy. *Obstetrics and Gynecology* 65 (1985):775.

Kaunitz, A. M., and D. A. Grimes. Good news about contraceptives and PID. *Contemporary OB/GYN* Vol. 27 (March 1986):153–57.

Krauss, R. M., et. al. Effects of two low-dose oral contraceptives on serum lipids and lipoproteins: Differential changes in high-density lipoprotein subclasses. *American Journal of Obstetrics and Gynecology* 145 (1983):446–51.

Mann, J. I., et. al. Myocardial infarction in young women with special reference to oral contraceptive practice. *British Medical Journal* 2 (1975):241–45.

Nora, J. J., and A. H. Nora. Birth defects and oral contraceptives. *Lancet* 1 (1973):941–42.

Notelovitz, M., C. Zauher, L. Mckenzie, et. al. The effect of low-dose oral contraceptives on cardiorespiratory function, coagulation, and lipids in exercising young women: a preliminary report. American Journal of Obstetrics and Gynecology, 156:591–598, 1987.

Ory, H. W., J. D. Forrest, and R. Lincoln. Making choices. Atlanta, Ga.: The Alan Guttmacher Institute, 1983.

Ory, H. W., et. al. Mortality among black women using contraceptives. *Journal of the American Medical Association* 251 (1984):1044–48.

Pike, M. C., et. al. Breast cancer in young women and use of oral contraceptives: Possible modifying effect of formulation and age of use. *Lancet* 2 (1983):926–30.

Porter, J. B., et. al. Oral contraceptives and nonfatal vascular disease—Recent experience. *Obstetrics and Gynecology* 59 (1982):299–302.

Rosenberg, L., et. al. Epithelial ovarian cancer and combination oral contraceptives. *Journal of the American Medical Association* 247 (1982):3210–12.

Rothman, K. J. Fetal loss, twinning, and birth weight after oral contraceptive use. *The New England Journal of Medicine* 297 (1977):468–71.

Rubin, G., P. M. Layde, and H. B. Peterson. Is this study valid? A closer look at the OC-breast cancer data. *Contemporary OB/GYN* Vol. 24 (July 1984):171–76.

Skolnick, J. L., et. al. Rifampin, oral contraceptives, and pregnancy. *Journal of the American Medical Association* 236 (1976):1382.

Skouby, S. O., et. al. Triphasic oral contraception: Metabolic effects in normal women and those with previous gestational diabetes. *American Journal of Obstetrics and Gynecology* 153 (1985):495–500.

Spellacy, W. N. Metabolic effects of oral contraceptives. *Clinical Obstetrics and Gynecology* 17 (March 1974):53–63.

Spellacy, W. N. et. al. Perspective carbohydrate metabolism studies in women using a low-estrogen oral contraceptive for one year. *The Journal of Reproductive Medicine* 26 (1981):295–98.

Spellacy, W. N., W. C. Buhi, and S. A. Birk. The effects of norgestrel on carbohydrate and lipid metabolism over one year. *The American Journal of Obstetrics and Gynecology* 125 (1976):984–86.

Speroff, L. PMS—looking for new answers to an old problem. *Contemporary OB/GYN* Vol. 22 (August 1983):102–24.

Stadel, B. B. National Institute of Child Health and Human Development, Bethesda, Md., Oral contraceptives and cardiovascular disease. *New England Journal of Medicine* 305 (1981):612–18.

Stadel, B. V., et. al. Oral contraceptives and breast cancer in young women. *The Lancet* 2 (1985):970–73.

Stern, E., et. al. Steroid contraceptive use and cervical dysplasia: Increased risk of progression. *Science* 196 (1977):1460–62.

Valente, P. T., and P. Hanjani. Endocervical neoplasia in long-term users of oral contraceptives: Clinical and pathologic observations. *Obstetrics and Gynecology* 67 (1986):695–704.

Vessey, M. T., and R. Doll. Investigation of relation between use of oral contraceptives and thromboembolic disease. *British Medical Journal* 2 (1968):199.

Vessey, M. P., et. al. An epidemiological study of oral contraceptives and breast cancer. *British Medical Journal* 1 (1979):1757.

Wilson, E. S. B., et. al. A prospective controlled study of the effect on blood pressure of contraception preparations containing different types and dosages of progestogen. *British Journal of Obstetrics and Gynaecology* 91 (1984):1254.

Invasive cervical cancer and combined oral contraceptives. *WHO Collaborative Study of Neoplasia and Steroid Contraceptives. British Medical Journal* 290 (1985):961–64.

Long-term oral contraceptive use and the risk of breast cancer. The Centers for Disease Control Cancer and Steroid Hormone Study, *Journal of the American Medical Association* 249 (1983):1591–95.

Oral contraceptive use and the risk of endometrial cancer. The Centers for Disease Control Cancer and Steroid Hormone Study, *Journal of the American Medical Association* 249 (1983):1600–1604.

Update on oral contraceptives. *The Journal of Reproductive Medicine* 29, no. 7 (Supplement, July 1984).

CHAPTER 3

Barrie, H. Congenital malformation associated with intrauterine contraceptive device. *British Medical Journal* 1 (1976):488–90.

Batzer, F. R., and S. L. Corson. Diagnostic techniques used for ectopic pregnancy. *The Journal of Reproductive Medicine* 31 (1986):86–92.

Cramer, D. W., et. al. Tubal infertility and the intrauterine device. *The New England Journal of Medicine* 312 (1985):941–47.

Cutler, P. Mitral valve prolapse, IUD insertion, and antibiotic prophylaxis. *The Journal of the American Medical Association* 247 (1982):687–88.

Daling, J. R., et. al. Primary tubal infertility in relation to the use of an intrauterine device. *The New England Journal of Medicine* 312 (1985):937–40.

Davies, A. J., B. M. Anderson, and A. C. Turnbull. Reduction by naproxen of excessive menstrual bleeding in women using intrauterine devices. *Obstetrics and Gynecology* 57 (1981):74–77.

Friberg, J., et. al. Chlamydia trachomatis attached to spermatozoa recovered from the peritoneal cavity of patients with salpingitis. *The Journal of Reproductive Medicine* 32 (1987):120–22.

Guderian, A. M., and G. E. Trobough. Residues of pelvic inflammatory disease in intrauterine device users: A result of the intrauterine device or Chlamydia trachomatis infection? *American Journal of Obstetrics and Gynecology* 154 (1986):497–503.

Haukkamaa, M., et. al. Bacterial flora of the cervix in women using different methods of contraception. *American Journal of Obstetrics and Gynecology* 154 (1986):520–24.

Heartwell, S. F., and S. Schlesselman. Risk of uterine perforation among users of intrauterine devices. *Obstetrics and Gynecology* 61 (1983):31–36.

Hill, J. A., E. Talledo, and J. Steele. Quantitative transcervical uterine cultures in asymptomatic women using an intrauterine contraceptive device. *Obstetrics and Gynecology* 68 (1986):700–703.

Kahn, H. S., and C. W. Tyler. IUD-related hospitalizations. *Journal of the American Medical Association* 234 (1975):53–56.

Kent, S. Therapeutic effects of Progestasert. *Contemporary OB/GYN* 10 (1977):33–40.

Kivijarvi, A., et. al. Iron deficiency in women using modern copper intrauterine devices. *Obstetrics and Gynecology* 67 (1986):95–98.

Larsson, B., O. Frankman, and L. Hamberger. Concentrations of copper in human secretions and weight of the copper wire during the four to seven years after insertion of a Cu-IUD. *Fertility and Sterility* 36 (1981):734–36.

Layde, P. M., et. al. Failed intrauterine device contraception and limb reduction deformities. *Fertility and Sterility* 31 (1979):18–20.

Lee, N. C., et. al. Type of intrauterine device and the risk of pelvic inflammatory disease. *Obstetrics and Gynecology* 62 (1983):1–6.

Loffer, F. D. The increasing problem of ectopic pregnancies and its impact on patients and physicians. *The Journal of Reproductive Medicine* 31 (1986):74–77.

Nelson, L. H., and J. B. Miller. Real-time ultrasound in locating intrauterine contraceptive devices. *Obstetrics and Gynecology* 54 (1979):711–14.

Randic, L., et. al. Return to fertility after IUD removal for planned pregnancy. *Contraception* 32 (1985):253.

Seiler, J. S. Laparoscopic tubal sterilization combined with removal of an intrauterine contraceptive device. *The Journal of Reproductive Medicine* 31 (1986):339–42.

Spellacy, W. N., W. C. Buhi, and S. A. Birk. Carbohydrate and lipid studies in women using the progesterone intrauterine device for one year. *Fertility and Sterility* 31 (1979):381–84.

Tatum, H. J., et. al. The Dalkon Shield controversy. *Journal of the American Medical Association* 231 (1975):711–17.

Valicenti, J. F., et. al. Detection and prevalence of IUD-associated actinomyces colonization and related morbidity. *The Journal of the American Medical Association* 247 (1982):1149–52.

Vessey, M., et. al. Outcome of pregnancy in women using different methods of contraception. *British Journal of Obstetrics and Gynecology* 86 (1979):548.

Yoonessi, M., et. al. Association of actinomyces and intrauterine contraceptive devices. *The Journal of Reproductive Medicine* 30 (1985):48–52.

Zakin, D., W. Z. Stern, and R. Rosenblatt. Complete and partial uterine perforation and embedding following insertion of intrauterine devices. *Obstetrical and Gynecological Survey* 36 (1981):401–13.

CHAPTER 4

Anderson, S. R., and L. S. Hyde. Toxic shock syndrome and the diaphragm. *Sexual Medicine Today* (February 1985):26–28.

Austin, H., W. C. Louv, and J. Alexander. A case-control study of spermicides and gonorrhea. *Journal of the American Medical Association* 251 (1984):2822–24.

Connell, E. D. Which contraceptives don't cause TSS? *Contemporary OB/GYN* (October 1985):127–37.

Cordero, J. F., and P. M. Layde. Vaginal spermicides, chromosomal abnormalities, and limb reduction defects. *Family Planning Perspectives* 15 (1983):16–18.

Darney, P. D. New developments in barrier methods of contraception. *Sexual Medicine Today* (March 1985):5–9.

Dent, T., and E. E. Brueschke. Barrier contraceptives. *The Female Patient* 6 (1981):57–62.

Duff, P. Recognizing and treating toxic shock. *Contemporary OB/GYN* (July 1983):43–59. Vol. 22.

Edelman, D. A., S. C. Smith, and S. McIntyre. Comparative trial of the contraceptive sponge and diaphragm. *The Journal of Reproductive Medicine* 11 (1983):781–84.

Eliot, J., L. Anderson, and S. Bernstein. Progress report on a study of the cervical cap. *The Journal of Reproductive Medicine* 30 (1985):753–59.

Faich, G., et. al. Toxic shock syndrome and the vaginal contraceptive sponge. *Journal of the American Medical Association* 225 (1986):216.

Fihn, S. D., et. al. Association between diaphragm use and urinary tract infection. *Journal of the American Medical Association* 254 (1985):240.

Jick, H., A. M. Walker, and K. J. Rothman. Vaginal spermicides and congenital disorders. *Journal of the American Medical Association* 245 (1981):1329–32.

Keith, L. G., G. S. Berger, and M. A. Jackson. Perspective on vaginal contraception: A method for the 1980s. *Contemporary OB/GYN* 19 (1982):63–82.

Kelaghan, J., et. al. Barrier-method contraceptives and pelvic inflammatory disease. *Journal of the American Medical Association* 248 (1982):184–87.

Lanes, S. F., et. al. Toxic shock syndrome, contraceptive methods, and vaginitis. *American Journal of Obstetrics and Gynecology* 154 (1986):989–91.

McBride, G. Putting a better cap on the cervix. *Journal of the American Medical Association* 243 (1980):1617–18.

Maine, D. Barrier methods: Renewed interest but more research needed. *Family Planning Perspectives* 11 (1979):237–40.

Melamed, M. R., et. al. Prevalence rates of uterine cervical carcinoma-in-situ for women using the diaphragm or contraceptive oral steroids. *British Medical Journal* 3 (1969):195–200.

North, B. B. The clinical background of a new contraceptive. *Sexual Medicine Today* (October 1983):24.

North, B. B., and B. W. Vorhauer. Use of the Today contraceptive sponge in the United States. *International Journal of Fertility* 30 (1985):81–84.

Powell, M. G., et. al. Contraception with the cervical cap: Effectiveness, safety, continuity of use, and user satisfaction. *Contraception* 33 (1986):215.

Prupes, K. Custom cervical cap reentering clinical trials. *Journal of the American Medical Association* 250 (1983):1946–52.

Remington, K. M., R. S. Buller, and J. R. Kelly. Effect of the Today contraceptive sponge on growth and toxic shock syndrome toxin-1 production by Staphylococcus aureus. *Obstetrics and Gynecology* 69 (1987):563–69.

Richardson, A. C., and J. B. Lyon. The effect of condom use on squamous cell cervical intraepithelial neoplasia. *American Journal of Obstetrics and Gynecology* 140 (1981):909–12.

Rosenberg, M. J., et. al. Effect of the contraceptive sponge on chlamydial infection, gonorrhea, and candidiasis. *Journal of the American Medical Association* 257 (1987):2308–12.

Shands, K. N., et. al. Toxic shock syndrome in menstruating women. *The New England Journal of Medicine* 303 (1980):1436–42.

Shapiro, S., et. al. Birth defects and vaginal spermicides. *Journal of the American Medical Association* 247 (1982):2381.

Stim, E. M. The Stim diaphragm method. *The Family Planning Alternative* (1979):1–15.

Stone, K. M., D. A. Grimes, and L. S. Magder. Primary prevention of sexually transmitted diseases. *Journal of the American Medical Association* 255 (1986):1763–66.

Toth, A. Alternative causes of pelvic inflammatory disease. *The Journal of Reproductive Medicine* 28 (1983):699–702.

Zaneveld, L. J. D., et. al. Primate model for the evaluation of vaginal contraceptives. *American Journal of Obstetrics and Gynecology* 129 (1977):368–72.

Tests confirm condoms block AIDS virus. *Medical World News* (January 30, 1986):7–8.

CHAPTER 5

Billings, E. L., et. al. Symptoms and hormonal changes accompanying ovulation. *Lancet* 1 (1972):282.

Chow, W. H. Vaginal douching as a potential risk factor for tubal ectopic pregnancy. *American Journal of Obstetrics and Gynecology* 153 (1985):727.

Elkind-Hirsch, K., et. al. Evaluation of the ovustick urinary luteinizing hormone kit in normal and stimulated menstrual cycles. *Obstetrics and Gynecology* 67 (1986):450–52.

Findlay, S. Natural family planning: Will it have a rebirth? *Ob. Gyn. News* 15, no. 2 (January 15, 1980): 8–10.

Hilgers, T. W., G. E. Abraham, and D. Cavanagh. Natural family planning. *Obstetrics and Gynecology* 52(1978):575–82.

Hilgers, T. W., and A. M. Prebil. The ovulation method—vulvar observations as an index of fertility/infertility. *Obstetrics and Gynecology* 53(1978):12–22.

Klein, T. A. Rhythm method of contraception. *Medical Aspects of Human Sexuality* 16(1982):113–17.

Levay, A. N., and A. B. Kagle. Overcoming premature ejaculation: "Stop and go" versus "squeeze" technique. *Medical Aspects of Human Sexuality* (June 1977): 105–12.

Marshall, J. A field trial of the basal-body temperature method of regulating births. *Lancet* 2(1968):8.

Masters, W. H., and V. E. Johnson. *Human sexual response* (Boston: Little, Brown, 1966), pp. 103–104.

Perez, A. Natural family planning: Postpartum period. *International Journal of Fertility* 26(1981):219.

Schumacher, G. F. B., et. al. Immunoglobulins, proteinase inhibitors, albumin, and lysozyme in human cervical mucus. *American Journal of Obstetrics and Gynecology* 129(1977):629–36.

Semans, J. H. Premature ejaculation: A new approach. *Southern Medical Journal* 49(1956):353–57.

Taylor, R. S., J. B. Woods, and M. Guapo. Correlation of vaginal hormonal cytograms with cervical mucus symptoms as observed by women using the ovulation method of natural family planning. *The Journal of Reproductive Medicine* 31(1986):167–72.

Vorherr, H. Contraception after abortion and postpartum. *American Journal of Obstetrics and Gynecology* 117(1973):1002–25.

Wade, M. E., et. al. A randomized prospective study of the use-effectiveness of two methods of natural family planning. *American Journal of Obstetrics and Gynecology* 141(1981):368–75.

Westoff, C. F., and E. F. Jones. The secularization of United States Catholic birth control practices. *Family Planning Perspectives* 9, no. 4(1977):153–57.

Zuspan, K. J., and F. P. Zuspan. Thermogenic alterations in the woman. *American Journal of Obstetrics and Gynecology* 120(1974):441–45.

Ovulation prediction in the treatment of infertility. *The Journal of Reproductive Medicine* 31, no. 8, Supp. (August 1986).

CHAPTER 6

Berger, M. J., and M. M. Alper. Intractable primary infertility in women exposed to diethylstilbestrol in utero. *The Journal of Reproductive Medicine* 31(1986):231–34.

Berger, M. J., and D. P. Goldstein. Impaired reproductive performance in DES-exposed women. *Obstetrics and Gynecology* 55(1980):25–27.

Bibbo, M., et. al. A twenty-five year follow-up study of women exposed to diethylstilbestrol during pregnancy. *The New England Journal of Medicine* 298(1978):763.

Brenner, W. E., and D. A. Edelman. Menstrual regulation: Risks and "abuses." *International Journal of Gynaecology and Obstetrics* 15(1977):177–83.

Conley, G. R., et. al. Seminoma and epididymal cysts in a young man with known diethylstilbestrol exposure in utero. *Journal of the American Medical Association* 249(1983):1325–26.

Cook, C. L., L. J. Wiist, and S. L. Kraft. Pregnancy prophylaxis: Parenteral postcoital estrogen. *Obstetrics and Gynecology* 67(1986):331–33.

Dixon, G. W., et. al. Ethinyl estradiol and conjugated estrogens as postcoital contraceptives. *Journal of the American Medical Association* 244(1980):1336–39.

Eisenberg, E. Fertility problems of DES daughters. *Contemporary OB/GYN* Vol. 21 (1983):197–99.

Gill, W. B., G. F. B. Schumacher, and M. Bibbo. Structural and functional abnormalities in the sex organs of male offspring of mothers treated with diethylstilbestrol (DES). *The Journal of Reproductive Medicine* 16(1976):147–53.

Gill, W. B., et. al. Association of diethylstilbestrol exposure in utero with cryptorchidism, testicular hypoplasia and semen abnormalities. *Journal of Urology* 122(1979):36–39.

Goldstein, D. P. Incompetent cervix in offspring exposed to diethylstilbestrol in utero. *Obstetrics and Gynecology* 52(1978):73s–75s.

Haspels, A. A., and R. Andriesse. *European Journal of Obstetrical and Reproductive Biology* 3(1973):113.

Herbst, A. L., et. al. Clear-cell adenocarcinoma of the vagina and cervix in young girls: Analysis of 170 registry cases. *American Journal of Obstetrics and Gynecology* 119(1974):713–28.

Herbst, A. L., et. al. Epidemiologic aspects and factors related to survival in 384 registry case of clear-cell adenocarcinoma of the vagina and cervix. *American Journal of Obstetrics and Gynecology* 135(1979):876.

Herbst, A. L., H. Ulfelder, and D. C. Poskanzer. Adenocarcinoma of the vagina: Association of maternal stilbestrol therapy with tumor appearance in young women. *The New England Journal of Medicine* 284(1971):878.

Irani, K. R., et. al. Menstrual induction: Its place in clinical practice. *Obstetrics and Gynecology* 46(1975):596–98.

Johnson, J. H. Contraception—the morning after. *Family Planning Perspectives* 16(1984):266–70.

Jukes, T. H. Estrogens in beefsteak. *Journal of the American Medical Association* 229(1974):1920–21.

Jukes, T. H. Diethylstilbestrol in beef production: What is the risk to consumers? *Preventive Medicine* 5(1976):438–53.

Kaufman, R. H., et. al. Upper genital tract changes and pregnancy outcome in offspring exposed in utero to diethylstilbestrol. *American Journal of Obstetrics and Gynecology* 137(1980):299–308.

Kaufman, R. H., et. al. Upper genital tract abnormalities and pregnancy outcome in diethylstilbestrol-exposed progeny. *American Journal of Obstetrics and Gynecology* 148(1984):973–84.

Kaunitz, A. M. Prescribing FDA-approved drugs in nonapproved ways. *Contemporary OB/GYN* 22(1983):27–36.

Lehfeldt, H. Postcoital contraception. *OB/GYN Digest* (1976):28–30.

Mattingly, R. F., and A. Stafl. Cancer risk in diethylstilbestrol-exposed offspring. *American Journal of Obstetrics and Gynecology* 126(1976):543–48.

Morris, J. M. Mechanisms involved in progesterone contraception and estrogen interception. *American Journal of Obstetrics and Gynecology* 117(1973):167–76.

Morrow, C. P., and D. E. Townsend. Management of adenosis and clear-cell adenocarcinoma of the vagina and cervix. *The Journal of Reproductive Medicine* 15(1975):25–26.

Notelovitz, M., and D. S. Bard. Conjugated estrogen as a postovulatory interceptive. *Contraception* 17(1978):443.

O'Brien, P. C., et. al. Vaginal epithelial changes in young women enrolled in the national cooperative diethylstilbestrol adenosis (DESAD) project. *Obstetrics and Gynecology* 53(1979):300–308.

Robboy, S. J., et. al. Increased incidence of cervical and vaginal dysplasia in 3,980 diethylstilbestrol-exposed women. *Journal of the American Medical Association* 252 (1984):2979–83.

Sandberg, E. C., et. al. Pregnancy outcome in women exposed to diethylstilbestrol in utero. *American Journal of Obstetrics and Gynecology* 140(1981):194–205.

Senekjian, E. K., and A. L. Herbst. Update on DES exposure. *Contemporary OB/GYN* (February 1987):29–46.

Stafl, A., and R. F. Mattingly. Vaginal adenosis: A precancerous lesion? *American Journal of Obstetrics and Gynecology* 120(1974):666–69.

Stenchever, M. A., et. al. Possible relationship between in utero diethylstilbestrol exposure and male fertility. *American Journal of Obstetrics and Gynecology* 140(1981):186–91.

Stillman, R. J. Pregnancy prospects of DES daughters. *Contemporary OB/GYN* Vol. 23 (1984):47–53.

Stringer, J., et. al. Very early termination of pregnancy (menstrual extraction). *British Medical Journal* 3(1975):7.

Yalom, I. D., R. Green, and N. Fish. Prenatal exposure to female hormones. Effect on psychosexual development in boys. *Archives of General Psychiatry* 28(1973):554.

DES daughters: The risks in their childbearing years. Vol. 26 Symposium, *Contemporary OB/GYN* (July 1985): 204–32.

CHAPTER 7

Anderson, G. G., and J. F. Steege. Clinical experience using prostaglandin F2$^\alpha$ for midtrimester abortion in 600 patients. *Journal of Obstetrics and Gynecology* 46 (1975):591–95.

Athanasiou, R. Psychological effects of abortion? *Contemporary OB/GYN* 3 (1974):54–55.

Berger, C., et. al. Repeat abortion: Is it a problem? *Family Planning Perspectives* 16 (1984):70–74.

Berry, F. N., and W. F. Peterson. D and E plus suction in midtrimester abortion. *The Female Patient* (1978):86–88.

Borten, M., and E. A. Friedman. Early pregnancy interruption with a single PGF2$^\alpha$ 15-methyl-analogue vaginal suppository. *The Journal of Reproductive Medicine* 30 (1985):741–44.

Buehler, J. W., et. al. The risk of serious complications from induced abortion: Do personal characteristics make a difference? *American Journal of Obstetrics and Gynecology* 153 (1985):14–20.

Burnett, L. S., A. C. Wentz, and T. M. King. Techniques of pregnancy termination. *Obstetrical and Gynecological Survey* 29 (1974):6–42.

Bygdeman, M. Comparison of prostaglandin and hypertonic saline for termination of pregnancy. *Obstetrics and Gynecology* 52 (1978):424–29.

Cates, W., Jr., and D. A. Grimes. Deaths from second trimester abortion by dilatation and evacuation: Causes, prevention, facilities. *Obstetrics and Gynecology* 58 (1981):401–7.

Cates, W., Jr., et. al. Dilatation and evacuation procedures and second-trimester abortions. *Journal of the American Medical Association* 248 (1982):559–63.

Darney, P. D. Dilatation—old and new techniques. *Contemporary OB/GYN* 26 (1985):41–54.

Donovan, P. The holy war. *Family Planning Perspectives* 17 (1985):5–9.

Foster, H. W., Jr., et. al. Postconception menses induction using prostaglandin vaginal suppositories. *Obstetrics and Gynecology* 65 (1985):682–85.

Freijka, T. Induced abortion and fertility. *Family Planning Perspectives* 17 (1985):230–34.

Goodlin, R. C., L. Reschl, and W. H. Clewell. Absence of maternal side effects from prostaglandins used for cervical ripening. *The Journal of Reproductive Medicine* 31 (1986): 1095–97.

Grimes, D. A. Second-trimester abortions in the United States. *Family Planning Perspectives* 16 (1984):260–66.

Grimes, D. A. Unplanned pregnancies in the United States. *Obstetrics and Gynecology* 67 (1986):438–42.

Grimes, D. A., and W. Cates, Jr. Deaths from paracervical anesthesia used for first-trimester abortion. *The New England Journal of Medicine* 295 (1976):1397–99.

Grimes, D. A., and W. Cates, Jr. The comparative efficacy and safety of intraamniotic prostaglandin F2$^\alpha$ and hypertonic saline for second-trimester abortion. *The Journal of Reproductive Medicine* 22 (1979):248–54.

Grimes, D. A., and K. F. Schulz. Morbidity and mortality from second-trimester abortions. *The Journal of Reproductive Medicine* 30 (1985):505–14.

Grimes, D. A., et. al. Midtrimester abortion by intraamniotic prostaglandin F2$^\alpha$. *Obstetrics and Gynecology* 49 (1976):612–16.

Grimes, D. A., et. al. Methods of midtrimester abortion: which is safest? *International Journal of Gynaecology and Obstetrics* 15 (1977):184–88.

Grimes, D. A., et. al. Local versus general anesthesia: Which is safer for performing suction curettage abortion? *American Journal of Obstetrics and Gynecology* 135 (1979):1030–35.

Grimes, D. A., K. F. Schulz, and W. J. Cates, Jr. Prevention of uterine perforation during curettage abortion. *Journal of the American Medical Association* 251 (1984):2108–11.

Henshaw, S. K. Observation: Contraceptive method use following an abortion. *Family Planning Perspectives* 16 (1974):75–77.

Hern, W. M. Serial multiple laminaria and adjunctive urea in late outpatient dilatation and evacuation abortion. *Obstetrics and Gynecology* 63 (1984):543–48.

Hogue, C. J. R., W. Cates, Jr., and C. Tietze. Impact of vacuum aspiration abortion on future childbearing: A review. *Family Planning Perspectives* 15 (1983):119.

Hulka, J. F., and M. Chepko. Vaginal prostaglandin El analogue (ONO-802) to soften the cervix in first trimester abortion. *Obstetrics and Gynecology* 69 (1987):57–60.

Kafrissen, M. E., et. al. Midtrimester abortion. *Journal of the American Medical Association* 251 (1984):916–19.

King, T. M., et. al. Intra-amniotic urea and prostaglandin F2$^\alpha$ for midtrimester abortion: Clinical and laboratory evaluation. *American Journal of Obstetrics and Gynecology* 129 (1977):817–24.

Lauersen, N. H., and Z. R. Graves. Preabortion cervical dilatation with a low-dose prostaglandin suppository. *The Journal of Reproductive Medicine* 29 (1984):133–35.

Lauersen, N. H., N. J. Secher, and K. H. Wilson. Mid-trimester abortion induced by intravaginal administration of prostaglandin E2 suppositories. *American Journal of Obstetrics and Gynecology* 122 (1975):947–53.

Mackay, H. T., K. F. Schulz, and D. A. Grimes. Safety of local versus general anesthesia for second-trimester dilatation and evacuation abortion. *Obstetrics and Gynecology* 66 (1985):661–64.

Nathanson, B. N. Ambulatory abortion: Experience with 26,000 cases. *The New England Journal of Medicine* 286 (1972):403–7.

Park, T., et. al. Preventing febrile complications of suction curettage abortion. *American Journal of Obstetrics and Gynecology* 152 (1985):252–55.

Peterson, H. B., et. al. Comparative risk of death from induced abortion at twelve weeks' gestation performed with local versus general anesthesia. *American Journal of Obstetrics and Gynecology* 141 (1981):763–68.

Robins, J., and E. J. Surrago. Early midtrimester pregnancy termination—A comparison of dilatation and evacuation and intravaginal prostaglandin E2. *The Journal of Reproductive Medicine* 27 (1982):415–18.

Schulz, K. F., D. A. Grimes, and W. Cates, Jr. Measures to prevent surgical injury during suction curettage abortion. *Lancet* 1 (1983):1182.

Schwallie, T. C., and K. R. Lamborn. Induction of abortion by intramuscular administration of (15S)-15-methyl PGF2$^\alpha$. *The Journal of Reproductive Medicine* 23 (1979):289–92.

Stubblefield, P. G., et. al. Fertility after induced abortion: A perspective follow-up study. *Obstetrics and Gynecology* 62 (1984):186.

Warren, T. M., and G. W. Ostheimer. A guide to complications of paracervical block. *Contemporary OB/GYN* 20 (1982):69–89.

Ying, U., J. Lin, and J. Robins. Acupuncture for the induction of cervical dilatation in preparation for first-trimester abortion and its influence on HCG. *The Journal of Reproductive Medicine* 30 (1985):530–34.

Prostaglandins and abortion. World Health Organization Task Force on the use of prostaglandins for the regulation of fertility. *American Journal of Obstetrics and Gynecology* 129 (1977):593–606.

CHAPTER 8

Frankel, M. S. Human-semen banking: Implications for medicine and society. *Connecticut Medicine* 39 (1975):313–17.

Goldachre, M. J., T. R. Holford, and M. P. Vessey. Cardiovascular disease and vasectomy: Findings from two epidemiologic studies. *The New England Journal of Medicine* 308 (1983):805–8.

Hussey, H. H. Vasectomy—a note of concern: Reprise. *Journal of the American Medical Association* 245 (1981):2333.

Lauersen, N. H., et. al. Vasectomy and atherosclerosis in Macaca fascicularis. *The Journal of Reproductive Medicine* 28 (1983):750–58.

Massey, F. J., et. al. Vasectomy and health—results from a large cohort study. *Journal of the American Medical Association* 252 (1984):1023–29.

Walker, A. M., et. al. Vasectomy and non-fatal myocardial infarction. *Lancet* 1 (1981):13.

Whitby, R. M., R. D. Gordon, and B. R. Blair. The endocrine effects of vasectomy: A prospective five-year study. *Fertility and Sterility* 31 (1979):518.

Wieland, R. G., et. al. Pituitary gonadal function before and after vasectomy. *Fertility and Sterility* 23 (1972):779.

Vasectomy . . . is it safe? *Sexual Medicine Today* (October 1982): 20–25.

Vasectomy, the nonreproductive effects. *Sexual Medicine Today* (June 1983): 21–23.

CHAPTER 9

Bernstein, I. C. Psychiatric aspects of sterilization. *The Journal of Reproductive Medicine* 22 (1979):97–100.

Bhiwandiwala, P. P., S. D. Mumford, and T. J. Feldblum. A comparison of different laparoscopic sterilization occlusion techniques in 24,439 procedures. *American Journal of Obstetrics and Gynecology* 144 (1982):319–21.

Bhiwandiwala, P. P., S. D. Mumford, and P. J. Feldblum. Menstrual pattern changes following laparoscopic sterilization with different occlusion techniques: A review of 10,004 cases. *American Journal of Obstetrics and Gynecology* 145 (1983):684–93.

Bhiwandiwala, P. P., S. D. Mumford, and K. I. Kennedy. Comparison of the safety of open and conventional laparoscopic sterilization. *Obstetrics and Gynecology* 66 (1985):391–94.

Brenner, W. E. Evaluation of contemporary female sterilization methods. *The Journal of Reproductive Medicine* 26 (1981):439–52.

Chi, I., and L. P. Cole. Incidence of pain among women undergoing laparoscopic sterilization by electrocoagulation, the spring-loaded clip, and the tubal ring. *American Journal of Obstetrics and Gynecology* 135 (1979):397–401.

DeStefano, F., et. al. Risk of ectopic pregnancy following tubal sterilization. *Obstetrics and Gynecology* 60 (1982):326–29.

DeStefano, F., et. al. Long-term risk of menstrual disturbances after tubal sterilization. *American Journal of Obstetrics and Gynecology* 152 (1985):835–41.

Divers, W. A., Jr. Characteristics of women requesting reversal of sterilization. *Fertility and Sterility* 41 (1984):233.

Domenzain, M. E. Advantages of the outpatient minilap for tubal occlusion. *Contemporary OB/GYN* Vol. 28 (August 1986):140–49.

Donnez, J., M. Wauters, and K. Thomas. Luteal function after tubal sterilization. *Obstetrics and Gynecology* 57 (1981):65.

Fishburn, J. I., et. al. Outpatient laparoscopic sterilization with therapeutic abortion versus abortion alone. *Journal of Obstetrics and Gynecology* 45 (1975):665–68.

Fortney, J. A., L. P. Cole, and K. I. Kennedy. A new approach to measuring menstrual pattern change after sterilization. *American Journal of Obstetrics and Gynecology* 149 (1983):830.

Gunning, J. E., J. P. Tomasulo, and T. Garite. Laparoscopic tubal sterilization using thermal coagulation. *Obstetrics and Gynecology* 54 (1979):505–10.

Hargrove, J. T., and G. E. Abraham. Endocrine profile of patients with post-tubal-ligation syndrome. *The Journal of Reproductive Medicine* 26 (1981):359–62.

Henderson, S. R. The reversibility of female sterilization with the use of microsurgery: A report on 102 patients with more than one year of follow-up. *American Journal of Obstetrics and Gynecology* 149 (1984):57–65.

Holtz, G. Laparoscopy in the massively obese female. *Obstetrics and Gynecology* 69 (1987):423–24.

Hulka, J. Female sterilization—how reversible? *Contemporary OB/GYN* Vol. 27 (April 1986):177–80.

Johnson, J. H. Tubal sterilization and hysterectomy. *Family Planning Perspectives* (1982):28–30.

Keith, L., et. al. Puerperal laparoscopy. *The Journal of Reproductive Medicine* 10 (1973):273–75.

Lawson, S., R. A. Cole, and A. A. Templeton. The effect of laparoscopic sterilization by diathermy or silastic bands on postoperative pain, menstrual symptoms, and sexuality. *British Journal of Obstetrics and Gynaecology* 86 (1979):659–63.

Leader, A., et. al. A comparison of definable traits in women requesting reversal of sterilization and women satisfied with sterilization. *American Journal of Obstetrics and Gynecology* 145 (1983):198–202.

Levy, D. A., R. M. Soderstrom, and D. H. Dail. Bowel injuries during laparoscopy. *The Journal of Reproductive Medicine* 30 (1985):168–72.

Loffer, F. D., and D. Pent. Indications, contraindications, and complications of laparoscopy. *Obstetrical and Gynecological Survey* 30 (1975):407.

Loffer, F. D., and D. Pent. Laparoscopy in the obese patient. *The American Journal of Obstetrics and Gynecology* 125 (1975):104–7.

Miesfeld, R. R., R. C. Giarratano, and T. G. Moyers. Vaginal tubal ligation—Is infection a significant risk? *American Journal of Obstetrics and Gynecology* 137 (1980):183–88.

Ocana, R., and W. McCormick. Open laparoscopy: Simple and direct. *Contemporary OB/GYN* Vol. 23 (February 1984):155–59.

Paterson, P. J. Factors influencing the success of microsurgical tuboplasty for sterilization reversal. *Clinical Reproduction and Fertility* 3 (1985):57.

Penfield, A. J. Minilaparotomy for female sterilization. *Obstetrics and Gynecology* 54 (1979):184–88.

Pent, D., and F. D. Loffer. Avoiding medical and surgical complications of laparoscopy. *Contemporary OB/GYN* 14 (1979):75–88.

Peterson, H. B., et. al. Deaths attributable to tubal sterilization in the United States, 1977 to 1981. *American Journal of Obstetrics and Gynecology* 146 (1983):131–36.

Phillips, J. M. Gynecologic Microsurgery. *The Journal of Reproductive Medicine* 22 (1979):135–43.

Rioux, J. E., and D. Cloutier. Bipolar cautery for sterilization by laparoscopy. *The Journal of Reproductive Medicine* 13 (1974):6–10.

Roe, R. E., R. K. Laros, and B. A. Work. Female sterilization. *American Journal of Obstetrics and Gynecology* 112 (1972):1031–36.

Soderstrom, R. N. Sterilization failures and their causes. *American Journal of Obstetrics and Gynecology* 152 (1985):395–403.

Soderstrom, R. M., and B. S. Levy. Bowel injuries during laparoscopy; Causes and medicolegal questions. *Contemporary OB/GYN* Vol. 27 (March 1986):41–45.

Spivak, M. M., C. L. Librach, and D. M. Rosenthal. Microsurgical reversal of sterilization: A six-year study. *American Journal of Obstetrics and Gynecology* 154 (1986):355–61.

Whitson, L. G., C. A. Ballard, and R. Israel. Laparoscopic tubal sterilization coincident with therapeutic abortion by suction curettage. *Obstetrics and Gynecology* 41 (1973):677–80.

Yoon, I. B., C. R. Wheeless, and T. M. King. A preliminary report on a new laparoscopic sterilization approach; The silicone rubber band technique. *American Journal of Obstetrics and Gynecology* 120 (1974):132–36.

Yuzpe, A. A., et. al. A review of 1,035 tubal sterilizations by posterior colpotomy under local anesthesia or by laparoscopy. *The Journal of Reproductive Medicine* 13 (1974):106–9.

Deaths following female sterilization with unipolar electrocoagulating devices. Centers for Disease Control, *Connecticut Medicine* (January 1982):31–32.

Minilaparotomy or laparoscopy for sterilization: A multicenter, multinational randomized study. World Health Organization Task Force on female sterilization. *American Journal of Obstetrics and Gynecology* 143 (1982):643–52.

CHAPTER 10

Ananth, J. Hysterectomy and depression. *Obstetrics and Gynecology* 52 (1978):724–29.

Ballard, C. A. Therapeutic abortion and sterilization by vaginal hysterectomy. *American Journal of Obstetrics and Gynecology* 118 (1974):891–96.

Barclay, D. L., et. al. Elective cesarean hysterectomy: A five-year comparison with cesarean section. *American Journal of Obstetrics and Gynecology* 124 (1976):900–910.

Christ, J. E., and E. C. Lotze. The residual ovary syndrome. *Journal of Obstetrics and Gynecology* 46 (1975):551–56.

Corson, S. L., et. al. Hormonal levels following sterilization and hysterectomy. *The Journal of Reproductive Medicine* 26 (1981):363–70.

Dicker, R. C., et. al. Hysterectomy among women of reproductive age—trends in the United States, 1970–1978. *Journal of the American Medical Association* 248 (1982):323–27.

Dyck, F. J., et. al. Effect of surveillance on the number of hysterectomies in the province of Saskatchewan. *The New England Journal of Medicine* 296 (1977):1326.

Goldrath, M. Laser ablation of the endometrium. 1986 review, Welcome Trends in *OB/GYN* 6, no. 4 (July 1986), 1–6.

Grimes, D. A. Declining surgical case-load of the obstetrician-gynecologist. *Obstetrics and Gynecology* 67 (1986):760–62.

Kaltreider, N. B., A. Wallace, and M. J. Horowitz. A field study of the stress response syndrome. *Journal of the American Medical Association* 242 (1979):1499–1503.

Laros, R. K., and B. A. Work. Female sterilization. *American Journal of Obstetrics and Gynecology* 122 (1975):693–97.

McGowan, L. Ovarian cancer after hysterectomy. *Obstetrics and Gynecology* 69 (1987):386–88.

O'Leary, J. A., and C. M. Steer. A ten-year review of cesarean hysterectomy. *American Journal of Obstetrics and Gynecology* 90 (1964):227–31.

Riedel, H., E. Lehmann-Willenbrock, and K. Semm. Ovarian failure phenomena after hysterectomy. *The Journal of Reproductive Medicine* 31 (1986):597–600.

Roeske, N. C. A. Evaluating hysterectomy's psychosocial impact. *Contemporary OB/GYN* 12 (1978):95–102.

Rutkow, I. M. Obstetric and gynecologic operations in the United States, 1979 to 1984. *Obstetrics and Gynecology* 67 (1986):755–59.

Schulman, H. Major surgery for abortion and sterilization. *Journal of Obstetrics and Gynecology* 40 (1972):738–39.

Sloan, D. The emotional and psychosexual aspects of hysterectomy. *American Journal of Obstetrics and Gynecology* 131 (1978):598–605.

Souza, A. Z., et. al. Ovarian histology and function after total abdominal hysterectomy. *Obstetrics and Gynecology* 68 (1986):847–49.

Wingo, P. A., et. al. The mortality risk associated with hysterectomy. *American Journal of Obstetrics and Gynecology* 152 (1985):803–8.

Hysterectomy in women aged 15–44, United States, 1970–1978. Centers for Disease Control. *Connecticut Medicine* (1981):663–64.

CHAPTER 11

Andreyko, J. L., et. al. Therapeutic uses of gonadotropin-releasing hormone analogs. *Obstetrical and Gynecological Survey* 42 (1987):1–16.

Asch, R. H., et. al. Mechanism of induction of luteal phase defects by danazol. *American Journal of Obstetrics and Gynecology* 136 (1980):932–35.

Atkinson, L. E., R. Lincoln, and J. D. Forrest. Worldwide trends in funding for contraceptive research and evaluation. *Family Planning Perspectives* 17 (1985):196–207.

Barber, H. R. K. GnRH agonists: No magic bullet, but . . . *The Female Patient* 12 (January 1987):8–14.

Beck, L. R., et. al. New long-acting injectable microcapsule contraceptive system. *American Journal of Obstetrics and Gynecology* 135 (1979):419–26.

Benditt, J. M. Current contraceptive research. *Family Planning Perspectives* 12 (1980):149–55.

Bennegard, D., B. Dennefors, and L. Hamberger. Interaction between catecholamines and prostaglandin F2$^\alpha$ in human lutealysis. *Acta Endocrinology* 106 (1984):532.

Bergquist, C., S. J. Nillius, and L. Wide. Intranasal gonadotropin-releasing hormone agonist as a contraceptive agent. *Lancet* (August 4, 1979):215–217.

Brenner, P. F., D. Shoupe, and D. R. Mishell, Jr. Ovulation inhibition with nafarelin acetate nasal administration for six months. *Contraception* 32 (1985):531.

Chari, S., et. al. Purification of "inhibin" from human ovarian follicular fluid. *Acta Endocrinology* 90 (1979):157.

Chaudhury, R. R. Current status of research on intrauterine devices. *Obstetrical and Gynecological Survey* 35 (1980):333–38.

Cole, L. P., et. al. Postpartum insertion of modified intrauterine devices. *The Journal of Reproductive Medicine* 29 (1984):677–82.

Corbin, A., A., F. J. Bex, and R. C. Jones. LH-RH and analogs: Contraceptive and therapeutic considerations. *International Journal of Fertility* 30 (1985):57–65.

Couzinet, B., et. al. Termination of early pregnancy by the progesterone antagonist RU-486 (Mifepristone). *New England Journal of Medicine* 315 (1986):1565–70.

Darney, P. D. Contraception? Are implants the answer? *Contemporary OB/GYN* Vol. 28 (July 1986):29–37.

Djerassi, C. What contraceptive revolution? *Family Planning Perspectives* 18 (1986):100.

Droegemueller, W., et. al. Cryocoagulation of the endometrium at the uterine cornua. *American Journal of Obstetrics and Gynecology* 131 (1978):1–10.

El Mahgoub, S. Body weight and cycle control of injectable contraceptives. *The Journal of Reproductive Medicine* 24 (1980):119–25.

Erb, R. A., and T. P. Reed. Hysteroscopic oviductal blocking with formed-in-place silicone rubber plugs. *The Journal of Reproductive Medicine* 23 (1979):65–72.

Gillard, R. C., et. al. RU-486 inhibits peripheral effects of glucocorticoids in humans. *Journal of Clinical Endocrinology and Metabolism* 61 (1985):1009.

Gold, R. B., and P. D. Wilson. Depo-Provera: New developments in a decade-old controversy. *Family Planning Perspectives* (1981):35–39.

Goldman, L. The injectable contraceptive debate; What are the pros and cons? *Modern Medicine* (December 1983):11–21.

Goldrath, M. H., T. A. Fuller, and S. Segal. Laser photovaporization of endometrium for the treatment of menorrhagia. *American Journal of Obstetrics and Gynecology* 140 (1981):14–19.

Greenblatt, R. B., et. al. Implantation of pure crystalline pellets of estradiol for conception control. *American Journal of Obstetrics and Gynecology* 127 (1977):520–24.

Gunning, J. E., J. P. Tomasulo, and T. Garite. Laparoscopic tubal sterilization using thermal coagulation. *Obstetrics and Gynecology* 54 (1979):505–9.

Hodgen, G. D. Pregnancy prevention by intravaginal delivery of a progesterone antagonist: RU-486 tampon for menstrual induction and absorption. *Fertility and Sterility* 44 (1985):263–67.

Huber, D. Update on techniques for voluntary sterilization. *Contemporary OB/GYN* Vol. 23 (April 1984):130–46.

Jacques, M., M. E. Olson, and J. W. Kosterton. Microbial colonization of tailed and tailless intrauterine contraceptive devices: Influence of the mode of insertion in the rabbit. *American Journal of Obstetrics and Gynecology* 154 (1986):648–55.

Kamada, M., et. al. Blocking of human fertilization in vitro by sera with sperm-immobilizing antibodies. *American Journal of Obstetrics and Gynecology* 153 (1985):328–31.

Klitsch, M. Sterilization without surgery. *Family Planning Perspectives* 14 (1982):324–27.

Klitsch, M. Hormonal implants: The next wave of contraceptives. *Family Planning Perspectives* 15 (1983):239–43.

Lauersen, N. H., and K. H. Wilson. Evaluation of danazol as an oral contraceptive. *Obstetrics and Gynecology* 50 (1976):91–96.

Liang, A. P., et. al. Risk of breast, uterine corpus, and ovarian cancer in women receiving medroxyprogesterone injections. *Journal of the American Medical Association* 249 (1983):2909–12.

Maheux, R. LH-RH agonists—How useful against uterine leiomyomas? *Contemporary OB/GYN* Vol. 28 (December 1986):66–77.

Marano, H. Key male hormone isolated; may curb sperm, keep libido. *Medical Tribune* (April 20, 1977):1, 10.

Minkler, D. The NORPLANT contraceptive system. *Connecticut Medicine* 50 (1986):309.

Mishell, D. R., Jr. New frontiers of contraception. *The Journal of Reproductive Medicine* 21 (1978):254–56.

Mishell, D. R., Jr., et. al. Clinical performance and endocrine profiles with contraceptive vaginal rings containing a combination of estradiol and d-norgestrel. *American Journal of Obstetrics and Gynecology* 130 (1978):55–62.

Moghissi, K. S. Cervical mucus changes and ovulation prediction and detection. *The Journal of Reproductive Medicine* 31 (1986):748–52.

Neuwirth, R. S. An alternative to hysterectomy for fibroids. *The Female Patient* (1979):54–56.

Nieman, L. K., et. al. The progesterone antagonist RU-486. *The New England Journal of Medicine* 316 (1987):187–91.

Ory, S. J., et. al. The effect of a biodegradable contraceptive capsule (Capronor) containing levonorgestrel on gonadotropin, estrogen, and progesterone levels. *American Journal of Obstetrics and Gynecology* 145 (1983):600–603.

Rioux, J. E., and A. Yuzpe. A guide to sterilization procedures. *Contemporary OB/GYN* 12 (1978):33–47.

Rosenfield, A. G. Contraception: Where are we in 1985? *Contemporary OB/GYN* Vol. 25 (February 1985): 79–94.

Rosenfield, A., et. al. The Food and Drug Administration and medroxyprogesterone acetate. What are the issues? *Journal of the American Medical Association* 249 (1983):2922–28.

Rosoff, J. I.: Some Organizational attitudes to increased support for reproductive and contraceptive research. Family Planning Perspectives, 16:pp 28–31, Jan–Feb, 1984.

Roy, S., et. al. Long-term reversible contraception with levonorgestrel-releasing Silastic rods. *American Journal of Obstetrics and Gynecology* 148 (1984):1006–13.

Segal, S. J. Contraception: What the future holds. *Drug Therapy* (June 1982):41–51.

Speidel, J. J. Steroidal contraception in the 80s—the role of current and new products. *The Journal of Reproductive Medicine* 28 (1983):759–68.

Tauber, T. F., et. al. Reduced menstrual blood loss by release of an antifibrinolytic agent from intrauterine contraceptive devices. *American Journal of Obstetrics and Gynecology* 140 (1981):322–27.

Toppozada, M. The clinical use of monthly injectable contraceptive preparations. *Obstetrical and Gynecological Survey* 32 (1977):335–47.

Zatuchni, G. I. Advances in fertility control. *The Female Patient* 9 (May 1984):17–27.

Zatuchni, G. New devices for intrauterine contraception. *Contemporary OB/GYN*, Technology Vol. 25 (1985):77–89.

Zatuchni, G. I. Contraceptive practices: Update and outlook. *The Female Patient* 11 (June 1986):97–99.

Zipper, J., et. al. Propanolol as a novel, effective spermicide: Preliminary findings. *British Medical Journal* 287 (1983):1245–46.

The search for male contraception. *MD* (May 1983):95–102.

INDEX

Abdominal hysterectomy, 239
Abdominal tubal ligation, 210–229; *see also*
    Laparoscopy/laparoscopic
    sterilization
  disadvantages of, 211–212
  minilaparotomy, 212–213
  postpartum sterilization, 212
  process of, 210–211
  vaginal tubal ligation compared with,
    208–209
Ablation of endometrium, 276
Abortion, 171–197; *see also* First-trimester
    abortion, Hypertonic saline abortion
  acupuncture to dilate cervix prior to,
    185
  choosing clinic and doctor to perform,
    185–186
  cost of, 186–187
  counseling regarding, 174
  decreasing risk of trauma to cervix and,
    183–185
  easy access to, effects of, 196–197
  ectopic pregnancy following, 182
  emotional problems following, 196
  fees for, 174
  husband's disapproval of, 173
  Hyde amendment, 171
  hysterotomy as means of, 195
  infertility following, 182
  IUD use after, resuming, 95–96
  for minor without parental consent,
    172–173
  political opposition to, 171
  prostaglandins in inducing, 190–191
  resuming birth-control pills after, 75
  return of fertility after, 152–153
  terminating pregnancy beyond twelve
    weeks, 187–188
Actinomyces israelii, 92
Adenocarcinoma, 160
Adenocarcinoma of cervix, 44
Adenomyosis, 245–246
Adenosis, 160
  diagnosing, 162
  patients with, and frequency of visits to
    doctor, 163
  treatment of, 162–163
  week of pregnancy DES is taken and, 162

Adolescents, *see* Teenagers
Adrenal glands, 48
AIDS
  condoms for prevention of, 127, 134
  nonoxynol-9 and, 114
Alcohol metabolism, birth-control pills and,
    67
Amenorrhea, 51
Antifibrinolytic agents, 268
Antithrombin III, 37
Appendicitis, birth-control pills and, 69
Arcing-spring diaphragm, 105
Atherosclerosis, 35, 204
Atropine, 209

Barrier contraception, 102–135; *see also*
    Cervical caps, Condoms,
    Diaphragms, TODAY sponge,
    Vaginal spermicides
  new methods of, 270
Bartholin's glands, 2
Bilateral salpingo-oophorectomy, 238
Billings method, 144
Biodegradable subdermal implants, 260
Biphasic (two-phase) formulations, 32
Bipolar cautery, 221
Birth-control pills, 14–77; *see also* Triphasic
    birth-control pills
  abnormal Pap smears caused by, 56–57
  for adolescents, parental consent and, 76
  adrenal glands and, 48
  alcohol metabolism and, 67
  altering date of period and, 55
  alternatives for woman who has difficulty
    swallowing pills, 261
  athletic performance by women and, 64
  birth defects due to using Pill early in
    pregnancy, 62–63
  black women and use of, 40
  blood clot risks in surgery and, 38
  blood clots caused by, 37
  blood sugar and effect of, 41
  breakthrough bleeding and, 55–56
  breast cancer and use of, 43
  breast milk and effect of, 32
  breasts and effects of, 412–413
  caffeine metabolism and, 67
  cervix and effects of, 43–44

Birth-control pills *(cont.)*
comparison of currently available pills, 15–23
current popularity of, 14
current research on, 251–252, 253
deaths and hospitalizations related to, 33–35
depression caused by, 65–66
diabetes developed while taking, 41, 42
escape ovulation and, 56
estrogens in, 15–23
complications and side effects of, 24–25
failure to experience withdrawal bleeding, 53–54
fertility and, 50
fibroids and, 63
folic acid deficiencies and, 56–57
forgetting a pill, 55–56
genital herpes simplex (HSV-III) and, 74
growth in teenagers stunted by, 63
hair loss and, 73–74
headaches and use of, 69
high blood pressure and, 39–40
increase in body's vitamins and minerals caused by, 58
infections and, 74
infertility caused by, 51
inhibin as, 277
interacting with other drugs, 66–67
intestinal ailments and, 68–69
irregular periods and use of, 52
IUD compared with, 79–80
length of time required to take effect, 66
lingering risks from using, 77
lipid content in blood and, 35–36
liver cancer and, 60–61
liver diseases and, 59–60
masculinization of female fetus genitals due to taking Pill while pregnant, 61
menopause and, 63
migraine headaches and use of, 70
mitral valve prolapse and use of, 40–41
new estrogens and progestins for, 252–253
obese women and use of, 64
ovarian cancer and, 46–47
ovarian cysts and, 46
PID and, 49–51
pigment of skin affected by, 47
PMS and, 59
as postcoital contraceptive, 69
pregnancy occuring while on, 61
progestogen in, 15–23
complications and side effects of, 25–26
prolactin and, 51
recommended corrections of side effects of, 28–30
resuming use after abortion or childbirth, 75
rheumatoid arthritis and, 49
sexual response in women and, 66–67
skin problems and, 48
smoking and, 33
stopping Pill three months before conception, 61–62

stroke and, 36–37
success of, compared with other contraceptives, 108
for teenagers with irregular menses, 52–53
temporary break from using, 51–52
thyroid glands and, 48
in treatment of endometriosis, 72–73
in treatment of primary dysmenorrhea, 71–72
urinary tract and effect of, 74–75
uterine cancer and, 45–46
varicose veins and use of, 38
vitamin deficiencies associated with use of, 57–58
vomiting and, 68
white-blood-cell count (WBC) and, 74
for women over thirty-five, 52
Blood clots
blood types and, 38
caused by birth-control pills, 37
vitamin K and, 58
Blood sugar, birth-control pills and, 41
Bounce test, 151
Breakthrough bleeding, 54–55
Breast cancer, birth-control pills and, 43
Breast milk, birth-control pills and, 32
Breasts, birth-control pills and, 412–413

Caffeine metabolism, birth-control pills and, 67
Calcium, birth-control pills and, 58
Carbonic anhydrase, 157
Carcinoma-in-situ, 44, 113, 254
Cervical adenocarcinoma, 160
Cervical cancer, 44
condoms for prevention of, 134
Depo-Provera and, 254
diaphragm as prevention of, 113–114
IUD use and, 99
Cervical caps, 119–122
access to, 120–121
compared to other barrier methods, 121
description of, 119–120
diaphragm compared with, 122
history of, 119–120
problems with, 120
TODAY sponge compared with, 122
Cervical os, 4
Cervix, 4–5
abnormalities of, and successful pregnancy, 160–162
acupuncture to dilate, prior to abortion, 185
decreasing trauma to, during elective abortions, 183
DES and changes of, 160
eversion of, 5
examining, 3
size of, 121
Cesarean hysterectomy, 238
Cesarean section, 249–250
Childbirth, resuming use of birth-control pills after, 75
Chlamydia, 49, 51

condoms for prevention of, 134
TODAY sponge in prevention of, 117
Chloasma, 47
"Chocolate cysts," 72
Cholecystitis, 49
Cholelithiasis, 49
Cholestatic pruritis, 48
Cimetidine, as male contraceptive, 279
Clear-cell adenocarcinoma, 162
Clitoris, 2
Coil-spring diaphragm, 105
Coitus interruptus, 136–138
  description, 136
  techniques for improving, 136–138
  unreliability of, 136
Colpotomy
  childbirth and, 230
  complications of, 230–231
Condoms, 127–135
  contouring of, 132
  current usage of, 127, 134–135
  description, 127
  determining size of, 128
  effectiveness of, 127–128
  history of, 127
  latex versus lamb membrane, 132, 135
  nonoxynol-9 in, 128, 132, 135
  pregnancy rates with, 133
  in prevention of sexually transmitted
    diseases, 133–134
  putting on, 128
  quality control testing of, 132
  success of, compared to other
    contraceptives, 108
  in treatment of infertility, 133
  types and brands of, 128–131
  withdrawal of penis after ejaculation, 133
Condyloma acuminata, 44
Contraceptive film, 126
Corpus luteum, 7, 9
Cryobanks, 206–207
Cryosurgery, of endometrium, 276
CUE Ovulation Predictor, 147–148
Culdoscopy, 231–232
Cyproterone acetate, 253
Cystocele, 240

D and C, *see* Dilatation and curettage
D and E, *see* Dilatation and evacuation
Dalkon Shield, 90
  reasons for higher infection rates with,
    91
Danazol
  as contraceptive, 260–261
  as male contraceptive, 279
Deep vein thrombophlebitis, 38
Deladroxate, 259
Delta Loop and Delta T IUDs, 267–268
Depo-Provera
  cancer and, 254–255
  disadvantages of, 255–256
  effectivesness as contraceptive, 253–254
  Food and Drug Administration (FDA)
    lack of approval for, 254
  women who would benefit from, 255
DES (Diethylstilbestrol)

benign cervical and vaginal changes
    caused by, 160
  effectiveness of, 158–159
  first pelvic examination and culposcopy
    of girls exposed to, 164
  as morning-after pill, and chances of
    malignancy, 165–166
  pregnancy in daughters of women
    exposed to, 160–162
  vaginal cancer and, 159–160
DES-exposed daughters
  abnormal Pap smears in, 164
  abnormalities of cervix and uterus in,
    160–162
  birth-control pill use by, 165
  carcinoma-in-situ in, 164
  dysplasia in, 164
  finding out if you are one, 165
  pregnancy in, 160–162
  vaginal cancer risk in, 159–160
DES-exposed men, 166–167
Diabetes, and use of birth-control pills, 41,
    42
Diabetic women, IUD use by, 98–99
Diaphragm inserter, 107
Diaphragms
  advantages of, 117
  being fitted for, 103
  cervical caps compared with, 122
  compared to other contraceptives, 108
  contraceptive jellies and creams used
    with, 111–113
  cost of, 113, 117
  description, 102
  determining size of, 103–104
  high pregnancy rates with, 109
  history of, 102–103
  insertion of, 104–105
  learning to use, 103
  medical problems associated with,
    110–111
  one-size-fits-all concept of using, 109
  pregnancy rates of TODAY sponge
    compared with, 115–116
  in preventing pregnancy, 107
  in preventing sexually transmitted
    diseases, 113–114
  reducing pregnancy rates of, 108–109
  toxic shock syndrome and, 118
  types of, 105
  women who should not use, 111
  women who will benefit from, 111
Diarrhea, birth-control pills and, 68
Diethylstilbestrol, *see* DES *entries*
Dilatation and curettage (D and C), 45, 52
Dilatation and evacuation (D and E),
    187–188
  compared with other methods of
    midtrimester abortions, 192–193
Douching, as contraceptive technique,
    154–155
Drugs, interaction of birth-control pills
    with, 66–67
Dysmenorrhea, 73
Dysplasia, 44, 113, 254
  in DES-exposed daughters, 164

Ectopic pregnancy, 61
  douching and, 155
  following abortion, 182
  tubal ligation and, 226
  in women using IUDs, 97–98
Endocarditis, IUDs worn by women with,
  100–101
Endometrial adenocarcinoma, 45
Endometrial cancer, 254–255
Endometrial hyperplasia, 45
Endometriosis
  birth-control pills in treatment of, 72–
  73
  dysmenorrhea due to, 73
Endometritis, after first-trimester abortion,
  178
Endometrium, 5
  ablation of, 276
  cryosurgery of, 276
  IUD use and, 99
  laser ablation of, 244
  in menstruation, 6
Epidermoid carcinoma, 44
Epididymis, 11
Epididymitis, 202
Estradiol, 253
  implanted below skin, 259
Estrogen, 4, 7
  complications and side effects of, 24–25
  blood clotting and, 37
  breasts and effects of, 42
  in HDL-C, 36
  in LDL-C, 36
Ethinyl estradiol, 24
External genitals (vulva), 1

Fallopian tubes, 6
  experimental methods for occlusion of,
  273–274
Falope Ring surgery, 223–224
Family planning, natural methods of, 139
Female sterilization, new techniques of,
  272–273
Fertility
  birth-control pills and, 50
  IUD used for enhancement of, 91–92
"Fertility awareness," 144
Fibroids
  birth-control pills and, 63
  hysterectomy for, 242–243
  myomyectomy for, 243–244
Fimbria, 6
Fimbriectomy, 234
First-trimester abortion
  chance of death following, 179
  complications of, 177–179
  complications of pregnancy following,
  182–183
  performed in hospital versus clinic or
  doctor's office, 181–182
  procedure of, 175–177
  procedures prior to, 173–174
  type of anesthesia for, 179–181
5-Thio-dextro-glucose, as male
  contraceptive, 279
Flat-spring diaphragm, 105

Floppy-valve syndrome, *see* Mitral valve
  prolapse
Focal nodular hyperplasia, 60
Folic acid deficiencies, 56–57
Follicle-stimulating hormone (FSH), 9, 12,
  24
Follicle-stimulating hormone-releasing
  protein (FRP), 279
Fraternal twins, 7
FSH, *see* Follicle-stimulating hormone

Gallbladder, birth-control pills and, 49
Genital herpes simplex (HSV-II), 74
Gestodene, 252–253
GnRH, *see* Gonadotropin-releasing
  hormone
Gonadotropin-releasing hormone (GnRH),
  9, 24
Gonorrhea, 49–51
  TODAY sponge in prevention of, 117
Gossypol, 270, 278
Graefenberg Ring, 266

Hair, birth-control pills and loss of, 73–74
HCG, *see* Human chorionic gonadotropin
HDL-C, *see* High density
  lipoprotein-cholesterol
Headaches, birth-control pills and, 69
Heart attacks, birth-control pills and, 33–34
Heart disease, vasectomy and, 204–205
Hematoma, 202
Hemorrhoids, birth-control pills and, 38
Hepatitis, 59–60
  transmitted via diaphragm rings, 110
Hepatocellular adenoma, 60
Herpes virus, 134
High-blood pressure, birth-control pills
  and, 39–40
High-density lipoprotein-cholesterol
  (HDL-C), 25, 35
  gestodene in, 252
  progestogens in, 35–36
  triphasic birth-control pills and, 31
HPV, *see* Human papilloma virus
HSV-II, *see* Genital herpes simplex
Human chorionic gonadotropin (HCG), 263
Human papilloma virus (HPV), 113
  condoms in prevention of, 134
  diaphragm in prevention of, 117
Hyaluronidase, 264
Hymen, 2
Hypernatremia, 189
Hyperplasia, 52
  Depo-Provera for, 255
Hypertension
  birth-control pills and, 39–40
  susceptibility of women to, 40
Hypertonic saline, 188
  PGF2$^\alpha$ compared with, 193
Hypertonic saline abortions, 189
  complications of, 189–190
Hypothalamus, 9
  malfunctioning of, 52–53
Hysterectomy, 237–250
  for adenomyosis, 245–246
  in benign disease of uterus, 248–249

for combined purpose of abortion and
  sterilization, 249
description, 238
for fibroids, 242–243
as method of sterilization, 238–239,
  241–242
number performed annually, 237–238
ovarian hormonal function following, 246
psychological problems after, 246–248
removing healthy ovaries, 248–249
at time of cesarean section, 249–250
Hysterosalpingogram, 160, 233
Hysteroscope, 269, 274–276
Hysteroscopy, 244
Hysterotomy, 195

ICD, *see* Intracervical device
Imperforate hymen, 3
Infertility
  condoms in treatment of, 133
  birth-control pills as cause of, 51
  DES and, 161
  IUDs and, 88–89
  related to type of IUD used, 90–91
Inhibin, 12, 127
Inner vagina, examining, 3
Interval abdominal tubal ligation
  minliaparotomy, 212–213
Interval sterilization, 208
Intestinal ailments, birth-control pills and,
  68–69
Intracervical device (ICD), 264–265
Intramural fibroid, 243
Intrauterine devices (IUDs), 78–101,
  265–269; *see also* Progestasert
  abnormal bleeding and replacement of,
    99
  actinomyces in Pap smears of wearers, 92
  birth-control pills compared with, 79–80
  cervical cancer and use of, 99
  as contraceptive, effectiveness of, 85
  of copper, 85–87, 98
  danger of becoming pregnant while
    using, 96–97
  for diabetic women, safety of, 98–99
  ectopic pregnancy in women using,
    97–98
  effectiveness of, after first year of use, 85
  endometrium and, 99
  expulsion of, 87–88, 268
  in fertility enhancement, 91–92
  future innovations in, 268–269
  heavy and prolonged period with use of,
    99–100
  history of, 78–79
  infection caused by, 88–90
  insertion of, 81–82
    immediately after delivery, 267–268
    precautions prior to, 83
    time to insert, during menstrual cycle,
      82
  intercourse or orgasm as cause of
    movement, 99
  levonorgestrel in, 266
  perforation of uterus by, 93–94
    treatment, 94–95

PID associated with, 267
of plastic, 87
process of preventing pregnancy, 84
prolonging contraceptive effectiveness of,
  265–266
reasonable fee for insertion of, 101
resuming use after abortion or full-term
  pregnancy, 95–96
status as contraceptive today, 78–79
strings of, inability to feel, 96
success of, compared to other
  contraceptives, 108
summary of effectiveness of, during one
  year of use, 86
tail of, 80–81, 99
tubal infection related to use of, 90–91
  reducing, 266–267
tubal sterilization and removal of, 101
vaginal discharge in women using, 99
various types of, 79
women who should not use, 84
women with heart disease and safety of,
  100–101
Iron, birth-control pills and, 58
IUDs, *see* Intrauterine devices

Jaundice, 48

Labia, 1–2
Lactic acid dehydrogenase C4 (LDH-C4),
  264
Lactotrophs, 9
Laminaria digitata, 183–184
Laparoscopy/laparoscopic sterilization
  advantages of, 228
  age when laparoscopy should no longer
    be performed, 229
  anesthesia for, 225
  bleeding complications of, 219
  complications of, 218–219
  discontinuing other methods of birth
    control prior to, 229
  electrical burns during, 221–222
  failure of, 225–226
  Falope Ring surgery for, 223–224
  finding good laparoscopist, 226–227
  immediately following childbirth, 228
  "open" versus "blind," 220
  perforations caused by trocar in, 219–220
  plastic clips for, 224–225
  postoperative infection following, 225
  resuming intercourse after, 229
  thermocoagulation method for, 222–223
  at time of abortion, 228
  women who should not undergo,
    227–228
Laser ablation of endometrium, 244
Laser hysteroscope, 276
Laser laparoscope, 273
LDH-C4, *see* Lactic acid dehydrogenase C4
LDL-C, *see* Low density
  lipoprotein-cholesterol
Leiomyomas, 63
  hysterectomy for, 242–243
Levonorgestrel, 259, 260
  in IUDs, 266

LH, *see* Luteinizing hormone
LH tests, *see* Luteinizing hormone-releasing hormone
Lipid content in blood, 35–36
Lipid metabolism, 35
Liver, birth-control pills and diseases of, 59–61
Low density lipoprotein-cholesterol (LDL-C), 31, 35–36
Luteinizing hormone (LH), 9, 12, 24
Luteinizing hormone-releasing hormone (LH-RH), 9
  agonist of, in fibroids and abnormal bleeding, 245
  analogs of, as contraceptive, 276–277
  analogs versus antagonists, 277
Luteinizing hormone (LH) tests, 146–147
Luteolytic effect of postcoital hormones, 157

Male contraceptives; *see also* Vasectomy
  of future, 279
  mechanical methods of, 280
  testosterone as, 279
Malignant melanoma, 47
MCA, *see* Methyl cyanoacrylate
Melanocyte-stimulating hormone (MSH), 47
Melasma, 47
Menfegol, 270
Menopause, 9–11
  birth-control pills and, 63
Mentrual cramps, *see* Primary dysmenorrhea
Menstrual cycle
  proliferative phase of, 7
  regulation of, 9
  secretory phase of, 7
  time to insert IUD during, 82
Menstrual extraction, 167–170
  description, 167
  injury to surviving fetus in, 169
  precautions following, 169–170
  process of, 167–168
  self-performance of, 170
  size of cannula used in, 168–169
  unnecessary performance of, 170
Menstrual period, tampon use during, 119
Mesosalpinx, 211
Mestranol, 24
Methyl cyanoacrylate (MCA), 273, 274
Microglandular hyperplasia, 44
Mifepristone, *see* RU-486
Migraine headaches, birth-control pills and, 70
Minihysteroscope, 275–276
Minilaparotomy ("minilap"), 212–213
Minipill, 31–32
  missing a pill, 56
  progestogens in, 32
Mitral valve prolapse, 100–101
Mittelschmerz, 151
Moniliasis, 261
Monophasic birth-control pills, 31
Mons pubis, 1
Morning-after hormonal preparations, 156–167

effect on developing fetus in unintercepted pregnancy, 159
  in preventing pregnancy, 157–158
MSH, *see* Melanocyte-stimulating hormone
Multiload Copper, 250, 265
Multiple sexual partners, effects of, 89
Myomectomy, 243–244
Myometrium, 5

Nabothian cysts, 43
New contraceptive methods, 176–177
Nonoxynol-9
  as carcinogenic agent, 115
  in condoms, 128, 132, 135
Nonspecific vaginitis (NSV), 133–134
Norethindrone enanthate (NET-EN), 259
Noresthisterone, 260
NORPLANT birth control system, 256–258
Nursing
  Billings method and, 154
  contraceptive effect of, 153, 154
  ovulation and, 75
  and risk of IUD perforation, 95–96

Obesity, laparoscopy and, 227–228
Oral contraceptives, *see* Birth-control pills
Orchitis, 202
Ortho-Novum 10/11, 32–33
Ovarian cancer, birth-control pills and, 46–47
Ovarian cysts, 242
  birth-control pills as cause of, 46
Ovaries, 7–9
Ovix Fertility Computer, 272
"Ovulation method," 144

Pap smears
  actinomyces in, 92
  birth-control pills and, 44–45, 56–57
Pelvic inflammatory disease (PID)
  birth-control pills and, 49–50
  IUDs and, 80, 88–89, 101, 267
Penis, 11
Pessaries, 105
PGE2 suppositories, *see* Prostaglandin (PGE2) suppositories
PID, *see* Pelvic inflammatory disease
PIF, *see* Prolactin-release inhibitory factor
Placenta previa, 183
PMS, *see* Premenstrual syndrome
Postcoital contraception, 156–170
  effectiveness of, 158–159
  morning-after hormonal preparations, 156–167
  side effects of, 158
Postcoital hormones, 157
Postcoital IUD, 167
Postpartum abdominal sterilization, 212
Postpartum and postabortal laparoscopy, 228
Postpartum hysterectomy, 238
Postpartum sterilization, 208
Post-sterilization syndrome, 232–233
Post-tubal ligation syndrome (PTLS), 232
Post-tubal sterilization syndrome (PTSS), 232–233

Pregnancy
  in adolescents, 76, 172
  resuming IUD use after, 95–96
Pregnancy vaccine
  by alteration of egg or sperm, 263–264
  as contraceptive, 263
Premature ejaculation, "squeeze technique"
      for treatment of, 137
Premenstrual syndrome (PMS), 59
Prepuce, 11
Primary dysmenorrhea, 71–72
Progestasert, 92–93, 101
  drawback of, 265–266
  safeguards before insertion, 101
Progesterone, 4, 7
Progestin-only pill, *see* Minipill
Progestins, *see also* Progesterone,
      Progestogens
  differences in strength of, 26–27
  side effects and complications of, 25–26
Progestogens
  in currently available birth-control pills,
      15–23
  in birth-control process, 24
  in HDL-C, 35–36
  in LDL-C, 35–36
  in Minipill, 32
  in triphasic birth-control pills, 27–31
Prolactin, production of, 9
Prolactin-release inhibitory factor (PIF), 9
Prolactinomas, 51
Propranolol hydrochloride, 270
Prostaglandin (PGE2) suppositories,
      190–191
  advantage of, over intra-amniotic
      injections, 188
  in inducing abortion between twelfth
      and sixteenth weeks of pregnancy,
      192
Prostaglandins
  in abortions, 190–191
  adverse reactions with, 193–194
  PGF2$^\alpha$ compared with hypertonic saline,
      193
  for women with sickle-cell trait, 194
PTLS, *see* Post-tubal ligation syndrome
PTSS, *see* Post-tubal sterilization syndrome
Puerperal sterilization, 208
Pulmonary embolus, 37, 38

Quinacrine hydrochloride, 269

Recanalization, 202
Rectocele, 240
Reproductive system, 1–13
Rheumatoid arthritis, birth-control pills
      and, 49
Rhythm method, 138–155, 270–272
  Billings cervical mucus method compared
      with sympto-thermal method, 146
  calculating safe period, 139–140
  categories of, 139
  cervical mucus and improvement of,
      144–145
  chances of conception with temperature
      method, 142–143

CUE Ovulation Predictor and, 147–148
  current use throughout world, 139
  daily temperature in determining unsafe
      days, 140–142
  description, 138–139
  Down's syndrome and use of, 151–152
  evaluating cervical mucus and, 270–271
  ferning and, 148–150
  future tests of women's saliva and urine,
      271
  improving temperature method of, 272
  new methods and devices for
      improvement of, 150–151, 272
  ovulation test kits for, 146
  pregnancy occurrence while using,
      151–152
  pregnancy rates for, 139
  problems with, 143
  taking temperature at different time of
      day, 144
RU-486 as contraceptive, 261–263
"Rubber condom" dermatitis, 135

Salpingitis, 49–51, 58
  IUDs and, 101
Sclerosing agents, 269
Scrotum, 11
Second-trimester abortion
  expense of, 195
  risks of incompetent cervix and
      premature birth following, 194–195
Semen, 11
Seminal vesicle, 11
Serotonin, 65
Sex chromosomes, 13
Sexually transmitted diseases (STDs)
  carried by speculums, 3
  condoms in prevention of, 133–134
  diaphragm in prevention of, 113–114
  nonoxynol-9 in prevention of, 114
  TODAY sponge in prevention of, 117
Skene's glands, 2
Smoking, birth-control pills and, 33
Speculum, 3
  performing "fern test" with, 148–150
Sperm banks, 206–207
Sperm granuloma, 203
Spermatozoa, 11, 12
Spermicidal agents, commonly used, 112
Spermicides, compared to other
      contraceptives, 108
Spinnbarkeit, 144–145
Spotting, *see* Breakthrough bleeding
Squamous cells, 46
"Squeeze technique" of Masters and
      Johnson, 137
STDs, *see* Sexually transmitted diseases
Stress incontinence, 240–241
Stroke, birth-control pills and, 36–37
Submucous fibroid, 243, 244
Suction curettage, 186–187
Sulfasalazine, 279
Superficial thrombophlebitis, 38–39
Supracervical hysterectomy, 238
Systolic click-murmur syndrome, *see* Mitral
      valve prolapse

Tampons, in menstrual period, 119
Teenagers
abortion for, 172–173
birth-control pills for, 76
growth stunted by, 63
with irregular menses, 52–53
pregnancy in, 76, 172
Telangiectasias, 48
Testosterone, 12
as male contraceptive, 278–279
vasectomy and, 203
Thrombophlebitis, 37
Thrombus, 37
Thyroid glands, birth-control pills and, 48
TODAY sponge, 114–119
advantages of, over diaphragm, 116–117
carcinogenic agents in, 115
cervical caps compared with, 122
cost for, 117
description, 114–115
manufacturers' number to report
problems with, 119
pregnancy rates of diaphragm compared
with, 115–116
in prevention of sexually transmitted
diseases, 117
process of preventing pregnancy,
114–115
toxic shock syndrome and, 118, 119
Toxic shock syndrome (TSS), 110
diaphragm and, 118
TODAY sponge and, 118, 119
Trichmoniasis, 133–134
Tri-cycle regimen of birth-control pills, 69
Triphasic birth-control pills, 27–31, 54
breakthrough bleeding and, 55
monophasic birth-control pills compared
with, 31
Tubal infection
associated with IUDs, reducing, 266–267
and type of IUD used, 90–91
Tubal ligation, 208–236; see also Abdominal
tubal ligation, Vaginal tubal ligation
abdominal versus vaginal, 208–209
anesthesia for, 209
current popularity of, 208
definition, 208
irregular period and abnormal vaginal
bleeding following, 232–233
pregnancy following, 226
procedures before, 209–210
reversal of, 233–236
Tubal pregnancy, 61
Tubal sterilization, as term, 208
Tubo-ovarian abscess, 90
Twins, 7

Unilateral salpingo-oophorectomy, 238
Urethra, 11
locating, 2
Urethrocele, 240
Urinary tract, birth-control pills and, 74–75
Urinary tract infections, diaphragm as cause
of, 110
Uterine atony, 177

Uterine cancer, 45–46
Uterine prolapse, 239
Uterus
abnormalities of, 160–162
anatomy of, 5
perforation of, by IUD, 93–95

Vagina
DES and changes of, 160
examining, 3
Vaginal adenocarcinoma, 160
Vaginal cancer, DES and, 159–160
Vaginal Contraceptive Film (VCF), 126
Vaginal contraceptive rings, 258–259
Vaginal hysterectomy
reasons for, 239–240
safety of, 239
ulterior motives for doctors to perform,
241
Vaginal spermicides, 122–126
and adverse pregnancy outcome, 126
contraceptive aerosol foam compared
with other types of, 123–124
cost of, 125
disadvantages of, 125
lowest possible pregnancy rates with, 123
Vaginal tubal ligation, 229–236
abdominal tuabl ligation contrasted with,
208–209
via culdoscopy, 231–232
complications of, 130–131
procedure for, 229–230
Varicose veins, birth-control pills and, 38
Vas deferens, 11
Vasectomy, 198–207
allergic reactions to sperm following, 203
complications of, 202–203
cost of, 206
current statistics on, 198
description, 199
diminished sexual drive due to, 203
female sterilization compared to, 199
history of, 199
later risk of heart disease and, 204–205
process of, 200–201
resuming coitus after, 202
steps following, 201–202
steps prior to, 199–200
storing semen prior to, 206–207
surgical efforts to reverse, 205
type of man likely to request, 205
Vasovasotomy, 205
VCF, see Vaginal Contraceptive Film
Venereal warts, condoms for prevention of,
134
Very low density lipoprotein-cholesterol
(VLDL-C), 31
Vitamin deficiencies, caused by
birth-control pills, 57–58
Vomiting
and effectiveness of birth-control pills, 68
after postcoital contraceptives, 158

White-blood-cell count (WBC),
birth-control pills and, 74